We ARE Stronger Together!

The Extraordinary Story of One Boy's Relentless Joy

Despite Fighting a Losing Battle

JULIE BAYLES

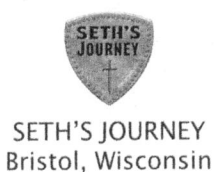

SETH'S JOURNEY
Bristol, Wisconsin

We ARE Stronger Together!

Copyright © 2024 Julie Bayles
Published by Seth's Journey, LLC

Editor, Cathy Harvey
Cover design by Hannah Linder Designs
Formatting and layout design by Catherine Posey
Photo editing by Lauren Hengeveld and Trisha Buster
Seth's Journey logo, marketing and creative design by Sherry Costello
All photos copyright Julie Bayles except the following:
Cover photo by Donna Roalkvan, back cover pop tab images by Drew Bayles

Chapter 1 - Artwork by Jessica Januszewski
Chapter 2 - Farmhouse photo by Mary Elizabeth Bacon-Benson
Chapter 3 - Chapter sketch photo taken by Donna Roalkvan
Chapter 6 - Julie and Seth in scrubs by Unknown
Chapter 8 - Stitches by Unknown; log cabin photo by Donna Roalkvan
Chapter 10 - Dr. Fischer photo originally taken by Encore Public Relations
Chapter 11 - Recess photo by Unknown
Chapter 13 - Group photo originally taken by Samaritan's Purse; Gala photo by Let Me Capture You Photography
Chapter 16 - Chapter sketch photo originally taken by Kim Allen
Chapter 18 - Groundbreaking photo by Dean Riggott Photography
Chapter 20 - Mt. Rushmore photo by Unknown
Chapter 21 - Chapter sketch photo originally taken by the late Dino Zagame; Flat Seth photo by Faith Rach; videographer by Nancy Switalla
Chapter 23 - Chapter sketch photo originally taken by Fagan Studios
Chapter 24 - Wristbands, football presentation by Nancy Switalla
Chapter 25 - Chapter sketch photo originally taken by Luke Bayles
Chapter 28 - Receiving diploma by Nancy Switalla
Chapter 30 - Chapter sketch photo originally taken by Matthias Academy
Epilogue - Low 5 by Nancy Switalla
Afterword photo by Janae Bayles

QR codes/videos used by permission from the following:
Ronald McDonald House Charities Midwest MN, WI, IA
Samaritan's Purse
Encore Public Relations, LLC

DEDICATION

To Uncle Bill - You've been there for me my entire life, my listening ear and biggest supporter. So much of who I am today can be attributed to you. Your unconditional love for me, Donnie, and the children is a priceless gift. "Guess what? I love you!"

To Donnie - Thank you for continuing to hold fast . . . for loving God, me, and our family fiercely. For putting up with endless hours at the computer needed to complete this. For never complaining about the mess or pizza for dinner again. You encouraged me to press on through exhaustion, because, in the end, it would all be worth it.

To the six sons and one daughter who call me mom - Your lives have shaped this journey. You all have taught me more about enduring difficulties with deep faith, resilience, kindness, joy, and perseverance than any humans I've ever known. The grace and love you have for me, an imperfect mom, is something I cherish.

To all those in the medical field who sacrifice so much - Thank you for devoting your lives to humanity, digging for causes and cures, and promoting and improving the field of medicine. Well done, faithful servants.

To all those living with invisible conditions, and those caring for them - You are not invisible.

To all the George Baileys out there who think your life doesn't matter, it does.

CONTENTS

1. The Storm of Our Life — 1
2. The Mystery Begins — 7
3. Not in Kansas Anymore — 15
4. Ramifications of Rare — 22
5. Mom on a Mission — 33
6. A Dresser Full of Junk — 46
7. From Snowflakes to Seizures — 61
8. The Plot Thickens — 77
9. Pain It Forward — 90
10. A Sling and a Handful of Rocks — 105
11. Learning to Cope — 114
12. The Need for Speed! — 129
13. When One Door Closes, Another Bursts Open — 142
14. Iron Sharpens Iron — 158
15. The Pop Tab Kid — 168
16. Not Rejection . . . Redirection — 183
17. The Pills Are Gone! — 194
18. In This Together — 209
19. Divine Providence — 223
20. The Big 18 — 232
21. The Adventures of Flat Seth — 245
22. With God All Things Are Possible — 258
23. Looks Can Be Deceiving — 267
24. Senior Year . . . It's Complicated — 275
25. Lessons from Quarantine — 288
26. Stuck! — 298
27. She's Not a Visitor, She's My Mom! — 308
28. From Hospital Gown to Cap and Gown — 320
29. "Just the Mom" Changing the Paradigm — 329
30. Grieving the Losses, Embracing the Calling — 342
31. Sorrowful Yet Always Rejoicing — 353
    Epilogue — 367

Afterword	371
List of References	377
Acknowledgements	383

All Scripture quotations, unless otherwise indicated, are taken from the *Holy Bible*, New Living Translation, copyright © 1996, 2004, 2015 by Tyndale House Foundation. Used by permission of Tyndale House Publishers, Inc., Carol Stream, Illinois 60188. All rights reserved.

The ESV® Bible (The Holy Bible, English Standard Version®). ESV® Text Edition: 2016. Copyright © 2001 by Crossway, a publishing ministry of Good News Publishers. The ESV® text has been reproduced in cooperation with and by permission of Good News Publishers.

The Holy Bible, New International Version®, NIV® Copyright © 1973, 1978, 1984, 2011 by Biblica, Inc.® Used by permission. All rights reserved worldwide.

All rights reserved. No part of this publication may be reproduced, stored in a retrieval system, or transmitted, in any form or by any means, electronic, mechanical, photocopying, recording, or otherwise, without the prior written permission in writing from the copyright owner.

ISBN: 979-8-9892821-0-4 (Paperback Edition)
ISBN: 979-8-9892821-1-1 (Ebook Edition)

Library of Congress Control Number: (LCCN) 2023922045

Disclaimer

Content in *We ARE Stronger Together!* is for the purpose of sharing Seth's journey. Some names, places, and/or minor details have been changed or withheld to protect privacy. This narrative nonfiction is a truthful recollection of actual events and experiences. Every effort has been made to ensure the accuracy of the content. Individuals spoken of may or may not agree with all of the views expressed.

Medical information in this book was taken from conversations with medical professionals and often compared to entries made in patient's medical files via notes, portal messages, results, and letters. The medical information throughout this book was correct and most accurate as it was divulged to us based upon Seth's age and particular circumstances.

The information is not intended to be a substitute for advice given by a physician, pharmacist, or other licensed healthcare professional. Please do not rely solely on the information presented in this book to make medical decisions, self-diagnose, or treat a health problem or disease.

The medical information throughout this book was correct and most accurate as it was divulged to us based upon Seth's particular extenuating circumstances. Seth's ever-changing medical needs and unknowns require ongoing research, treatment, and intervention based on the most current and relevant information and resources available at the time.

The practice of medicine is not an exact science. Information and statements regarding dietary supplements, alternative therapies, complementary and alternative medicine have not been evaluated by the Food and Drug Administration and are not intended to diagnose, treat, cure, or prevent any disease or health condition.

The publisher, author, medical facilities, or their providers assume no liability for inaccuracies or misstatements about medical information. This includes, but is not limited to, various medical opinions, hypotheses, educated guesses, experimental medicine, and individualized care. Everyone's situation is unique and may respond differently to various interventions or lack thereof.

CHAPTER ONE
THE STORM OF OUR LIFE

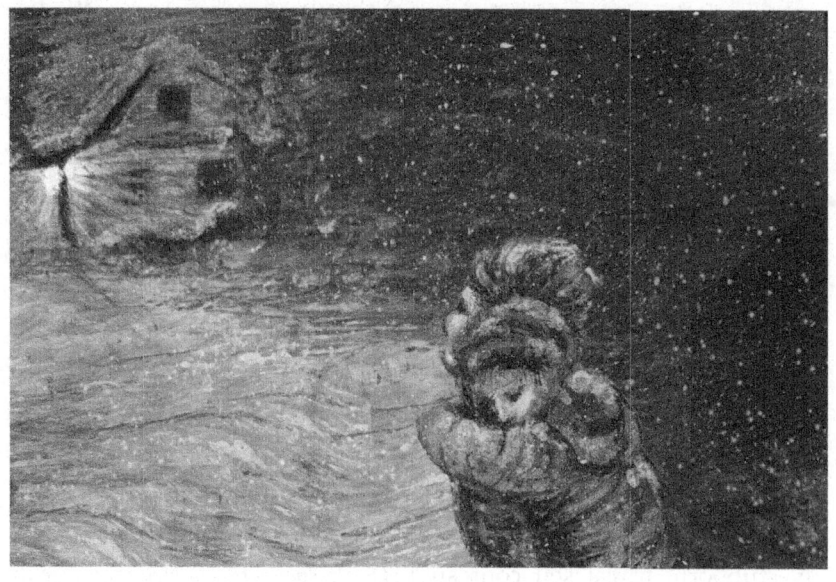

In order to realize the worth of the anchor,
we need to feel the stress of the storm.
–Corrie Ten Boom

The catastrophic storm earned many titles: The Groundhog Day Blizzard of 2011, Snowmageddon, Snowzilla, or Snowpocalypse. For us, God used the blizzard to teach us a life lesson that would carry us through our own storms.

On an overcast day in February, my ten-year-old son, Seth, and I had just finished his latest round of medical treatments at Mayo Clinic in Rochester, Minnesota. Commuting for all of Seth's appointments for the last two years had us exhausted, not only physically, but mentally, emotionally, and financially. I contemplated staying in Rochester for another night, but Seth was anxious to get home. The radio broadcasted bits and pieces about a blizzard, but I didn't pay close attention.

Living in the Midwest, I'd become used to reports of snow emergencies. I had driven through countless snowstorms on our trips to and from Minne*snow*ta for Seth's care. We had some close calls, but God faithfully protected us. I had no clue of the severity of this powerful storm system moving toward us–or the impact it would have on us.

The conditions continued to worsen as we approached central Wisconsin, but it was bearable. I had both hands on the steering wheel as fierce winds battered our vehicle and roared across the open fields. Winds blasted fifty to sixty miles per hour and crescendoed with gusts up to seventy miles per hour. Heading east, we made our way toward Milwaukee. As we approached the west side of the city, visibility deteriorated quickly. The radio blared lake effect snow warnings. When cold, below-freezing air passes over Lake Michigan's warmer waters, the clash dumps a heavy accumulation of wet snow.

My gut instinct told me to get off the expressway and find a hotel. My stubborn, frugal self contested, *Don't spend the money, you're only forty-five minutes from home. You can do this!* My frugal voice won and I kept going. After coming to my senses, I realized that I should have trusted my gut. Too late now. Suddenly, the snow seemed to swallow us. In complete white-out conditions, I could not see out any of my windows.

"This is dangerous, we need to pray, Buddy," I said to Seth in the back seat.

He prayed out loud, "Dear God, help us, please, help us get home!"

I found comfort in his simple, child-like faith spoken with confidence. What I didn't know was this storm system was dumping two feet of snow on the two counties to the south of us directly in our path. I had never experienced anything like this. Crazy lightning. Eerie. It was like entering a vortex but also hitting a wall. The exit ramps proved inaccessible due to snow drifts at their entrances making it nearly impossible to leave the freeway. I now found myself and my son trapped on the interstate.

Driving blind, my hearing sharpened. I could hear a snowplow but couldn't see it. I was sure it was ahead of us, which made me feel safer. I heard scraping on the road and needed to stay in its wake wherever that was. I saw flashing lights and thought it was the plow. Perplexed at the flashing lights on the sides, I quickly realized those were cars' hazard lights. They were not moving with me. They were stalled on either side of the freeway in the ditches. I gripped the steering wheel petrified I would hit them or veer off the side of the road.

My husband Donnie's light, two-wheel-drive truck lacked traction. We cruised around Florida in it for three years, but it was ill-equipped for our move to the Midwest. I was in trouble, and I didn't know what to do. I knew if I stopped, I wouldn't be able to gain momentum.

"I don't know where the road is! I don't know where the road is!"

"Mom, look at the GPS!"

I dared to take my eyes from the windshield for a split second toward the GPS. The cartoon image of my car moved slowly up the screen. It was ludicrous to look at it as a sole means to navigate, but I was out of options, and it was just crazy enough to work. At least the GPS showed the bends in the road and the approaching exits. Up until that point, I couldn't even tell where I was. It was the only way to keep going. My eyes watched the navigation screen as my ears followed the sound of the plow. *O God, O God, please help me not run into the back of it!* I thought as I heard Seth continue to pray out loud.

My brain flew into overdrive with scenarios and potential solutions. Should I call for help? Rational thoughts discouraged it. I couldn't take my eyes off the screen even for a moment. If I slowed down enough to focus on dialing, I might lose traction and start spinning tires. Besides, what could anyone do? Even if I called my husband, and he did come out to help us, he would have to leave six children at home, and then *both* parents would be out in this mess.

I knew if I pulled over and tried to wait things out, I was a sitting duck, risking getting hit by another car. I remembered reports of families trapped in blizzard conditions, pulling over only to be found dead from carbon monoxide poisoning from clogged tailpipes. How I regretted not spending the money on a hotel room!

Simultaneously driving and praying, it seemed miraculous we were still moving. We stared at the GPS screen. The only time I looked away was when blinking hazard lights caught my peripheral vision, and I needed to correct to avoid contact with the stationary cars. The fierce winds blew drifts of snow from five to seven to over ten feet high. As each exit approached on the screen, my heart pounded in my ears. I had no idea how I was going to get off the highway. I feared I might have no choice but to follow the plow and have to miss my snow-blocked exit.

It wouldn't be long before the highway took us to the Wisconsin/Illinois border. I didn't want to leave our home state and head into Illinois, but our exit was quickly approaching. Finally, I could see the vague outline of a wall of snow blocking our exit under the lights of the businesses nearby. No way could my vehicle clear it. Decision time: go straight and head into Illinois or head west toward the exit. My heart raced and vision grew blurry as tears filled my eyes realizing the danger we were in.

All of a sudden, out of nowhere, a huge farm truck with a plow fully engaged came up behind us. Its bright lights penetrated my obstructed window. The huge vehicle maneuvered beside me, around me, in front of me, and then—darted off toward my exit. Without thinking, I immediately swerved into the path the truck cleared.

It happened in seconds. Snow, wind, ice, and slush splashed everywhere. I could hardly believe what just took place. There was no doubt in my mind that God himself sent that truck driver as an answer to our cries for help. After seven hours of driving on the interstate, we were finally off it. This angel cleared a path from the highway all the way to the road we lived on–then disappeared into the night. My brain struggled to process what happened, yet still focused on the end goal: *Get home!*

Now, after 1:00 a.m. on an abandoned country road, I felt a new terror–isolation. The silence in our rural corner of the world was deafening. Nearly pressing my face to the glass, I squinted to see through the snowy windshield. Even though the wipers couldn't keep up with the weight of the wet snow, I could make out a faint green light ahead. It had to be our intersection's stoplight. My shoulders were locked as they had been for hours, but now we were in the home stretch.

I drove as close as possible to our corner, which was completely snowed in. I floored the truck to drive it as far off the road as I could until one of the snowbanks consumed it. We bolted to a jarring halt, but I didn't care. I finally knew exactly where I was, on our farm property, within walking distance of the house. *Oh, sweet victory! Thank you, God!* I turned off the truck and told Seth I would carry him the rest of the way. Seth bundled up and climbed over the seat.

"Seth, when I open the door, get on my back and hang on tight, and do not let go, no matter what."

He was scared but listened and obeyed. I grabbed only the bare essentials, my purse and his medical bag. Away from the intersection lights, the trek to our house was pitch black. *Oh, God, please help me not drop Seth!* As I trudged through deep snow, the full weight of his ten-year-old body with disabled legs flopped against the back of my legs. Seth buried his nose in the nape of my neck as the wind stung our faces. At last–through squinted eyes–our front porch lights. We made it *home.*

We would not fully appreciate how God answered our prayers until we saw the aerial footage on the news at daybreak. Bumper-to-bumper vehicles were deserted everywhere the storm hit. Cars scattered down the interstate like a parade from Milwaukee all the way to Chicago.

Reporters referred to it as one of the most iconic winter storms. CBS Chicago reported about nine hundred cars abandoned on Lake Shore Drive that night alone.

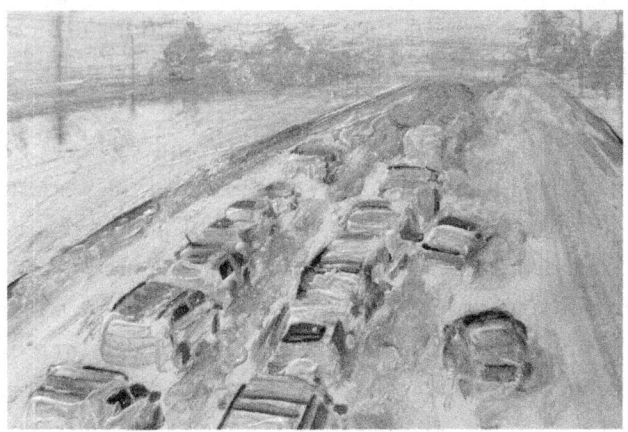

We felt a great loss for several who didn't make it home. We realized things could have ended differently for us. We were humbled and immensely grateful for answered prayer. We thanked God for making a way for us to get home when there seemed to be no way.

Before this, the five-hour drive home had become so mundane. I never again wanted to take for granted returning home safely. The experience reminded me that tomorrow is never promised. My faith was strengthened by that anything-but-routine drive home from Mayo Clinic on February 1 and 2.

This blizzard, one of the deadliest in US history, deserved all the titles it earned. Whatever title by which people recall it, for us, it will always be remembered as a lesson in faith over fear. This storm was temporary, a physical blizzard lasting only a couple of days. Our family would endure greater storms in life, as days turned into weeks, weeks into months, and months into years. How we navigated, and all who supported us through the seemingly never-ending blizzard of suffering, is our story. We began to see a unique plan and purpose unfold for us beyond what we could have ever imagined.

Here's how it all began . . .

CHAPTER TWO
THE MYSTERY BEGINS

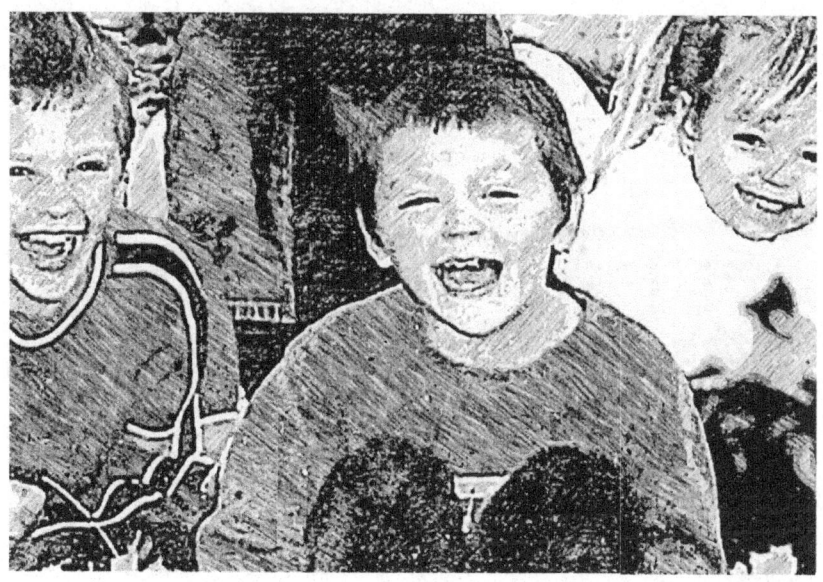

I will choose to believe that the good story and
the hard story can be the same story.
–Katherine & Jay Wolf, *Suffer Strong*

Nine Years Earlier, December 2002

Donnie and I packed up our four boys, the pick-up truck, and a moving van and said *adios* to Palm Beach County, Florida. How crazy to leave behind the house we had built just two years earlier in a newly developed area called "The Acreage." It broke our hearts to leave our loved ones, church, jobs, beaches, and never-ending sunshine. However, we couldn't deny the desire to return to our family roots. Donnie had moved to Florida from West Virginia and I from Wisconsin, two places where we left our hearts. Now, we were starting the twenty-one-hour journey northwest to Wisconsin, more specifically, where I spent the first years of my life, Wil-Mar Farm.

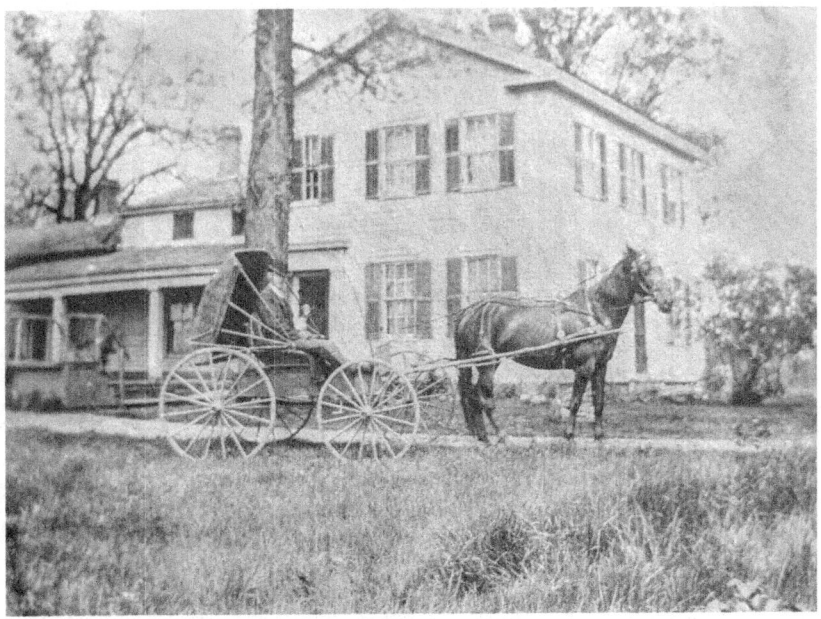

"Good to be home" said it all and was worth every sacrifice. The creek running through eighty acres of wooded property provided the ideal playground for wildlife and four active boys ages ten and under. The towering oak trees I climbed as a girl proved perfect for our boys to climb and swing on or to build a fort. Our children could run, play,

THE MYSTERY BEGINS

and explore the same land that cradled the best memories of my childhood.

We crammed our family of six into the back half of the 1832 family farmhouse built sixteen years before Wisconsin became a state. Seth and his siblings became the eighth generation of our family to live here. If only these walls could talk, right? Although I was excited to make this old house work for us, farmhouses from the eighteen hundreds lacked, among other things, the storage needed for a large family in the twenty-first century.

Springtime blossomed into much cleaning and organizing. While Donnie and our three older boys tackled yard work, I decided to run to town for totes and shelving units with our youngest son, Seth. Constantly on the move, our adventurous two-year-old wanted everything he saw in the store. I quickly filled multiple carts and headed to the checkout. As I unloaded bulky items onto the conveyor from the first of two carts, I turned for a moment to see Seth standing on his tippy toes leaning for an item from the seat of the cart. I dropped the items in my hands and lunged. I stretched as far as I could to grab any part of him, but I missed just as he lost his balance.

To my horror, Seth fell several feet *headfirst* onto the store floor. The sound of his head hitting was horrific. Time stopped. I tried to process what just happened. People were talking, but I heard everything in muffled tones and saw the scene in slow motion. The sight of him lying motionless shook me to the core. I dropped to my knees calling out his name. "Seth, wake up, Mama's right here! Seth!"

He didn't move. An employee approached and asked if she should call 9-1-1. I was trying to speak but couldn't form sentences. All I could muster was, "Jesus! Please, Jesus!" A crowd circled around us; every register stopped.

Someone said, "The ambulance is on the way."

I knew not to move someone after a fall, but the mama bear in me couldn't wait. I scooped my limp baby up off the floor and ran to the car. I put him in his car seat in the back and sped off to the hospital. *It's just a few miles away,* I thought, as I drove as fast as I could. Holding the steering wheel with my left hand while reaching back with my right to grab his toes, I shouted repeatedly, "Seth, wake up! God, please help my baby!" I pinched his toes again and again. I finally got a slight response showing he had regained consciousness even though he wasn't attempting to speak or cry. I swerved in and out of traffic, refusing to stop. Throwing the car into park, I flew into the emergency room with Seth in my arms.

"Please, help my son! He fell headfirst. He lost consciousness!"

Grabbing a gurney, a nurse said, "We need to take him for a CT scan to check for bleeding and swelling in the brain."

I watched helplessly as they whisked my baby boy down the hall. It was nearly as painful as seeing him fall. In a blink, the doors closed behind them. My legs gave way as I dropped to the chair and buried my face in my hands. With my mind racing and body trembling, tears came pouring out. *If only I could have caught him. If only I had paid closer attention to him. If only we had stayed home for his naptime as I contemplated earlier. If only . . .*

As I prayed, I felt a peace settle over me. Over half an hour passed before the ER doctor returned. I jumped to my feet.

"He's going to be okay. It's quite remarkable, actually. We can see that his skull is fractured, but there's no swelling or bleeding on the brain. This is good. He's very lucky. It should heal on its own but keep your eye on him closely. Don't hesitate to call or come back if things get worse. Follow up with his pediatrician in two days. The nurse will give you information on what to look for with this type of injury."

Seth was discharged, but for the next couple of days, I stayed at his bedside praying, reflecting, and feeling thankful. I promised God that I would do everything I could to teach Seth about His truth and encourage him to serve God all the days of his life. Now and then, Seth would wake up, cry for a bit, vomit, then fall back asleep. I called the hospital and learned that this was normal after a traumatic injury. I continued to monitor him and gave his body the time it needed to heal. It broke my heart to see him like this, but I chose to focus on the fact that things could have been much worse.

I accepted each day of improvement as a gift and a sign of hope that he was healing. With our hearts full of praise Seth made a full recovery. I believed God had protected him. Within a week, Seth was back to his spunky, silly, happy self.

We learned that life can change in an instant. Our faith and family bond strengthened and renewed as he healed. A follow-up visit to the doctor revealed no areas of concern, and he was pleased with how well Seth had bounced back.

Our family was blessed to have other members in several residences living on the same property. As the years went by, we cherished the time spent together. Seth woke up excited and ready to take on each day. He loved to run, play with his siblings, and climb trees. He rode on the tractor with his dad, jumped on the golf cart with his Uncle Bill, and worked on projects in the barn with Uncle Lee and Uncle Rich. He loved to press wildflowers from the field with Grandma Sue.

Four years went by, and we added three more children to the Bayles bunch. At six years old, Seth happily embraced the role of "middle child." He loved hanging out with the three older boys yet loved being "big bro" to the younger three. A family with seven children rarely knows boredom. Seth and his siblings never lacked for something to do with built-in playmates and best friends. He always had a smile, was funny, and loved to make people laugh.

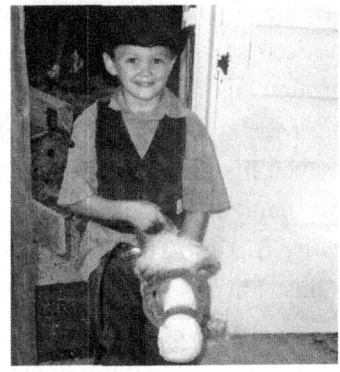

Seth also loved watching old black-and-white westerns. Roy Rogers, Gene Autry, Annie Oakley, and the Lone Ranger were his favorites. He would gallop around the farm on his stick horse, named "Trigger." Outfitted in his cowboy hat, boots, chaps, holster, and leather vest, we often heard him singing the chorus of Dale Evans' "Happy Trails."

Early September 2007

Shortly after Seth's seventh birthday, I began to notice a change in him. At first, I couldn't put my finger on it, but his demeanor changed. He became withdrawn. He didn't run like he used to. In fact, he didn't even stand for very long. He seemed tired most of the time. The little boy I often found up in his tree fort stopped trying to climb.

"What's going on, Buddy?" I asked.

"Nothing. My legs just hurt."

How peculiar, I thought to myself. I couldn't see any outward injury. Over the next couple of weeks, Seth's physical activities declined. He started going to bed earlier, woke up later, and described constant pain in both legs. I figured he was having a growth spurt. Was this a form of "growing pains?" I never saw this with my other three boys.

Autumn slipped around the corner and the ground grew cooler. Seth had always loved the change of seasons. With the help of his siblings, we encouraged him to go outdoors and rake leaves. He looked forward to jumping in mounds of fall colors every year. He reluctantly put on a pair of boots and headed out. My little man lacked joy and motivation. This was so not like him.

After he returned, he plunked down by the doorway exhausted. He struggled to take off his boots, so I helped him. It was then that I noticed something I had never seen before–red lumps under his skin around his ankles, but they were different from a typical rash. *How bizarre. They're perfectly symmetrical on both outer legs.* At first, I thought maybe his ankles had rubbed the inside of his boots. When I placed my hand inside the boots, I found nothing protruding that would cause friction. The liner was soft and intact. His skin revealed no abrasions, blisters, or open sores. The nodules appeared to be *under* the skin's surface.

When I rubbed my finger lightly over the bumps, Seth winced and drew in a breath.

I called to my husband, "Donnie, look at this!"

He was just as puzzled as I was. Neither of us had ever seen anything like it. Although I had never been one who runs to the doctor for every ailment, in my gut I *knew* something wasn't right. Donnie agreed. It was time to see Seth's doctor.

There were no appointments available with Seth's regular pediatrician for weeks. Since I was eager to get answers, I opted to schedule an appointment in October with a doctor who had immediate openings. When the new doctor looked at Seth's ankles, I spoke up.

"I have tried to make sense of every possible explanation, like his boots rubbing."

"Yes, that is likely the cause." the doctor responded.

Thank you, Captain Obvious. That was so worth the twenty-five-dollar co-payment–not. Good thing she couldn't read my thoughts. Forgive me, Lord.

"I feel there's more to it. That's why I'm here."

The doctor shook her head, not convinced.

"Seth's not my only child. I wouldn't be here wasting your time if I truly believed that it was caused by his boots rubbing. Plus, his whole demeanor has changed. There's got to be something more to this."

"I don't see any reason for concern. This will more than likely resolve on its own. Feel free to return if it persists."

The appointment was not only disappointing but frustrating. I did not feel heard. We left the office with a pricey co-pay and no answers. Although I hoped she was right, my maternal instincts told me otherwise. I couldn't shake the thought that there was something going on deep beneath the skin, but who was I? Just the mom, not a medical expert. Shut down by the doctor's comments, we were forced to wait and see. In the meantime, I was determined to prove this wasn't caused by his boots or shoes rubbing.

For the next few weeks, I made sure Seth didn't wear anything on his feet but socks. If we left the house and it was raining, I carried him. It seemed ridiculous to carry a seven-year-old, but for the short term, I needed to eliminate possible triggers. Despite all my measures, his legs and feet got worse. By now, the bumps linked together to create a ridge of dark red nodules beneath the skin. It was puzzling and disconcerting. Seth told me repeatedly that his legs hurt.

By November, I called for an appointment and insisted on seeing his regular pediatrician. Nearly eight weeks had passed since I first noticed a change in his demeanor. Our family pediatrician was as perplexed and concerned as I was. She suggested it may be some type of bone malformation. That made sense to me since the "ridge" was hard and seemed to be growing. She made a referral to an orthopedic specialist at a children's hospital. Unfortunately, we couldn't get a consultation until the first week of January, four months after our first observation.

For Seth, the pain never stopped unless he was in a very warm bath. As a typical boy, he wasn't fond of baths. Yet, he started asking to take a bath several times a day. His only relief came when he laid flat in the tub, legs floating until his skin was pruney.

By December, the ridge on Seth's ankles resembled the edge of a volcano ready to break through his skin. The skin started to peel, and the pain was relentless. Seth sat in agony and rocked back and forth rubbing his legs. Nothing comforted him. Over-the-counter pain meds did nothing. I felt so helpless. My heart broke that my son had to endure this.

Then, I realized the ridges around his ankles had changed and moved. Previously, they outlined each ankle bone resembling the letter C. Although they were still mirror images on both sides, the formation had changed. The ridges spread and grew up the front and back of his legs, across the tops of his feet, and continued to increase toward the sides. The area next to the ridges looked sunken in.

What the heck is this?

CHAPTER THREE
NOT IN KANSAS ANYMORE

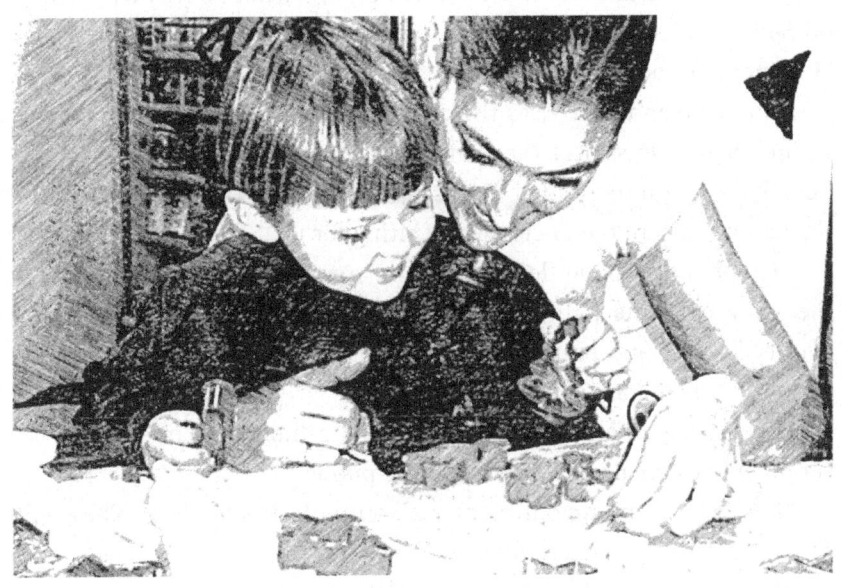

How we walk with the broken speaks louder
than how we sit with the great.
–Bill Bennot

January 2008

Finally, the long-awaited appointment with the specialist arrived. Standing outside the children's hospital complex in his stocking feet, my seven-year-old gazed up at the twelve-story building towering over us. Seth drew close to me and squeezed my hand. As we walked into the vestibule, we were directed to check in with security for a visitor's badge. This was nothing like the pediatrician's office in the little blue house two miles from our farm. *Something tells me we're not in Kansas anymore. Focus, Mama, you're here to find answers.* I had so much hope riding on this appointment. Certainly, the professionals here would figure things out. I was confident we'd leave with a plan and get some relief for Seth at last.

After the examination, the orthopedic specialist looked perplexed. He confessed he had never seen anything like what he was witnessing on Seth's limbs. He was not convinced this represented a bone issue. He sent us to radiology for x-rays.

"Hurry up and wait" was the common theme. As we waited for the results, Seth leaned over the arm of the wheelchair and fell asleep. An hour later, the nurse called Seth's name. I pushed him to the end of the hallway where the doctor was waiting for us.

"This is not a bone deformity," the specialist explained as he slid the x-ray onto the lightbox. He traced meticulously with his finger over each layer and pointed to a ridge. "Whatever this is, it seems to be in the subcutaneous fatty tissue."

His urgency in grabbing the phone and calling another department set my nerves on alert. He hung up the phone.

"I scheduled an appointment for you with dermatology. They will fit you in. You can head there right now."

"Doesn't dermatology specialize in the skin?"

"Dermatologists specialize in the skin, deep tissues, and fatty layers . . . They are often on the front lines of disease. Many diseases can first manifest themselves in these layers."

Although taken aback by the word disease, I really didn't want to leave without answers. *Disease? My kid has a disease?* I was grateful he pulled some strings to get us in to see the next specialist right away. I wasted no time finding the way to dermatology.

My hopes were dashed, however, when a young female dermatologist came in and barely glanced at Seth's legs. She didn't even look at the x-rays. She immediately started to write on his chart.

She spoke as she wrote, "This is *granuloma annulare*."

"Are you sure?" I wondered how she could be so confident.

"I am 99.9% sure! It's a harmless skin rash that just has to run its course."

"How long is that course expected to take?"

"Could be two to three years." She didn't make eye contact but continued to write.

I touched Seth's legs. "But it seems much deeper than the skin. It actually looks like his flesh has been eaten away." His poor legs looked angry and crude.

"It's merely an optical illusion. Because this area is so high, it only *looks* like the other is sunken in." She continued to write.

"What about the pain?"

"This is *not* a painful condition."

"But he *is* in pain. He is not participating in his normal activities, his *favorite* activities."

The doctor seemed annoyed at my persistence. Still looking down at Seth's chart she said, "I see here you have six other children. Maybe he's not getting the attention he needs at home and by saying he is in pain, he feels he can get the attention that he lacks. Maybe you should ignore him when he says he's in pain and focus on positive reinforcement."

I continued to look in her direction, but our eyes never connected. Then, as quickly as she entered the room, she got up and walked out. I tried to process her accusations and apathy, but her response had taken my breath away. I started to question everything that had happened over the last few months.

The doctor peeked back in and asked if her medical students could come in and observe. Seth turned to look at me and shrugged. I must have nodded because soon a room full of strangers was staring at my son's legs. Seth's big, brown sad eyes looked to me for comfort. I wondered what he thought of everyone coming in to stare at his mangled legs. He didn't say a word.

"This is a remarkable example of *granuloma annulare*," the dermatologist explained to the students.

Someone asked for permission to take photos, and I was given a form on a clipboard to sign. After a few quick clicks of the camera, everyone filed out of the room. Seth and I waited in awkward silence for the doctor to return as I tried to process the brief conversation. I tried to see things from the doctor's perspective. *Surely, she sees a vast array of cases. Do some people really go through all of this for attention? Do people really have nothing better to do with their time and money than run to doctors for nothing?*

A long time passed. I opened the door and asked a nurse if the doctor was coming back.

"No, you are free to go." The nurse pointed to the hallway leading to the lobby.

I thought to myself, *That's it? Wait two to three years? Ignore him?*

The ride home was a long one. The conversation was branded in my brain.

"What did the doctor say about my legs? Can she fix them?"

"The doctor said there is nothing wrong with you."

"But, Mama, it hurts–"

"You need to stop."

Those words pierced my heart as they rolled off my tongue. I bit my lip as my nose and eyes stung trying to fight back tears. I felt like a failure as a parent. I was torn. Deep in my heart, I believed my son, but I needed to take the doctor's advice. *Right? Who am I? After all, I'm just a mom.* Like all moms, I wanted the very best for my son. If only I knew what that was. I glanced in the rearview mirror to see him close his eyes and drift off to sleep.

The next couple of months were rough. Seth didn't complain, but the family could see the anguish on his face. I took the doctor's advice and tried to ignore what was happening. Every time I saw Seth wince in pain, I would not acknowledge the negative but redirect to a positive.

Seth began to sit for most activities. I tried to divert attention away from his lack of participation. As a family, we tried to go on as if nothing was wrong, but it was nearly impossible. We missed the old Seth. I know he did too.

APRIL 2008

The weather began to break after a long winter. We welcomed the warmer weather and more time outside. One afternoon, I invited a friend and her children over. We sat in the yard with our babies and watched the older children play a game of softball.

My friend asked, "What's going on with Seth? Why isn't he playing?"

"He's got somethin' goin' on with his legs. They're hurting him."

"I was gonna ask what the red marks all over his legs were but didn't want to be rude."

I was embarrassed. It was too painful to talk about, so I let it go. I realized at that moment how obvious it was to others. Seth's legs were spotty and erratic-looking. Some areas were deep red, angry, and inflamed as though the fat under his skin was badly mauled. Other areas had a normal skin color but were clearly recessed. I no longer bought the doctor's "optical illusion" theory. *But what's goin' on?* The fear of the unknown was the worst. Whatever it was, it was growing more pronounced. Although each leg looked unsightly in its disfigurement, both legs were mirror images of each other. *How bizarre.*

I never stopped thinking about the details of the whole situation. The conversation with the doctor at the children's hospital replayed in my head as did the conversation with Seth on the way home. I regretted not being a better advocate for him. I believed him, and he was counting on me to help him. That's my job as a parent. Even if everyone else thought we were crazy, I was determined to get answers.

The next day I called local dermatologists. I explained the situation and how painful it was for my son. I could tell by the tone of several of the offices, they were hesitant. When I spoke of the unusual circumstances we found ourselves in, one after another said their doctors were booked far in advance. I moved on to the next number and explained our situation again. I started to get discouraged. Before I dialed again, I prayed, "God, lead us to someone who can help. We need you!"

How grateful I was to find an office that listened and seemed to have compassion for our predicament. They graciously agreed to schedule a consultation at a facility close to our home. At our first visit, Dr. Mart's demeanor exuded kindness. She *looked* me and Seth in the eyes and listened. Until this point, Seth seemed to be talked *about* rather than talked *to*. We shared our experiences, thoughts, and fears. She acknowledged all our concerns as valid.

She placed her hand gently above my knee and said, "Don't worry, I'm going to help your son."

Dr. Mart prescribed several different steroid creams. I tried ever so gently to rub the creams in, but Seth's pain level and sensitivity to touch escalated. He tried hard to tough it out, but it caused more pain to try and relieve it. His walking became painstakingly slow and labored. As we were getting ready to leave the house one afternoon, Seth changed out of his shorts and put on flannel pants.

I asked, "Why are you putting on pajama pants to go outside? It's warm out."

"I don't want anyone to see my legs. They just stare at them."

"Why don't you wear your jeans instead? Real cowboys do."

"They scrape my legs, Mom, and it hurts. These are soft."

His legs were now completely red and swollen from his knees down. His toes looked like little sausages. I feared infection.

"Mom, it feels like my legs have fire in them."

I called Dr. Mart's office, and they told us to come immediately. I felt my lungs exhale with relief when Dr. Mart walked into the room. I remembered her earlier promise and knew help was on the way. When she lifted Seth's pant leg, I saw her eyes open wide and her brows raise. I read her concern before she said a word.

"This could be a very serious bacterial infection like MRSA or cellulitis. We need to take a biopsy."

She started to prepare the room. My anxiety returned. I wasn't clear on what those infections were but needed to remain calm for Seth. He looked me in the eyes, and I faked a big smile. I plunked him on my lap and talked to him as a distraction.

"When we're all done, Buddy, we'll stop n' get some Superman ice cream," I promised.

Seth looked at the doctor. "That's my favorite."

The doctor nodded and said, "Seth, I need you to be as still as a statue. You'll feel a little pinch."

She stuck him with a needle full of numbing medicine. He did better than we expected. I saw the tension in his tiny body relax as the injection took effect. Her gentle tone reassured him.

"Seth, you are a brave young man and doing a great job being so still. I need to get out the *special* treasure chest reserved for my very *best* patients."

Seth managed to crack a half smile. He watched as Dr. Mart pulled the thick black thread of each suture taut until his flesh closed. She put the tissue sample in a container labeled with Seth's name.

"We can't wait for the results. We need to start treating this now," Dr. Mart said to me. She wrote a prescription for a hefty dose of antibiotics. "Start the first dose immediately, and if things get worse, go to the ER and have them page me right away. I will call you as soon as I know anything."

CHAPTER FOUR
RAMIFICATIONS OF RARE

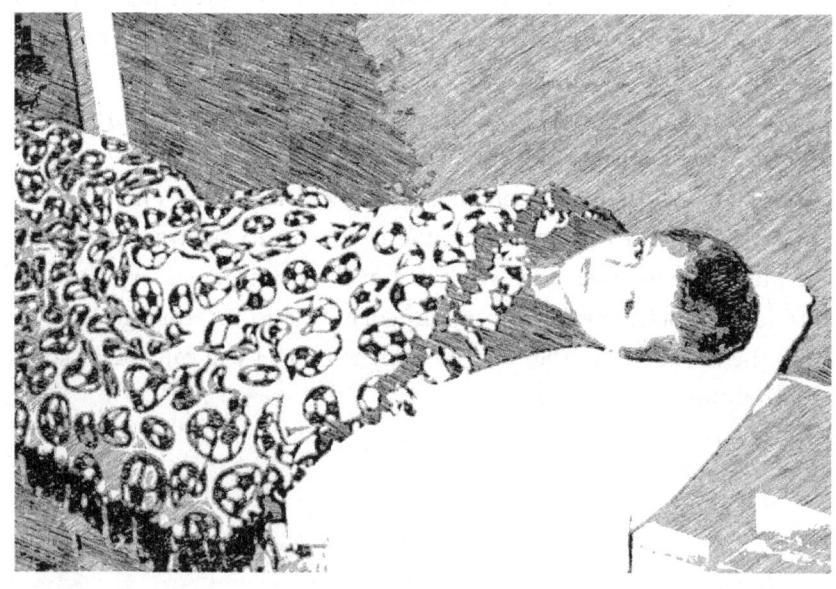

Difficult roads often lead to beautiful destinations.
–Zig Ziglar

For a week and a half, my heart raced every time the phone rang. Finally, I saw the doctor's name pop up on the caller ID and snatched the phone off the charger.

"Hello?"

"Hi, Julie, this is Dr. Mart. I just got Seth's results back. Are you sitting down? Do you want the good news or the bad news?"

I couldn't speak. After what felt like an eternity, the doctor continued.

"The good news is the biopsy revealed no bacteria, so Seth can stop taking the antibiotics. The biopsy also revealed no viruses, fungus, or parasites known to man." She took a deep breath then continued in a soft, serious tone. "The bad news is, *we don't know what this is*. At this point, we need you to come back as soon as possible to perform more biopsies. We've exhausted the sample."

The next day we headed back to Dr. Mart's office. Seth climbed up on the exam table.

"Come over here, Mom. Seth, why don't you hop up on your mom's lap."

I sat on the table and pulled Seth onto my lap.

Dr. Mart looked at Seth. "Seth, your mom's going to give you a nice big hug."

I thought it was clever how she masked the procedure to come. I wrapped my arms around Seth and held him close. Because of that, Seth wasn't scared.

Once again, Dr. Mart numbed his legs. It didn't bother him–he was an old pro this time around. The doctor performed a handful of punch biopsies along the ridges and other areas. The tool looked like a straw with a metal edge on one end to penetrate the epidermis, dermis, and into the subcutaneous fat layer. She rotated the circular blade while applying pressure. Seth's little fingers squeezed my forearm. He surprised Dr. Mart by remaining calm.

She commented, "Most kids would be kicking and crying."

Soon there were black knotted threads with wispy ends trailing down both legs from the sutures.

Seth offered his seven-year-old opinion. "Mama, it looks like spiders are all over my legs."

Dr. Mart chuckled. "You're right, it does."

After we left the hospital, I knew I couldn't continue to carry Seth, so I stopped at an outlet store to find shoes he could wear.

"Mom, do I hav'ta go in? Everybody will stare at me. I look like a mummy with my legs wrapped like this."

"I can't leave you in the car, Seth. You have to try them on. We have to make sure they fit and don't rub your ankles."

I scoured the aisles for a pair of the most comfortable shoes I could find. Because of the swelling, Seth tried several sizes. He sat surrounded by a sea of shoe boxes. We were getting frustrated, so I told Seth to stay there while I looked for help.

"Excuse me. Can you help me?" I asked a young sales clerk. "We have a special situation."

He followed me as I led him back to Seth. I lifted Seth's soft flannel pajama pants with a simple explanation of what we were looking for. The clerk looked empathetic but still had a difficult time understanding what we needed. I felt, as I had on many occasions, like I was trying to explain something that was unexplainable.

"Do you have something open in the back but soft? This is painful," I said as I looked toward Seth's wrapped legs.

The clerk left and returned with open-backed, fur-lined, clog-type shoes. They were perfect. Seth perked up. He really liked the army green color. However, as we walked slowly to the register, he felt the weight of people's stares. I wondered, *how am I gonna pay for this?* I sighed. *Donnie and I will figure it out later.* The clerk followed us to the register, and I noticed him lean in toward the cashier. I heard him tell her to give us his (employee) discount, which cut our cost in half. My eyes filled with tears as I mouthed "thank you" to the clerk who had helped us.

One evening soon after we bought the shoes, our family was walking through a parking lot when Seth fell. He tried to get up but couldn't. As I bent down to help him, his ankles stuck out from beneath his flannel pants. They were the size of grapefruits! His legs were red and warm to the touch. I tried not to show my concern, but inside I was panicking. My son was lying in the middle of a parking lot and couldn't get up. He looked into my eyes for reassurance that he was going to be okay. I laughed it off as I scooped him up.

"Let's see if we can catch up with the others," I joked.

I gave him a piggyback ride as we hurried to join his siblings. I knew I needed to call the doctor and get him into the office as soon as possible, but we also needed to enjoy time together as a family. I pretended, for the moment, all was well.

As soon as I called the doctor's office, they told us to go to the hospital immediately to have labs drawn and then come to Dr. Mart's office. The doctors would mark the orders *stat*, so she could get the results ASAP. The physician's assistant was waiting for us.

"I just wanted you to know the doctor has been working tirelessly on your son's case," the assistant assured me. "Dr. Mart has a long-standing rule that no charts are allowed on her desk. When she is in her office, she's off-duty. For as long as I've worked here–thirteen years–that's always been a rule–until now. I see her working late at night with your son's file open on her desk. She is certainly committed to his case."

This moved me deeply–and yet I had mixed emotions. Although grateful for her efforts, I also felt frustrated that such a brilliant doctor was having trouble figuring this out. It was a heavy load for all of us. But there was no time for tears or pity. We needed to get to the bottom of this. The doctor came in with the results of the latest blood-work and biopsies and got right down to business.

"Seth's blood levels are alarming. I have *never* seen an inflammatory marker this high . . . His white blood counts are abnormally low. His platelet count is off the charts . . . We can see his entire body is under attack, but there is no explanation why."

Dr. Mart flipped through the chart, then looked up and said, "We're going to have to take some rather aggressive measures, including starting Seth on a substantial dose of steroids to reduce the inflammation. As far as the biopsies, they did reveal nodular panniculitis and lipoatrophy."

"What?" These words were foreign to me, a language I didn't understand. "That's the name of this?

"Unfortunately, it's not the name or a diagnosis, but rather several medical terms describing the series of inflammatory and destructive processes happening inside your son's body."

"What exactly does this mean? What's triggering this? How do we stop it?"

"I wish I knew. In an instance like this (where the disease or condition arises spontaneously or for which the cause is unknown), we add another medical term, idiopathic."

The doctor asked all kinds of questions, many of which seemed random to me.

Has Seth ever been given blood products?
What is your water source?
Could your soil possibly be contaminated?
You said you live on a farm, are there pesticides used?
Do you hunt/eat wild game?
Have you recently been swimming in what could have been contaminated water?
Do you remember Seth getting any kind of bites followed by a rash?

I listened intently and answered the questions to the best of my ability. I tried to identify any red flags, but nothing jumped out at me.

I asked Dr. Mart, "If it was something environmental or genetic, why wouldn't the other six children be affected? They all have the same mother and father, all are living in the same house, living off the same land, and eating the same foods. Why Seth and not them?"

"That's a valid point."

Seth and all the children had been remarkably healthy until this point. I could not remember the last time they were sick. Not even so much as the common cold. When the annual flu spread around the community, we never caught it. When our friend's children were getting their tonsils/adenoids removed and tubes put into their ears, ours never had so much as a sore throat or an ear infection. Our children never had to take antibiotics. We felt profoundly grateful and blessed. My mind was trying to make sense of this new world we were whisked into. I wasn't one to cave into fear, but I felt myself being consumed.

Consulting doctors ran every kind of test they could think of on Seth. They sent labs out-of-state to specialty facilities. More than once, Seth and I were sent into a hospital restroom with containers to collect urine and stool samples.

"Mom, why do we have to do this?"

"These doctors are trying to solve the mystery of why you are feeling so bad."

"This is so gross!"

We were hopeful the doctors would find answers eventually, but the testing seemed endless, from cancers to immunodeficiency diseases. More tests meant more days at the clinic. Although we were grateful for each negative result, we grew frustrated at the lack of insight and answers. *Abnormal* and *inconclusive* were added to the results. We prayed for a light-bulb moment when all of this would make sense. We just wanted to get back to our lives minus a calendar full of appointments. We were no closer to knowing what this was, only what this was *not*, by process of elimination. The medical team shared our frustration.

Although there were outward manifestations, medical terminology categorized the disease wreaking havoc on my son's body as "invisible." It was terrifying to watch this unfold. We were trying to put out fires while, at the same time, trying to determine the cause of them. Our family watched helplessly as Seth's life deteriorated before our eyes. He now complained of stomach pain, had blood in his stools, was losing weight, and had relentless headaches. His legs couldn't be touched. They were red, swollen, and the lesions on both legs were traveling rapidly and destroying aggressively.

The doctor that we had grown so close to sat us down. I could see Dr. Mart had something heavy on her heart. After a bit of hesitation, she got to the point.

"This is no longer fair to Seth. You need to get him to a bigger facility."

I was shocked and crushed. This was the doctor we had come to respect and trust. She had such compassion. She went above and beyond. She saw us after hours. She waived her fees. She called while on vacation to check up on Seth.

I sat heartbroken, yet grateful. Dr. Mart cared enough to let her patient go where he could take advantage of more abundant resources and a larger team of professionals. She was sending us back to the previous children's hospital. I started to cry.

"I-I can't go back there. We were misdiagnosed and treated so callously. They didn't believe him and wouldn't help us. H-how are they going to help us now?"

Dr. Mart looked directly at me and spoke confidently. "But *now*, you have hard evidence, and the evidence doesn't lie. If anything good can come from his legs looking as horrific as they do, it's that now they have to believe him. The seriousness of this can no longer be denied. Your son is only getting worse, and he needs help that I can't give. I've already done much of the work for them. His records will be sent. You don't have to start over."

This amazing doctor was just as frustrated. She responded warmly when I reached my arms out for a hug. She kept her emotions at bay when she said it was people like us who inspired her to study medicine. We were sad to part ways, but we both wanted the best for Seth.

"I can't thank you enough for helping my son when he needed you most. You've done *so much* for him. We'll never forget you."

"I'm not going anywhere. The new team can always contact me, and I'll be monitoring the progress. I'm better because our paths crossed. I wish you the very best."

After that day, we never saw Dr. Mart again.

June 2008

With the evidence from Dr. Mart and a new team in place, I decided to call the doctor in dermatology who had originally seen Seth and diagnosed him with granuloma annulare. Part of me wanted her to know her diagnosis (and accusations) were incorrect and had cost us valuable time. But that desire was overshadowed by my concern that she would publish the photos and teach future medical students incorrect information. I opted to leave a message for her staff, asking them to retract the photos and data.

Moving forward, I got a crash course in specialized medicine. Gastroenterology was our first stop for the stomach pain and traces of blood. The pediatric gastroenterology waiting room was cheerful and full of bright colors. Toys around the room kept children distracted. In the past, Seth would have been eager to play with them. Instead, he rested his head on my lap as I filled out yet another patient medical history form. When the nurse called Seth's name, we made our way into the exam room. Since it had now been eight months since this nightmare began, Seth had become familiar with the routine.

"Mom, can we please just go home? I won't complain, I promise." Seth pleaded.

"After we talk with the new doctor, maybe we can stop on the way home and get a sundae."

I had hoped the promise of ice cream would cheer him up. He had lost weight and lost interest in eating. If he would eat an ice cream sundae, I'd consider it a win.

The doctor walked in and after a quick introduction opened Seth's chart.

"I agree we need to get in and see what's going on, but I see he's on prednisolone. I don't like to do scopes with patients on this. It's too risky. Besides, any inflammation that would be helpful to see would be masked because the steroids reduce the inflammation, therefore, defeating the purpose. The only way we would move forward is if we discontinue the medication immediately."

I realized steroids were hard on the gut, but we needed them. The doctors and I kept a close vigil on the risks versus the benefits of each medicine or treatment. I learned it's not an exact science, and no two patients are the same or respond in the same way. Because Seth's case was uncharted territory, treatments were tweaked as his condition improved or declined. His journey required constant management and oversight. This became our life routine in managing his chronic disease(s).

With each doctor visit, I grew convinced that as the parent, I was my son's primary advocate. It was a team effort between parent, patient, doctors, departments, and staff. We were all between a rock and a hard place. As a mom, I was especially cautious about chemicals going into my children. I knew I had to remain vigilant over his care.

Seth had been on a substantial dose of steroids for six weeks already. They're miraculous but meant for short-term use. Steroids reduce inflammation, but they have ugly side effects: can cause weakness, lower immune response, and make a person irritable. If we could find the root cause, then we could wean Seth off of them, I hoped.

We started the process of weaning him off the medication, but Seth quickly got worse, and the inflammation came back with a vengeance. The side effects were better than a relapse. High doses of steroids were essential for now. No doubt something problematic was going on, but what? Gastroenterology referred us to immunology.

The immunologist requested more vials of blood than I thought possible to draw at one time. Again, we received good and bad news, inconclusive, and more unknowns. He came to explain.

"The good news is your son is not immunodeficient. His immune system is replenishing what it needs. It's actually quite strong. I am going to go out on a limb and say this looks like an autoimmune disorder."

This was the first time I had heard this term. I asked a lot of questions. I didn't realize our immune systems could malfunction but still be strong, aggressive, and effective at stopping infection.

He continued, "The bad news is a good fight response may be

targeted at the wrong things, like healthy cells, tissues, and organs. I'm sending you to rheumatology for further evaluation."

Rheumatology was a specialty I had never heard of before. At the time, I didn't know how many different conditions were covered by this subspecialty of internal medicine. However, I was optimistic that *this* doctor would be the one to figure things out, but it was not to be. My hopes quickly faded at our next department stop.

I don't know if it was because of this unknown "thing" attacking his limbs, but the way we were treated by the doctor and medical staff during this phase was humiliating and dehumanizing. Even though his chart noted nothing contagious, they acted as if Seth had an infectious disease. Sadly, he picked up on that.

A nurse entered the room carrying a blue pair of disposable shorts.

"Put these on," the nurse ordered.

Avoiding contact with Seth, she dropped the shorts on the exam table. No greeting or small talk, no smile, just awkward silence. She left the room to let Seth change. When she reentered, her eyes fixated on Seth's legs. I understood her shock. At this point, if I held his ankle with my thumb and index finger, they would touch. Seth felt the weight of her stare. He jumped off the table and hurried toward me.

"Wait!" Her command startled us.

She grabbed the exam table paper to put down a barrier before he sat on the bench beside me. I had a sudden glimpse of what people with leprosy must have felt like in biblical times. Shunned, degraded, isolated. I wanted to tell her he wasn't contagious, that he couldn't contaminate the room, but I couldn't speak. The raw, painful weight of it all overwhelmed me. Seth was on the verge of tears. *Oh, my son . . . my heart.*

Soon the doctor walked in and stated matter-of-factly, "I've looked over his chart, and I have never seen anything like this. Frankly, I don't see how I can help." As if to appease my disappointment, he attempted to soften the blow with words that will forever be etched in my mind. "I mean, I could accept him as a patient out of *default* because no one else *wants* him, but quite frankly, I don't know what to do with him."

Holding back tears, I looked at Seth and then again at the doctor.

"Wh-w-what would you do if this was your s-son?" I didn't know what to do or where to go.

"I don't answer rhetorical questions!" He stood up, grabbed Seth's chart, and walked out.

CHAPTER FIVE
MOM ON A MISSION

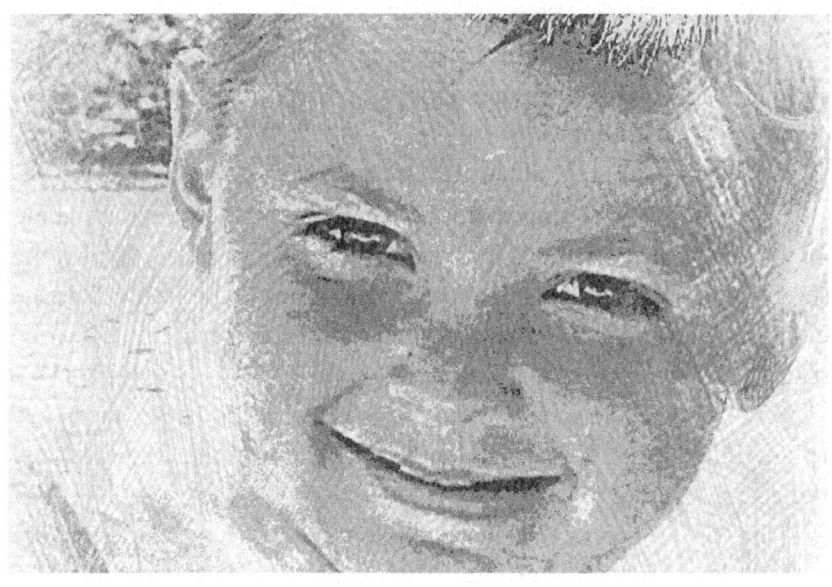

A worried mother does better research than the FBI.
–Author Unknown

The doctor's brutal honesty struck a tough blow. It didn't matter that I felt frustrated and defeated. I could not allow this to continue. My son was counting on adults to help him, and so far, most involved in his care had failed him. I looked at Seth hoping he had not understood the doctor's insensitive words. I tried to act like it never happened.

I faked a smile and said, "Okay, Seth, it's time to get your clothes back on." I fought to keep my composure as I gathered our belongings.

All of a sudden, Seth let out a wail.

"What? What happened?"

I never heard this level of anguish: prolonged, mournful, high-pitched. He struggled to catch his breath. Tears covered his face. He tried to speak, but I couldn't decipher the words.

"Seth, calm down. What's wrong?"

"M-Mom, huh-huh, what's wrong, huh, with me!" He sobbed bits and pieces that he heard the doctors say, "No one else wants me. He didn't know what to do with me."

Seth's words pierced my heart. I looked him straight in the eye.

"There's *nothing* wrong with *you*! There is something wrong going on inside of you. And I'm going to get to the bottom of it." I pulled my seven-year-old up onto my lap and let him release the frustrations he didn't have words to express. I assured him, "I'm gonna find someone that will know what to do, I promise."

Seth was not one to cry. In fact, he was always so happy and rarely let anything bother him. The relentless pain, fear of the unknown, and the doctor's words took their toll.

This was *the* pivotal moment that ignited in me a new boldness not to back down and never give up. The mama bear claws were out. The way Seth was treated was unacceptable. I could and would do better for him. I walked out of the exam room, holding my head high. The old mom, identified as "just the mom," was being transformed. I might not have had a medical degree, but I knew my son. I approached the check-out desk with confidence.

"I would like all of my son's records back, please."

The gal behind the counter looked puzzled. I had just handed over a slew of paperwork when I came in.

"They haven't been scanned yet. Would you like me to make you copies?"

"That will not be necessary. You don't even need to create a file. We will *not* be back."

I would not look back except to learn from this experience. With God's help, I was evolving into an unwavering, unapologetic patient advocate. I left the facility that day in 2008 a different parent and caregiver.

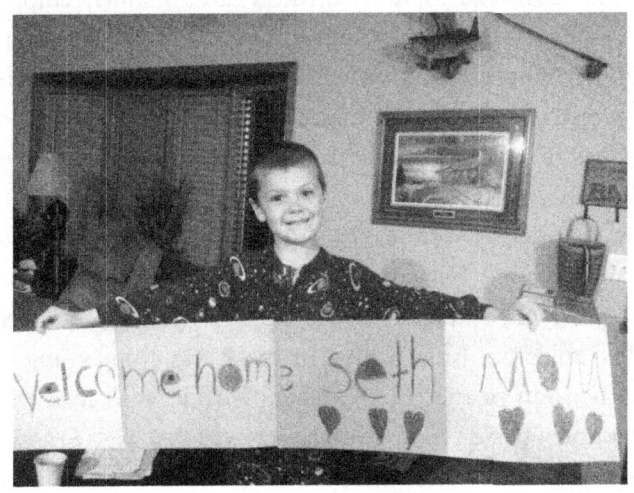

When we arrived at home, I saw little Luke waiting by the door. His arms spread out proudly displaying a banner he and his siblings had created. My four-year-old beamed with love and excitement. They had taped pink, green, red, and orange sheets of construction paper together. The kids used markers to print the words "Welcome home Seth Mom" across all four sections and colored three large hearts underneath each of our names. I hugged Luke tighter and longer than I had before. And in that moment, all of the week's tension melted away.

It was so good to be home. Being together as a family meant everything. When Seth and I were away, our thoughts were focused on the goal–get home as soon as possible. Donnie and I and our seven children enjoyed the simple things again. I had a new appreciation for the "normal" interactions, smiles, and hugs of our daily home life. Our three youngest children were one, two, and three years old when Seth first developed symptoms. We never saw it coming. One day all was fine, and the next, rare disease struck our family. No family can prepare for this. God was revealing to us what was important in life. Without our faith, we could have succumbed to the destruction this type of trauma brought to our family life. We were determined to fight not only for our son's life but also for our marriage and family.

Every time Seth and I left for medical care, it slowly chipped away at a piece of my heart. But I knew it wasn't only my heart involved. One day, our youngest son showed me how my absence affected him. As I was preparing to leave for another trip to the hospital, I couldn't find my shoes. I searched and searched to no avail. We were going to be late for Seth's appointment.

"Has anyone seen my shoes?" I shouted throughout the house.

Soon, our precious Luke appeared with hands behind his back. His sad, dark eyes looked up at me. Our eyes locked. He hesitated. Then brought his hands out from behind his back. He dropped my shoes on the floor, then ran to the couch and buried his head in the cushion. When I sat down beside him, he started to cry.

"Luke, where were my shoes?" I asked, trying to piece the mystery together.

Tears slid off his cheeks onto his Batman pajama shirt.

"I'm sorry, Mama. I didn't mean to take them. I thought. I th-thought," his crying became more intense, "if I hid your shoes, you couldn't leave."

There are days when being a mom to multiple children, one of which requires specialized, time-intensive care, can feel like a losing battle. Being torn between the one child at the hospital and the other children who also needed–and deserved–my attention at home was gut-wrenching. The guilt permeated every fiber of my being. The grieving of time lost and not spent together regularly occupied my thoughts, but I learned to stuff it because there was too much required of me. God hand-selected each of these children to complete our family, and we loved them all. I clung to God's plan, even though we had no idea what it was.

Seth's siblings rarely complained. Their joy in the little things was a constant reminder for me to be thankful in everything, even the hard stuff. Their attitude reminded me we were a team, just like Luke displaying that banner of support for our family. Sometimes we played at home, and sometimes we played away, but we never quit the team. When there was a win, we celebrated the victory together. When there was a loss, we rallied around each other. The deep faith, love, sacrifice, and support of Team Bayles enabled me to keep moving forward.

I was a mom on a mission. I needed to navigate a system with which I had no experience. I opened the phone book and started dialing. With each call, I was learning. I wrote extensive notes and absorbed details like a sponge. I spent an exorbitant amount of time on hold, but I was home and could hold my babies and enjoy the older children while I waited. I would start early in the morning and stop at 5:00 p.m. Then, I got up and did it all over again.

It wasn't long before my dining room table was converted into a "command center" covered with sticky notes, names, extensions, titles, phone numbers, and to-do lists of follow-up calls for the next day. This demanded organization, documentation, and persistence. I learned the good, the bad, and the ugly of the healthcare system. Days were spent cutting through the red tape and jumping through hoops. I saw the power that medical insurance has on a patient's care.

Looking ahead, I knew it was going to get worse before it got better. The more testing he needed, the more treatments, the more time off of work, the more bills . . . "More" exhausted my energy for the future. Mounting medical bills fanned the flames of despair. *How in the world are we ever going to get out from underneath this?*

Meals? Donnie took care of them and taught the children how to cook as well. Self-care? Non-existent. Schooling? We took advantage of curriculum videos and homeschool co-op. Sleep? A luxury. After the kids went to bed, I stayed up studying Seth's medical files, researching, and cross-referencing medical terms. I needed to understand this new world, this new language.

From then on, when I made phone calls, I asked a ton of questions. Sometimes I was told they were good questions, but they had no answers. I politely asked for someone who could give me an answer. I gained strength as a patient advocate. My son needed me to be his voice, so he could secure the care he desperately needed. Filing paperwork, addressing insurance companies, and initiating the grievance process became second nature.

Call after call, it became apparent that my son didn't fit into any one specialty or category. Talk about trying to fit a square peg into a round hole. He had things going on in many parts of his body that were still a mystery. I "cold-called" dozens of offices who reiterated the same theme, "I don't think our office is the right fit for you."

I was down but not out. I couldn't quit. Finally, after weeks of calling, I found the right person who listened and kindly explained. What we needed was a pediatric diagnostician, a medical doctor with specialized training and rigorous study in unraveling medical mysteries. In fact, she offered to give me the name and number of the best doctor she knew of in this field. Oh, how I appreciated this lead.

Hope! The doctor practiced in Madison, Wisconsin. This university hospital had a stellar reputation and was well within a day's drive to and from our home. Filled with anticipation, I dialed the number. Excitement turned to despair when we discussed insurance.

"Dr. Ned is *in network,* but according to your insurance, our facility is *out of network.*"

Ok, where else does he practice? I'll drive anywhere."

"He only sees patients here. I'm sorry."

What? It must be a misunderstanding. I contacted the insurance, and sure enough, we were caught in a loophole. I was devastated. We were so close!

With my three-year-old on my hip and phone propped on the opposite shoulder, I looked over at my two babies in their high chair and playpen and broke down.

"I can't do this."

Before long, I realized how true that was. *I* can't do this, but *God* can. Like Seth's failing body, my strength was long gone. Doubt, fear, and frustration filled my head. I prayed. It wasn't much of a prayer, but the Lord knew my heart. I needed to take a break and just love on the children that God so graciously blessed us with. I held them all a little tighter that night.

The following day, I woke up before the rest of the family. I took some quiet time to reflect and pray. I sat down with my coffee at the table of organized chaos. I looked out the patio door as the first rays of sun crept above the horizon. *God's mercies are new each morning.*

I called the insurance company to ask how I could proceed with our dilemma. The voice on the other end stated in a monotone, "I understand how you feel, but there's nothing we can do."

I said, "I'm sorry, but *no*, you *don't* understand. Unless you are walking in my shoes and have a child in this situation, then you don't understand."

Regardless of whether something could be done, I needed to be heard. I wanted someone to know there were real people behind the health ID number on their screen. I know representatives are just doing their job, but my son . . .

Time was running out as Seth continued to decline. I faxed papers and filed grievances and appeals to go before a board for review. After much anticipation, I received word that a final decision was made: Denied.

I hung up the phone and broke down. I prayed, "God, we need you! I cannot stand back and watch my son waste away! I know you want the best for him. I need you to intervene and fight for my son."

Donnie walked in and set down the mail. Enclosed in one particular envelope, I discovered a pamphlet. It mentioned the state "Ombudsman" located in Madison. This word I had never heard of before intrigued me. It meant "one who resolves disputes from a neutral, independent viewpoint." I called the number on the brochure expecting to get transferred and leave a voicemail. Instead, I actually got through to a live person who happened to be the exact person I needed to talk to! That was an answer to prayer.

I explained in depth our frustrating journey. My voice cracked as I said, "I don't know if my son would make it through another appeal process or denial of services. This doctor is our only hope, and we need to see him now."

There was silence on the other end. I had a split second of doubt. *Maybe she thinks I'm crazy. Had we been disconnected?*

"Hello?" I asked.

"I'm here. I have a son that age, and this hits close to home. I cannot imagine what you are going through. I am changing your status in our system. You will now be able to go to the facility. The only contingency is that your status for continuity of care will need to be recertified and reviewed annually. But I will be here for you when that time comes. In the meantime, if you have any trouble of any kind, please, don't hesitate to call me."

I engraved that lady's name in my mind. After thanking her profusely, I got off the phone and prayed again. This time I thanked God for sending a helper. I immediately dialed that doctor's phone number. I had won the lottery and was calling to claim my prize! Within days, Donnie, Seth, and I piled into our truck and headed to Madison. My heart beat with thankfulness.

August 2008

We stepped into a friendly, inviting office. Seth watched neon-colored fish swim around in a saltwater tank. We heard Seth's name as a cheerful nurse greeted us. When we first met Dr. Ned, he made eye contact with me. When I spoke, I felt heard. He gave me ample time to express my concerns and addressed them thoroughly. Dr. Ned had done his homework. He already knew the details of Seth's case. He spoke compassionately and with great conviction.

"If this was my son, I couldn't just sit by and do nothing."

He continued to explain what he would do, but my mind heard Charlie Brown's teacher, "Wah wah wah, wah wah." My brain was trying to process, "If this was *my* son." I hadn't asked him what he would do if it was his son. He *answered* it on his own, and his answer was genuine. I knew–he was the one.

This doctor spent *four* hours with us. He examined Seth head to toe. He secured a photographer who was waiting in a special studio. Everything was documented extensively. The staff carefully tended to all of Seth's needs with compassion and respect. Dr. Ned asked Seth a lot of questions. At just seven years old, Seth was engaging in his own care. They gave him a neat glow-in-the-dark astronomy set for being the "perfect model patient." Dr. Ned looked at Donnie and me.

> I need you to understand how rare this case is. The research I've done showed similarities to Weber-Christian Disease, but even that is considered an abandoned term, and there are different distinctions to Seth's case. Seth's case is more serious, aggressive, systemic, and mysterious. The isolated cases of Weber-Christian Disease don't have enough documentation to be helpful. Clinical trials will not be available because his case is too rare to warrant it. Treatment will be experimental. There is a chance it won't work, but we will tweak things together until we get it right. I will talk to colleagues and pull resources from many different specialties to come up with a treatment plan.

I was so grateful for this new "team" approach and already felt stronger knowing we were in this together. I thanked God for the men and women we hadn't even met yet. Dr. Ned looked solemn yet hopeful. At least he had a plan. I managed to pull off a smile while trying not to fall apart. Seth looked at me, needing reassurance. By the end of the consultation, Dr. Ned, Donnie, and I were all on the same page. He called several days later, and I put him on speaker, so Donnie and I could listen together.

"I wanted you to know I have been working on Seth's case since our last office visit. I have arranged an extensive collaborative meeting with some of the most qualified specialists in rare disease."

Donnie and I asked others to cover that meeting in prayer. A large group gathered after church the following Sunday. Wall-to-wall people packed into one of the Sunday School rooms. Our Big Ask: that doctors could *stop* the progression of this destructive disease as quickly as possible–Seth's life depended on it. I lifted Seth up on one of the desks so that they could see him. Too exhausted to explain our prayer request, I lifted his pant leg. Some people gasped. Some moaned. Others started to cry. When I put him back on the floor, our Christian brothers and sisters rallied around him. We united in a powerful time of prayer. They helped bear our burden and refreshed our faith. They held up weary parents when our strength waned. Community support proved essential for the road ahead. We had no idea of the journey looming before us.

We headed back to Madison to start the process of the recommended tests. Seth and I attended consultations with departments and specialties I never knew existed. Our schedule was packed every day. When one test was completed, Seth was wheeled to the next department waiting for him. Nearly every part of his body was tested, scanned, and investigated. With each test result, we grew used to the words abnormal, idiopathic, negative, and inconclusive. The doctors were left scratching their heads as things with Seth intensified.

On top of debilitating headaches, gut pain, and internal bleeding that had been going on, Seth mentioned his wrist hurt. In hindsight, I noticed he stopped using it. Two new red spots had appeared overnight on it. "*Nooo!*" I silently screamed. The familiarity of the lesions that marked the first indicators of this evil disease terrified me. But even more terrifying, within forty-eight hours, inches of his fat were gone–eaten away!

"Mom, what's happening to me?"

My son needed answers and treatment *now*. Determined to get it, I called Dr. Ned. He told me to drive Seth to Madison right away. I got off the phone, grabbed Seth, jumped into the truck, and took off.

As soon as we arrived, one of the nurses offered to take Seth to look at the fish, so Dr. Ned and I could discuss important findings.

Your son has what we believe to be an extremely rare, very aggressive autoimmune disease or disorder that is targeting and destroying his subcutaneous fat cells. Think of your immune system as a security guard, your body as a warehouse. The immune system is in charge of keeping things secure and protected (keeping intruders out). The guard is constantly making its rounds, monitoring the state of affairs. When your immune system senses a threat, its job is to eliminate that threat. In the case of an auto (self) immune disorder, instead of recognizing a true threat (whether it be a foreign invader, virus, parasite, bacteria, cancer cells, fungi, etcetera), healthy cells and tissues are mistakenly perceived as a threat and set for destruction.

"So, is there a name for this?" I asked. It was all too complex to wrap my brain around. I just needed a name.

"There is no name, only medical terms for what has and is taking place. The deep nodules below the surface are inflammation of the fat cell itself, called panniculitis. The medical term for fat is lipo. The stage of active destruction is called phagia, meaning eating or devouring (lipophagia), ultimately resulting in atrophy (death, decrease, lack), meaning the cell is gone (lipoatrophy). Scrambling for some good news, I asked, "Okay, so if he gained weight, the fat could return, right?"

The doctor took a deep breath and exhaled slowly before delivering the bad news. "Unfortunately, the answer is no. Once the cell is destroyed, it's impossible to house fat there again because there is no cell to hold it."

What a gut-wrenching blow. The ugly truth meant this disease was eating away parts of my son, leaving him permanently disfigured and possibly disabled. As I tried to process this, Dr. Ned gave me worse news.

"As we have witnessed, this disease is not only *aggressive* but seems to be *progressive*. We can see the wave of destruction outwardly, but I am more concerned about what's going on internally. Organs are composed of fat. If this spreads to his internal organs–" He paused. "We all know what that means. We have to stop this."

Dr. Ned spoke frankly. We faced a life-or-death situation with many unknowns. I was glad they had the foresight to take Seth out of the office. He always knew when I was upset, and I didn't want him to be scared. I needed time to process this.

Dr. Ned couldn't define Seth's prognosis. The doctors' research frustrated them at the lack of available documentation. Seth's multiple conditions fell under uncharted territory. Dr. Ned walked me through every step of the process as if he was discussing his own child. That alone comforted me. He explained the risks of the experimental cocktail of medications the medical team recommended to try and halt the progression. It wouldn't be cured, but it would be his best chance. Weekly low-dose chemo injections could stunt his growth and make his hair fall out. This level of medicine scared me, but losing Seth would be more than we could bear.

I asked, "How long will Seth need to endure this treatment? A month? Twelve months?"

"To tell you the truth, it's hard to say. If I was to guess, a couple of years at minimum, plus at least a year or more for a taper off."

I felt sick to my stomach. How could I allow someone to inject my son with poison every single week for several years? How could I have peace signing papers for this? The mental wrestling tore at my heart and kept me awake nights. *It's too much, Lord, too much.* But losing my son? Not an option.

I appreciated Dr. Ned's thoroughness, patience, and frequently pausing to answer my questions. His bedside manner reflected a perfect balance of empathy for what Seth had already endured as well as an honest look forward to the projected battles.

He explained that because this wasn't a foreign invader, we were, instead, fighting Seth's *own* body by suppressing the immune system from working so aggressively. Everything depended on how long Seth's body continued to fight against itself. Seth had previously been tested for everything possible that could provoke his immune system. As frustrating as it was not to know, we needed to come to terms with the word idiopathic (cause unknown), which would now precede medical terms in his chart.

Dr. Ned continued. "I need to warn you. This fight will not be pretty. It will be a long road, and your lives will never be the same. I know this is hard to think about right now, but you need to get things in order in preparation. Do everything you all want to do now. Take Seth away and spend some quality time as a family."

"Seth's eighth birthday is this month. We had plans with extended family to spend the week at the Lake Katherine cottage up north."

"That's perfect. Take some time together and make memories. We don't know where your son will be for his ninth birthday. When you return, we'll start the first phase of aggressive treatment."

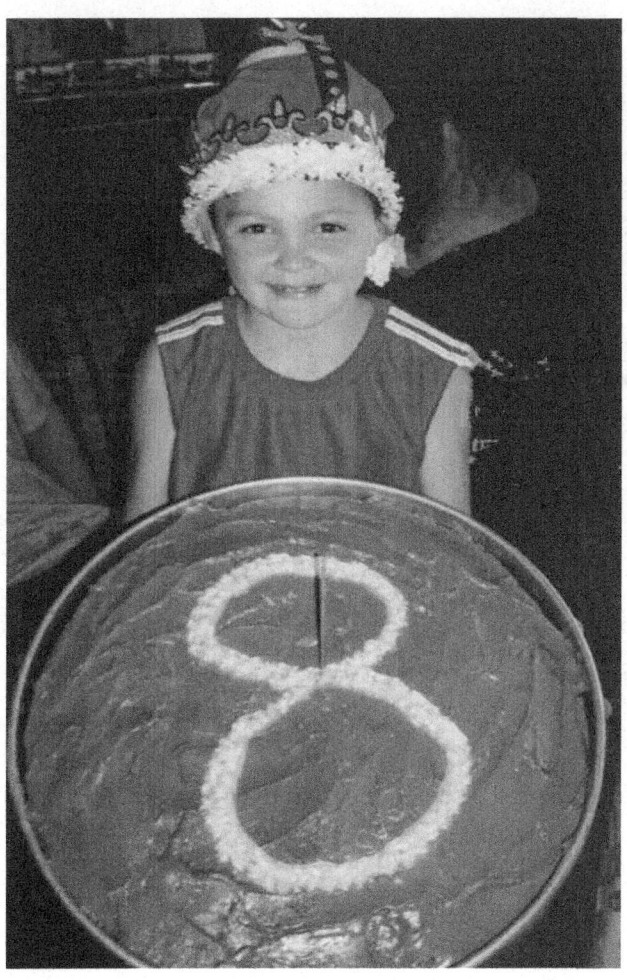

CHAPTER SIX
A DRESSER FULL OF JUNK

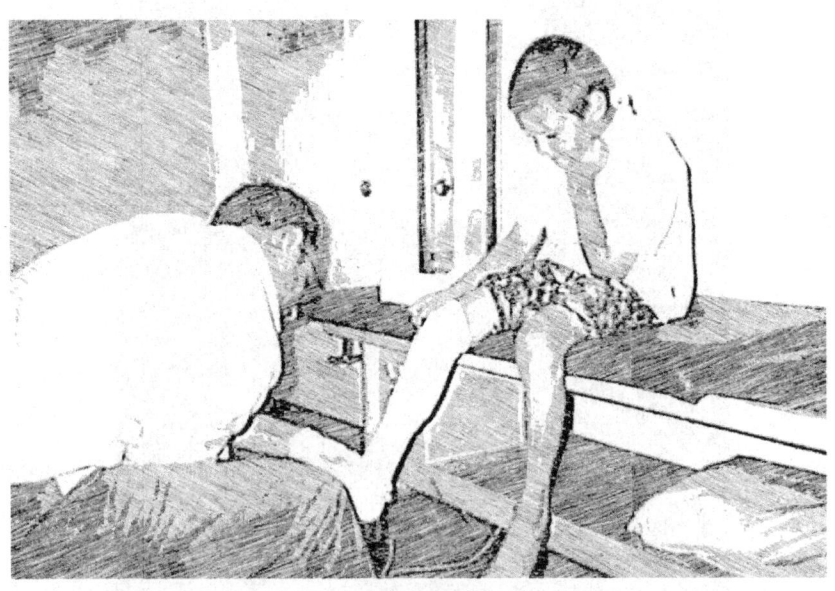

Medicine is a science of uncertainty and an art of probability.
–William Osler

August 2008

I drove the five hours home from the cabin on Lake Katherine. The family slept soundly and comfortably stretched out in the back seats of our fifteen-passenger van. With one hand on the steering wheel, the other wiped the tears that streamed down my face. We were driving away from our favorite place on earth, our happy place, where stress and problems didn't exist. I wanted to rewind time to the carefree activities and laughter of the previous week. My heart breathed prayers of thanks for all of it.

Now . . . silence. My mind replayed the events from the last few months. The *what-ifs* poked and pierced me. Pushing aside the spirit of thanks, the what-ifs fought to consume my thoughts. *Dear God, please, calm my fears. Give us strength for the unknown journey ahead.*

Monday morning, before sunrise, I dropped off six of the children at my best friend Pam's house. She had been praying for our family and was eager to help. I thanked God for her. Knowing Seth's siblings would be well cared for in my absence was a huge comfort. Now, I could focus on the task at hand.

Donnie, Seth, and I traveled two hours to the University of Wisconsin health clinic. Dr. Ned read aloud and explained to us the potential risks of the treatment plan. It seemed surreal, like it wasn't even our family. The decisions we faced weighed us down. We had built trust in this man through our time together in honest conversations. I believed Dr. Ned was an answer to prayer. I needed to stop second-guessing. I needed to step out in faith, and I needed to trust that God would continue to direct our path.

We signed the paperwork to begin treatment. The medical team detailed a well-written plan of the medications for treatments in a list from least to most aggressive. If the lesser didn't work, the next medicine would be added to the existing cocktail of meds. They sent us home with the understanding that Dr. Ned was available by phone and would closely monitor everything.

Grateful that Dr. Ned stayed in regular communication with us, I acted as his eyes and ears to inform him of what Seth was going through. In return, Dr. Ned provided the knowledge and direction we needed to understand our next steps. When Seth started to experience excruciating abdominal pain and bloody stools, Dr. Ned told us to head to our local emergency department. To our dismay, the local ER staff was reluctant to provide any care. They informed us they had no experience with lipoatrophy even from a non-immune standpoint. Due to the rarity of his case, they referred us back to Dr. Ned. So, Seth and I had no choice but to drive back to Madison while Donnie stayed home with the other six children.

As soon as we arrived at the university clinic, they were waiting for us in one of the exam rooms. Seth climbed up on the exam table and curled up in the fetal position holding his stomach. Dr. Ned furrowed his brow.

"I am concerned that we could now also be dealing with mesenteric panniculitis."

"What's that?"

"It's another rare disease that affects the mesentery. It's like a web to hold organs in place. It's made of fat."

This made sense since Seth's body was already attacking and destroying his fat cells. The danger of this spreading *inside him* worried everyone, but doctors had no easy way to investigate. Seth came home on pain meds. Exasperating.

We saw Dr. Ned in his office a week later for a follow-up. Medical personnel taught Seth to point to a series of "pain faces" on a chart to describe his pain level. But understanding the location and type of pain he was experiencing (stabbing, shooting, burning, throbbing, etc.) was harder to decipher. At Seth's young age, he didn't possess the vocabulary for describing pain. Dr. Ned asked Seth if his legs still hurt. Seth responded matter-of-factly.

"They don't really hurt, I guess. It just feels like there's a dresser full of junk laying on them. And then someone is holding the dresser on my legs with rubber bands and banging it with a hammer. That's all." He continued to play with a toy from the treasure chest.

"How often does it feel like that, Seth?" Dr. Ned asked.

Seth shrugged as he moved a colorful slinky back and forth in the palms of his hands.

"Umm, when I wake up and the daytime, and at night, and sometimes in the middle of the night. It feels like needles poking my legs."

My eyes met the doctor's. Neither of us realized the full extent of pain that had become normal for Seth. Dr. Ned ordered an MRI of both legs. The results left the team wondering how Seth could even walk.

The MRI revealed abnormalities in both legs, including bone marrow lesions, swelling, and inflammation. He had multiple stress fractures. Both legs lit up (increased signals) like a Christmas tree confirming the constant pain.

Every time Seth bumped into something, such as a leg of a chair, or backed into the open dishwasher door, he dropped to the floor in debilitating pain. For us, bumping into something might create a bruise. But for Seth, it created much more.

"I am referring you to a pediatric oncologist specializing in pain management."

"Wait. With all due respect, Dr. Ned, why would you send my son to oncology when he doesn't have cancer?"

"There is pain, and then there is deep, penetrating, destructive, cell-destroying, inner-core disease pain that pediatric oncologists know how to deal with best. The pain medicine I usually prescribe won't touch this."

I protested, "But I don't want my son on narcotics. I don't want him to get addicted. He's only eight years old!"

"I understand your concerns, Mrs. Bayles. I wouldn't have you go this route if I didn't think it was absolutely necessary. In this case, I feel it's cruel not to."

That sentence hit me like a ton of bricks. *Cruel not to.* Also, the lesser medications were not working as well as they had hoped. Therefore, they added the chemotherapy agent we had hoped to avoid. I was scared and anxious, but the addition gave him a fighting chance. Dr. Ned could see how much I was struggling.

With my voice quivering at the brink of tears, I said, "We rarely even give our kids Tylenol."

He sincerely empathized. He had the foresight to prescribe preservative-free methotrexate injections. This variation of the drug, not typically used, meant one less foreign ingredient Seth's already malfunctioning immune system would have to battle. I felt better about this.

They could do little to prevent the trauma caused by walking without the shock-absorbing layer of fat with which everyone is born. This was not the way the body was designed. Dr. Ned explained further that there was a "mechanical breakdown" due to areas being shifted into places that weren't meant to deal with extra torque. This resulted in chronic Achilles tendonitis. In a domino effect, Seth's body also suffered deep tissue trauma and nerve damage. A tidal wave of problems was overwhelming his little body.

Doctors told us the constant "electricity jolts" Seth described as "hitting my funny bone, but really bad, prickly, and matches with fire on them" was Seth's way of describing damaged nerves. To make matters worse, his nerves and veins were now superficial, closer to the surface, without the God-designed fatty layer of protection. Seth had the perfect storm for pain receptors to torment him relentlessly.

This wave of destruction wasn't just a few spots here and there. The disease was *systemic* meaning it involved the entire system. His immune system was sending messages of destruction internally like a tsunami through both sides of his body at once from the inside out. It would be quite impressive if it weren't so horrific. The team of doctors were observing combined conditions not seen anywhere else. They broadened their search to the Internet looking for any documentation to help illuminate this medical mystery.

Having nothing to compare Seth's case to, Team Seth put their minds together to think outside of the box. Seth needed the natural God-given layer of fat that he now lacked. In the interim, Dr. Ned suggested soccer-like shin guards, on the front and back of Seth's legs. I scoured a sports store and purchased tall socks and several plastic guards. Seth wore them even though they were uncomfortable and didn't stay in place. This mission was to protect Seth's tibias, calves, areas of lipoatrophy, and superficial veins. To also support his traumatized Achilles tendons would be ideal.

Dr. Ned found a professional outside of Madison at a prosthetic clinic willing to take on this challenge. They made a cast of Seth's legs to create custom ankle foot orthotics (AFOs) for his specific needs. Unlike anything of its kind, the braces covered a large surface yet moved just like legs via discrete hinges molded into the virtually indestructible shell for optimal protection. They gave Seth a full range of motion without hindering the growth or function of any muscle groups. The braces were revolutionary as a two-part clamshell-like interlocking protection for the front and back of both legs. A special thick, spongy inner padding was added to ease the pain.

In the process of being fitted for the braces, Seth mentioned he was a huge Pittsburgh Steelers football fan. When the orthotist asked if he could create the new leg braces with the team emblem embedded, Seth's whole demeanor changed!

From that point on, everywhere we went, we got feedback on the one-of-a-kind design. No one had seen anything like them. They were used as a model for personalized care. This professional went above and beyond to make Seth exactly what he needed and added a personal touch. The orthotist was so gracious, kind, and empathetic. He genuinely wanted to help make Seth's situation better. This was a huge win for Seth's quality of life and mobility. Every time someone mentioned the Steelers design, Seth broke into a smile and made a new friend. Steelers all the way, Baby!

Everyone was impressed–except the insurance company (government healthcare). Since Seth's condition was so rare, requiring extras specific to him, insurance had trouble making fiscal sense of it. The medical team provided a case for the reason and need for every nut and bolt. It was satisfying to think we were a part of changing what patients needed, not only to survive but to thrive. We did battle not only for ourselves but for others after us who needed custom orthotics or prosthetics.

This propelled me toward gaining confidence as a patient advocate.

I quickly realized that advocating and taking on the insurance giant to prove "medical necessity" for a disease without a name would be a constant uphill battle. Mama Bear did not back down, and we fought until we were heard. Whether through multiple attempts for coverage or the appeals process, we pressed forward. A system doesn't change unless–and until–someone challenges it. Clawing and scratching for medical needs seemed like such an injustice. I was unaware that an almost robotic insurance system existed. A patient either fit into their box or got denied. My son would prove that people are not one-size-fits-all.

We would now live outside the box in unknown and unpredictable territory. Dr. Ned was wise to precede with caution. He handed Seth a box of surgical masks. "From now on, have Seth wear one of these whenever he's indoors around others. The drugs he is on will suppress his immune system making him more vulnerable to infection."

As we were leaving, there was a Halloween-themed event going on for children in the lobby. There were costumes, balloons, toys, and face painting. Seth looked down as we walked past the face-painting area.

"Did you want your mask painted?" a young girl shouted.

Seth stopped in his tracks and turned toward her.

"You can do that?"

"Sure! What would you like?"

"Could you do a spider?"

"You betcha!"

The young girl painted a black spider with beady red eyes. Then, she gave Seth a mirror to approve her work. He beamed at his reflection.

"That's so cool! Thanks!"

Seth walked out of that medical facility with a different outlook. All because someone took the time to see him, not as a boy with a mask, but simply as a boy who wanted to fit in.

2009, Eight Years Old

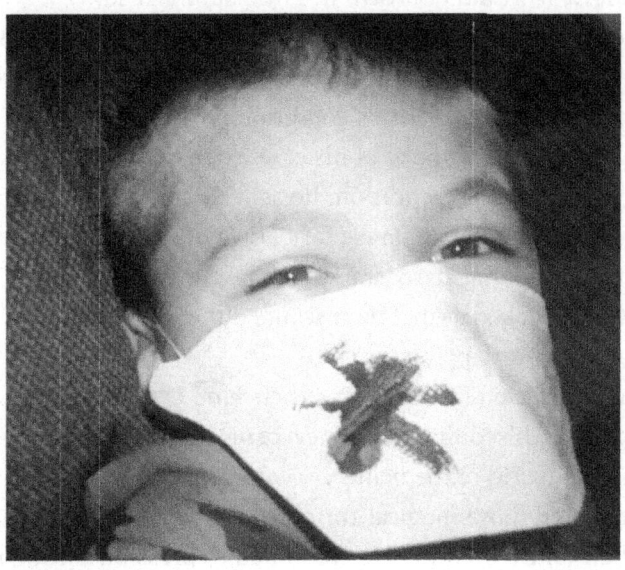

Dr. Ned asked if he could present Seth's case at an annual convention of physicians that the University of Wisconsin would be hosting. It would offer physicians from all over the country and worldwide an important opportunity to raise awareness for such a rare disease.

Seth and I met with over 150 doctors, a few at a time, over a full day. They came to see, inspect, ask questions, and attempt to weigh in on his rare, mysterious conditions. Dr. Ned led the event. He told me his biggest frustration had been the lack of solid documentation on what Seth's condition could be. I remember him saying he found a case of a woman from decades ago with *one* similar characteristic. However, no follow-up information was documented. What treatments did they try? Did this woman live? He wanted to ensure this case was well-reported in permanent medical documentation for years to come.

We agreed Seth's case needed to be thoroughly documented to pave the way for others. At first, it was awkward for Seth to have so many physicians coming in to stare at his body in only a hospital gown. I kept reminding him that they were learning from him. If we could save the next patient and parent from the painful journey we had to endure, it would be worth it. Little Seth agreed.

Dr. Ned asked if we would like to join the conference. We headed to the vast auditorium and quietly grabbed a seat in the back of the room. We saw pictures of Seth's condition on the big screen. Then, Dr. Ned took the stage and spoke of his case extensively.

At the end of the presentation, he said, "Let's give this young man and his mom a round of applause for being with us today."

Seth was encouraged to stand as the crowd turned and rose to their feet. Seth looked at me, then scanned the room.

I said, "They're clapping for you!"

His mouth turned into a grin as their kind eyes met his. It was the beginning of Seth's difficult journey being used for good to initiate changes in the world of medicine.

Seth endured more medical turmoil as an eight-year-old than most have in their entire lifetime. He continued to press on through all that was expected of him but grew lethargic, and his blood work continued to have many abnormal flags. Cells were low, high, and abnormally shaped. Was this the disease progression? The treatments? So many unknowns.

Meanwhile, our hometown pediatrician Dr. Billingsley was retiring. What a loss to our family. We had developed great love and respect for her many years of care for all our children. She was very concerned about her little patient. She wanted to make sure he was taken care of long-term before she closed this chapter in her career. She suggested we think about Mayo Clinic in Rochester, Minnesota. Even though I didn't know much about Mayo, I knew they had a stellar reputation. She told me they specialize in "mysterious" conditions.

I was torn. I had grown to have a great deal of respect for the medical team in Wisconsin, but I needed to consider that this might be all they could do. Knowing Mayo Clinic had a year-long waiting list for an initial assessment, our dear pediatrician wrote a letter of referral detailing the dire situation. We owe her a debt of gratitude. She was a game-changer for us. Without her suggestion and letter, we may never have explored Mayo as a possibility.

I will never forget the call I received from the Mayo Clinic in the summer of 2009 from the admissions office. It seemed we were being prioritized. They asked if we could be there for ten days to meet with various specialists. I was excited but hesitant. Ten days? For a mother of seven, that seemed like an eternity to be out of state with one child. I asked if they could use some of the old testing and condense the time we would be required to stay. However, and understandably, they preferred to do their own investigation and draw their own conclusions. It made sense. After all, if we were completely satisfied with the answers we had, we wouldn't ask for their input.

I answered a resounding "Yes!" Then hung up the phone and cried my eyes out. I didn't realize the full weight I had been carrying.

THE WORLD-RENOWNED MAYO CLINIC, OCTOBER 2009, SETH IS NINE YEARS OLD

The fact that we were approved to go out of state marked a huge victory. The burden of proof had fallen on me to demonstrate why we needed to go out of state for his care. I compiled all the documentation from the last eighteen months detailing every ER visit, every misdiagnosis, and record of his continued decline. I hand-carried the paperwork to the health department to prove how Wisconsin was ill-equipped to continue servicing the complex challenges of Seth's unique case. Mayo Clinic, on the other hand, was known for its work with medical mysteries.

It was hard for me to believe *we* were finally here. Rochester, Minnesota, seemed like another world. I felt nervous and overwhelmed, sick to my stomach. I was out of my comfort zone. I'd never been to Minnesota. I felt uncomfortable not knowing anyone. Seth teared up and told me how much he wanted to go home. Having just arrived, we were already counting down the nearly two weeks we needed to be there.

Our hotel stood a mere twenty-five feet away from the entrance of the main hospital. As the bellhop unloaded our bags, we gazed up at the world-renowned Mayo Clinic. We watched as people took photos of themselves in front of the hospital. At first, I wondered why anyone would document a photo in front of a hospital. But then, it hit me. Mayo represented hope. Arriving here erased the hopelessness of having exhausted all other resources.

The city of Rochester seemed very fast-paced. We didn't know one single person. Oh, how I longed to have just one connection in this vast city. Giant architectural masterpieces and bronze statues reminded us we were far from our small, rural hometown. I asked questions wherever we went. Everyone was gracious and kind.

Mayo Clinic operated like a well-oiled machine. Our schedule was booked from clinic open to close. Staff scheduled appointments for Seth at all three campuses. I pushed Seth in a wheelchair with all of our stuff, schedule in hand, and toggled between the three. We dashed for the shuttles trying not to be late. We learned as we went. I was told there were "checkers" waiting to claim a slot if someone didn't show. I needed to make sure if a department had to keep us longer than anticipated, the next department was notified. We were grateful they respected our time and packed as much as they could into our preliminary visit, but the hustle wore us out. "Hurry up and wait" all day long exhausted us mentally and physically.

Someone suggested we eat at the Canadian Honker restaurant. It would be a wonderful distraction from the hospital food. Seth told me he wasn't hungry. I ordered him a milkshake anyway, hoping to get something into his stomach. He took one sip to appease me, then put his head down on the table and immediately fell asleep.

Hotel room life was depressing and isolating. Seth would stare blankly at the cartoons on the television trying to be interested. He would say, "I wonder what the kids are doing." And then he'd name his siblings one by one. I wondered why God allowed our family to be separated. I knew he loved children and families. Had we made the right decision? Maybe we should have stayed in Wisconsin. I questioned everything but my faith.

One day as we headed through the Gonda building, we suddenly heard the sweetest sound imaginable. I felt chills from head to toe. It was the lovely sound of a piano with voices singing a classic hymn. "How Great Thou Art" floated through the air. I couldn't believe my ears! We looked over the balcony to see a crowd enjoying the musical medicine like balm on an open wound. As we left the elevator, angelic voices sang, "Then sings my soul, my Savior God to Thee . . ." As we drew closer, I realized the singers huddled around the piano were Mayo Clinic employees. Tears filled my eyes as I looked around at so many with their eyes closed, soaking it in and mouthing the words. Seth couldn't take his eyes off of the pianist, a lady with big glasses and an even bigger smile. We would later learn she was a volunteer lovingly referred to as "Piano Jane." I pushed Seth close to the big black grand piano as her hands flowed effortlessly across the keys. She warmly acknowledged his appearance.

The piano, strategically placed in the center of the Gonda building, looked similar to my beloved Uncle Bill's piano. Since I grew up listening to him play, it was like a piece of home. The building's design supported the acoustics so that the sound flowed throughout the corridors wrapping everyone within earshot in peace.

I reflected on the 1400-mile journey that led us to move back to the Midwest. Long before Seth developed this disease, God directed us in our move home, which would play a vital role in one day saving his life. I sat in the moment and let the music melt my fears. Overwhelmed with gratitude, I felt a new, undeniable confirmation: this was where Seth and I were supposed to be.

PORTRAIT OF A HOT MESS

In layman's terms, except for the manifestations on Seth's disfigured legs, most of his conditions were invisible, impossible to see on his exterior. In order to solve the mysteries of his abnormal test results, doctors needed to do exploratory surgery. I had been sitting at my son's bedside for days watching him wince in pain even in his sleep. I hated that they had put my little boy on narcotics for pain, but I also didn't want him to suffer. I cried out day and night praying for answers, so we could go home. I was physically, mentally, and spiritually stretched beyond natural limits.

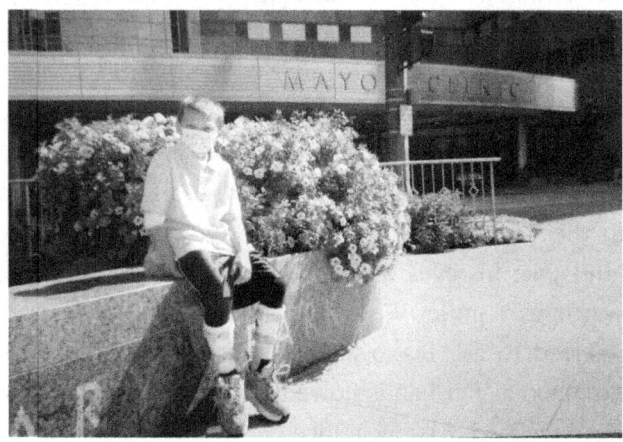

I called Donnie hoping for some sense of normalcy. Several of the children got on the phone and talked about happenings on the farm. It was bittersweet as I affirmed them. I handed Seth the phone, and soon he giggled like old times. I wanted to press pause and take a snapshot in my mind of this treasured moment.

I didn't want to face the reality to come. I wanted to go back to the way things were before. I dreaded more time away from my precious family. At this point, I wasn't sure I wanted to know what they might find through exploratory surgery.

With all of these thoughts running through my brain, I felt the need to escape. I couldn't show Seth any sign of weakness, fear, or doubt, so I motioned that I was going to the bathroom. I looked in the mirror at eyes I barely recognized. I splashed water on my face that reflected the portrait of a hot mess: exhaustion, weariness, and the weight I bore as a mama bear stared back at me. Finally, I dried my face and pulled myself together. I returned with a smile and reassurance because that's what moms do. My son needed to see confidence in my eyes. We would be stronger by God's mercy, grace, and strength.

A PICTURE PAINTS A THOUSAND WORDS

They scheduled Seth for the first surgery of the day. Before I had my first cup of coffee, a young aide walked into our room full of energy. She was bubbly and engaging and asked if she could take a photo of the two of us. *Before coffee?* Secretly wanting to run, I politely declined. I suggested she take a picture of Seth alone. She insisted that I get in the photo also. My eyes gazed at her, imploring that she take the photograph of Seth alone in his scrubs.

Her tone changed as she set me straight. "Mom, you will look back at this photo one day and be glad you were in it. But, if not, you can tear it up." She giggled as she prepared her camera.

Whatever she has in her coffee cup, I want it. I couldn't even begin to match her energy. I said, "I must be a sight," as I attempted to run my fingers through my hair that hadn't been washed in days.

She looked me in the eyes and said with wisdom beyond her years, "None of us are guaranteed a tomorrow. You will look back at this memory, and the only thing that will matter is that you were there with your son." She snapped the picture and disappeared.

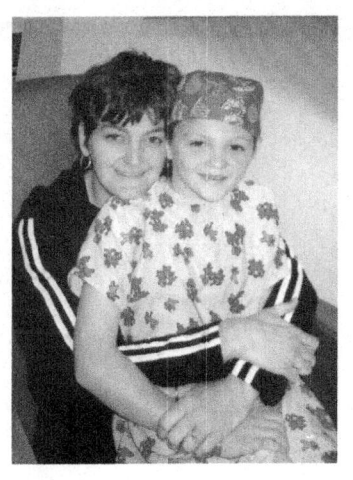

I felt ashamed for being so vain. She was 100 percent correct, and I needed to hear it. Before I knew it, attendants wheeled Seth off to surgery, and I was alone. As tears filled my weary eyes, the aide reappeared and handed me the photograph she had just printed. It was indeed a precious gift! I thanked her for her persistence.

"If I may give you some advice since you are just starting this journey - this comes from the experience of witnessing regret: Take pictures. Get in the pictures. And tell your story!"

She offered her arms for a hug, and I warmly accepted. I was such a hot mess. Tears flowed as she said, "You are a good mama!"

She walked out of the room, and I never saw her again. I didn't even catch her name. I don't know who she was or why she walked into our room that morning. This was the first of many sweet connections that would burst from hard places.

From that point on, I took photos every chance I could. It has meant so much looking back to have those tangible reminders. My photo journal helps me revisit the feelings, the lessons, and the blessings. The photos bring into focus the people whose paths crossed ours. I believe God sent them to walk beside us, and we were stronger because of them.

CHAPTER SEVEN
FROM SNOWFLAKES TO SEIZURES

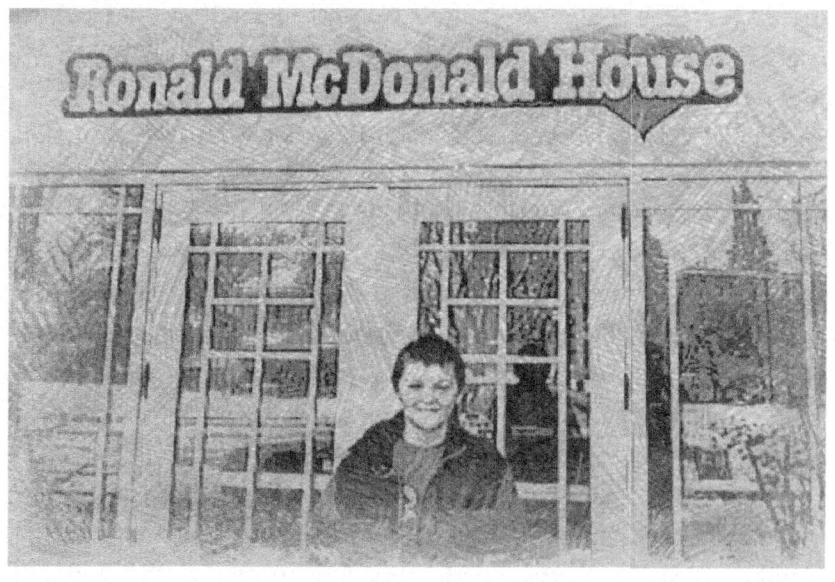

Life is 10% what happens to you and 90% how you react to it.
–Charles R. Swindoll

When asked about Seth's ultra-rare case, a Mayo Clinic pediatric expert in rare disorders who knew Seth's case well gave his perspective. "I've been doing pediatrics for about thirty years, taking care of complicated kids, and I don't know that I've seen anyone else with his condition. The fat cells underneath his skin just wilt away. He's, in a sense, trying to destroy himself . . . . He's got a lot going on every day, which makes his smile a lot more powerful."

At this point, the aggressive treatment plan had successfully suppressed Seth's immune system enough to keep it from destroying him. We were grateful, no doubt, but it came at a cost. Among other things, Seth developed sores and blisters inside his mouth, including oral thrush. He lost interest in eating and drinking. His smile disappeared. Scabs on the corners of his mouth made the simplest functions painful. His doctor expected it, but we did not. We had taken that sweet "Seth smile" for granted. Concerned and heavy-hearted, we realized we were in for a physical, mental, and emotional battle. We would need to fight for smiles, laughter, and joy.

Donnie decided to take Seth and Drew out for a lake excursion. Seth loved fishing and anything having to do with water. My phone beeped. Donnie sent a text with a photo of Seth in the boat. The excitement and joy on his face was bittersweet. I stared at the image and wept with a sweet release. I didn't realize the weight I was carrying: the second-guessing, the questioning, the treatment plan, the unknowns, the frustration, and the fear. The "Seth smile" was back! Like a sign of hope moving us forward, his smile brought a beautiful confirmation that joy and suffering can coexist. We could do this.

Since Seth's complications required more visits to Mayo Clinic, we began to feel the effects. My heart broke for what Seth was enduring. Simultaneously, I was grieving the time away from my other children. Donnie told me that Luke had lost his first tooth. After I hung up the phone, I cried. I would never get that time back.

The divide-and-conquer life we had grown accustomed to affected the entire family. Donnie and I made a pact early on in Seth's health crisis. He would hold down the fort while Seth and I were away, so I could focus all my attention on helping Seth get well. Neither of us got the easier end of the deal. Both roles were demanding. I felt like we went from a close-knit family living in a carefree comfort zone to survival mode in a combat zone.

HOLDING ONTO HOPE

Our nurse in the Pediatric Infusion Therapy Center at Mayo's Saint Marys Hospital campus made small talk while she prepared to give Seth his methotrexate injection.

"So, where's home, Seth?"

"About a five-hour car ride."

"How long are you here for?" She put on the two layers of gloves, a gown, and face shield required to administer a chemotherapy drug.

"This time, only three days, but we go back and forth regularly. We're scheduled to stay for several weeks soon."

"Do you stay at the Ronald McDonald House®?"

"No."

"That place is amazing! Little poke here, Seth."

I interrupted, "Do you think we would qualify to stay there?"

"Absolutely!" The nurse flashed me a confident smile.

Until then, we were spending a small fortune on hotel bills. I had heard of the Ronald McDonald House before, but I visualized it for really sick kids and their families. *Were we now one of those families?* Everything in me contested the reality. The nurse encouraged us to pursue this provision. I knew my son would benefit, so I humbly accepted her suggestion.

Upon inquiring, the clinic's administration initiated our request through the proper channels. After several days on the waiting list, we received a call that a room was available with our name on it. We adopted the Ronald McDonald House as our new "home away from home." I never imagined how this place would change our lives!

From the moment we entered the Ronald McDonald House, we felt the warmth of that extraordinary place through the smiles and genuine care that exuded from those who represented the house. We didn't have to explain anything. It was as if they already knew.

After check-in, a staff member invited Seth to pick out a blanket. She brought us to a room where stacks of fuzzy fleece blankets lined the walls in every conceivable design. A Wisconsin Badger blanket caught Seth's eyes, reminding him of home. Seth was thankful for this gift of comfort. He also chose a hand-crocheted hat, perfect for indoors. The hat was crocheted with purple and gold stripes of the Minnesota Vikings. Although, as a huge Pittsburgh Steelers fan, Seth chuckled that it would be better if it were black and gold. Nevertheless, he was grateful. The Minnesota winters were brutal, and Seth often felt chilled, so he regularly wore the hat.

The Christmas season, our favorite time of year, was upon us. The decor at the Ronald McDonald House glowed cheery and festive. Beautifully decorated Christmas trees in different themes graced every floor. Despite the beauty, the harsh reality remained–we were stuck out of state for the holidays. My thoughts drifted to home with family and simpler times.

Seth picked up a pillow and sat in a chair next to the Christmas tree outside our room. I looked at the pillow inscribed with the word HOPE. I wanted to capture the visual, "Holding on to HOPE," as exactly what encompassed us this year. It was a Christmas gift to have this place of retreat and support despite a horrific disease. We saw the Ronald McDonald House exemplify hope for everyone who stayed there.

Our older children were pretty self-sufficient and comfortable being at home with Donnie on the farm. But it was much harder on the younger children, especially emotionally. Unlike hospitals and clinics, our new home away from home provided a place the entire family could visit. Seth's whole demeanor changed when his three younger siblings made the trip on several occasions. Instead of dreading the hospital, he relished the distraction of showing them around.

It was important for them to see how we spent our days. They realized how much of our time was spent talking with adults and waiting.

It wasn't a fun time away but a difficult life for Seth. I think they found a new appreciation for being blessed with health.

Our family also made memories at the Ronald McDonald House. Rather than remaining confined to our room, we spent a lot of time down in the lobby. The clinic offered pet therapy. Seth's younger brothers gravitated toward the "train table," where they spent hours playing. His sister preferred the playroom on our floor with a play kitchen set. My favorite was the evening meal that volunteers prepared and served to families. After a long day at the clinic, what a blessing to have a hot meal for the entire family to enjoy together.

Through the exhausting schedule day after day, it was easy to grow weary and discouraged. But I didn't have to look very far to see people all around us committed to helping us on this journey. It occurred to me how much stronger we were together.

Immersed in the lights and candy canes, I reflected on the long-standing traditions that were important to us. Three, in particular, stood out. Ever since our children were little, we participated in a local live nativity. For decades, our friends the Gillmores, whom we had grown to love dearly, hosted it on their farm. Our family played minor roles: from shepherd boys to wise men, from an angel to singing in the choir. Another long-standing tradition was Christmas Eve at my Uncle Bill's House. It was something I had anticipated every year since childhood. He'd play Christmas music on the piano, and I got goosebumps every time he played *O Holy Night*. Without fail, one of our children would read the Christmas story from the book of Luke in the Bible.

Seth asked, "Mom, how will we be able to do any Christmas things this year?"

"I'm not sure, Buddy."

Seth was scheduled for treatment at the clinic three times each week into the new year. He received treatments on Mondays, Wednesdays, and Fridays. Sometimes, we drove the ten hours back and forth on the weekends, but everything was getting more complicated. *How could we afford, or even be able to shop for, Christmas gifts this year or even be able to make it home?* I prayed we could keep our family traditions even if things looked different.

One morning, a Ronald McDonald House staff member approached Seth and said it was his turn to visit the enchanting Snowflake Room. We had no idea what she was referring to, but as we often said, "Christmas isn't the time for asking questions." The staffer whisked Seth away with instructions that I relax with a cup of coffee and cookies while I waited. While sipping my second cup of coffee, Seth rejoined me with a huge smile and a big black trash bag slung over his shoulder.

"Mom, you wouldn't believe it. This room was filled with aisles of toys and gifts, just like a store! The lady told me I could pick out a gift I wanted for Christmas—anything I wanted!" With eyes wide and voice raised, he continued. "Then, she said, 'You can pick out something for your siblings too!' Then, we went into another room and wrapped all the gifts. I can't wait to give these to everybody for Christmas!"

The new sparkle in Seth's eyes boosted my spirit with thankfulness and renewed anticipation. Christmas Eve morning, we waited in the lobby for the patient shuttle to take us to the clinic. Suddenly, Seth pulled his Bible out of his backpack and started to read the Christmas story aloud. Soon, many gathered around to listen, creating a beautiful Christmas moment.

After we finished our day at the clinic, Seth talked about how excited he was to give the gifts he picked out. So, on a snowy Christmas Eve, we left the Ronald McDonald House and headed five hours southeast to Uncle Bill's to surprise the family.

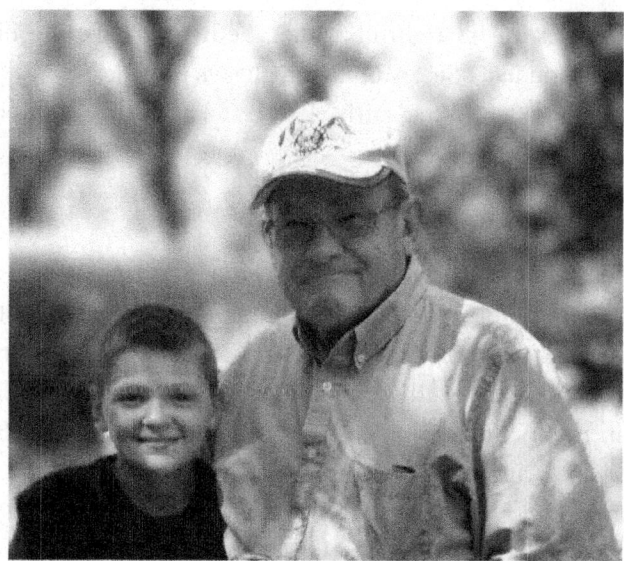

Seth and Uncle Bill

As we exchanged gifts, Seth proudly handed me a beautifully wrapped gift with a bright green bow.

"You do so much for me, Mom. This is for you."

I was shocked. *But how*–then I pieced it together. Seth had not only picked out gifts in the Snowflake Room for his siblings but for me as well. His smile was beaming as he shared how he selected just the right travel-size lotion to pack for our trips. It's hard to put into words how much I treasured that gift and family time together.

Traveling back to Minnesota on Christmas Day, we stopped at several fast-food restaurants, but they were closed for the holiday. We finally found a McDonald's with a lit sign.

As we waited in line, Seth said, "Here, Mom. I heard you tell Dad you didn't have much money for gas. I want you to have this."

He handed me a twenty-dollar bill that he had just gotten as a Christmas gift from his Grandma Sue. I didn't want to take my son's money, but he insisted.

When we inched our way to the drive-up window, the cashier said, "Your order has already been paid for–Merry Christmas!"

With immense gratitude, I reached into the back seat and handed the money back to its rightful owner. Seth received the bill with a smile and responded, "See, Mom, God always provides."

The wisdom of child-like faith . . .

POP TABS

As we spent time in the lobby of the House, we noticed a constant stream of community visitors dropping off items. Seth noticed, in particular, milk cartons, boxes, and ice cream pail containers. He watched as they dumped little pieces of metal into a plexiglass "house" in the lobby. Upon closer investigation, he noticed they were tabs from cans. Curiosity got the best of him.

"What are these used for?"

Staff explained the "Pull for the House" tab program was one of their main fundraisers held year-round. The money from recycling those tabs helped to offset the expense of running the house.

Seth immediately piped up, "I want to do that, Mom!"

It had been months since I had seen that level of excitement in Seth's eyes. I saw how important this new mission was to him.

He said to me with confidence, "Every time we come back, we're going to bring pop tabs!"

Back home, Seth immediately started telling everyone to pull the tabs from their cans. He asked his school administrator if he could send home a letter to every student in his grade school. We attached a sandwich bag to the letter explaining what he was doing. We turned a tall pickle jar into a permanent pop tab collection jar and put it on the counter of The Benson Corners Antique Mall with the owner's permission. Word spread, and seven days a week, people came in to drop off tabs for Seth. The Bristol Fire and Rescue station became a permanent drop-off site and more.

Everyone could sense how much the Ronald McDonald House meant to Seth and how important it was for him to give back. His passion for these little pieces of metal was contagious! The local newspaper ran a story about him collecting them and included our post office box number. A few days later, the post office called and asked us to come and get the overflowing amounts of pop tabs.

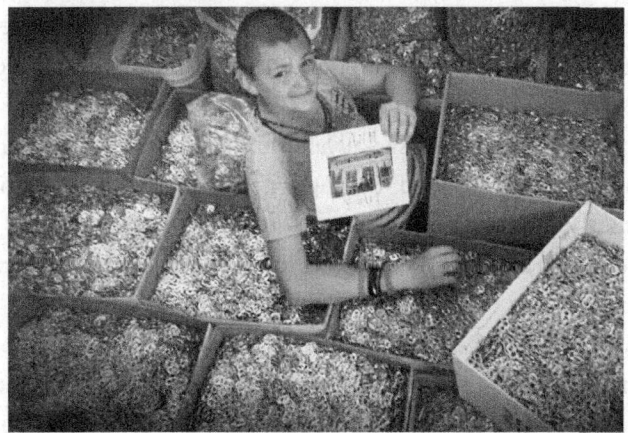

Surrounded by pop tabs, Seth holds a note of thanks to his community.

INDIVIDUALIZED EDUCATIONAL PLAN (IEP)

Seth was falling behind more and more in school, and it became apparent that it was due to more than his absences from appointments at the clinic. Teachers noticed the widening learning gap between him and his peers. The school psychologist suggested I initiate a request for an Individualized Education Plan (IEP) evaluation. I had never heard of this.

Seth went through extensive testing with several professionals. I didn't realize at the time how important it would be to have this in place. As his health declined, the qualifying assessment would be vital to enable the school to plan and provide staff and services specific to Seth's needs. It took time, effort, and a lot of dialogue, but it was worth it. Such a worthwhile mission to be on together! We counted it a blessing to give Seth a shot at normalcy (whatever that means).

I attended my first IEP meeting. How hard could it be? Like a teacher's conference, right? I was not prepared for a room full of professionals. They seemed to be talking *at* me, everyone sharing their professional input. Seth did *not* meet all of the legal markers required for special education services but *would* qualify under the Other Health Impairment (OHI) category. Just as I had to learn the language doctors used, I now had to learn the language, legalities, rights, and responsibilities of the special education system. I would build relationships, and I would learn.

With each meeting, the talks went smoother, became more interactive and productive. Seth's situation and needs were unique and regularly changing. We learned through a lot of trial and error. Since certain methods didn't work for Seth, I learned how to balance looking out for my son's best interests while extending grace and understanding.

Donnie and I decided to move Seth from the smaller parochial school to a school with a full-time nurse and a Special Ed department. This way, he would receive services based on the IEP at our local public school. The transition wasn't easy. Seth's case was unique and required an investment of time, resources, and numerous meetings. As we got to know each other, both sides learned to express empathy and understanding, enabling us to collaborate and decide what Seth needed. The school staff built an extraordinary team. Seth loved going to school, and they loved having him. The staff's dedicated teamwork enabled Seth to attend school every day that he wasn't at the clinic.

Seth's physical therapy team at Mayo Clinic communicated their expectations and goals to the local director of the school-based physical therapy team. Everyone committed to working toward giving Seth the best quality of life. The school district, guided by Seth's medical providers, purchased specialty equipment. I learned this was not usually the norm, but thankfully, our school and district were eager to meet his needs. They even hired an aide to support him with one-on-one therapy and other needs throughout the week. We all collaborated to think outside the box, which Seth didn't fit into, and implemented ways to help Seth and future students. We all worked hard and sacrificed to accomplish this vital goal.

I was working a part-time job at the time to try and make ends meet while the kids were in school. But, our doctor explained this responsibility could not fall solely on the school. So, I quit my job to make myself readily available to work with the school nurse in a moment's notice. We wrote an emergency plan, so everyone was on the same page. This made everyone feel more confident.

One of Seth's doctors wrote an extensive report of Seth's individualized, rare neurological findings, probably a dozen pages long. It was part of the IEP with resources for the best way Seth could learn. The team said they had never seen anything like it and found it highly informative. Having that first neuropsychological baseline evaluation on record proved most helpful. Seth's educational team could more easily monitor and track gains and declines. With this baseline, they could immediately address any cognitive decline as it presented.

Being a squeaky wheel, a voice and advocate, and staying on top of my son's unique needs was a never-ending job, but it was necessary for the best outcome. I was forever grateful for our tribe. They helped me hold on to hope and my faith when the journey was tiresome. I became convinced no person was an island. We needed each other, and we were better together. We saw first-hand the life-changing effects of both receiving help and giving back.

NOVEMBER-DECEMBER 2009, CHALLENGING COMPLEXITIES

The damaged nerves known as peripheral neuropathy caused Seth shooting and stabbing pain like electrical shocks. This never-ending torment affected every area of his life. Because walking was so painful, we focused on his legs. For my nine-year-old, mobility represented independence.

Once again, a specialist referred us to another specialist, who referred us to yet another and another. Each examination left professionals bewildered as they noted extraordinary distinctions of this ultra-rare condition. As doctors analyzed Seth's intriguing case, they voiced diverse opinions on how to proceed to bring relief. More than nine doctors discussed a plethora of possibilities in terms I had never heard of before.

- The first doctor suggested the possibility of "fat reinjection" into the areas of lipoatrophy, depending if his skin were adherent to the underlying bone or tendon. He referred us to another specialist for a complete assessment.
- The second doctor weighed in to say reinjections were unlikely to "take" since the disease had destroyed the cell which holds the fat.
- A third communicated that Seth's condition was more layered and complex than any of them had seen. He did not feel reintroducing fat into those areas was a viable option. . . There were too many variables and facets to this disease, unknowns about its path and ramifications of its destruction.
- A fourth doctor suggested they take live fat cells from another part of Seth's body and redistribute them to the needed area. However, there was no way to tell if the particular cell they would harvest had been already targeted (by his immune system) for destruction. Therefore, the redistributed cell would eventually be destroyed anyway.
- A fifth doctor was concerned about the localized and mechanical pressure on nerve structures and/or nerve tracts. Since the nerves cross either a fascial border or an artery with loss of padding, this would produce chronic and repeated trauma to the nerve.
- The sixth doctor then suggested Seth see another specialist concerning whether he would be a candidate for peripheral nerve transposition/release.
- The seventh doctor chimed in and said he would prefer to see a peripheral nerve decompression *and* micro lipo-grafting in order to pad the nerves from their contact with fascia and blood vessels.
- An eighth doctor was very suggestive of a certain syndrome, yet recorded in his notes, "the problem, in this case, would be to confirm the diagnosis which currently there are no available tests to speak of at the Mayo Clinic." He

recommended I think about connecting with a certain doctor at an institute in Baltimore, Maryland.
- Finally, another doctor insisted all of the invasive options were too risky. He insisted the consequences of doing something in haste could have dire consequences. Surgically manipulating and injecting into the area increased the chance of reactivating the disease. This could trigger his immune system to start destroying new cells in different places. If this did happen and came back with a vengeance, they might not be able to stop it.

I was receiving a crash course in medical terminology that would be difficult to explain to anyone outside the medical field. Through these meetings, I learned more about the human body than I ever thought I would need to learn in a lifetime. I *wanted and needed* to learn their language.

In the past, I felt patronized and dismissed as "just a mom." It was discomforting to keep asking doctors to put things in layman's terms. So, I listened, asked questions, took notes, and went home and studied. I read the post-visit summaries and cross-referenced medical terms. I prayed for wisdom, and God answered. I began to soak up and retain things like a sponge. All of a sudden, it started to make sense! This mama was now equipped to effectively carry an intelligent conversation with doctors, nurses, and ER personnel in order to be my cub's best advocate.

Empowering!

Having studied Seth's case in depth made all the difference when we met a new doctor. Oftentimes, they didn't have time to do a deep study of his case and were only scheduled for a short time slot. Being an active contributor to the conversations regarding my son's care was a win-win for all involved.

Meanwhile, a repeat MRI revealed more stress reactions above where the ankle foot orthotics ended. Annually, insurance allowed Seth to have a new set of leg braces cast if he outgrew the old ones. Each year they were able to make much-needed improvements. The shells would now be higher with more surface area to accommodate for growth and to prevent fractures. The braces proved their efficacy.

Unfortunately, his lower extremities had to take a back burner for the time being. Seth was developing more fires internally that would need to be extinguished immediately.

Nine Years Old - Epilepsy

Seth and I had not had a full night's rest in quite some time. He began exhibiting strange things in the middle of the night, causing me to sleep with "one eye open." Sometimes, I would awake to hear him mumble gibberish. Sometimes, I found him hitting the wall with his body. Other times, I would find him on the floor, but he wouldn't wake up or try to get back into bed. He didn't respond to my voice.

Clearly, something was wrong. He had not fallen out of bed since he was a toddler. Now nine-and-a-half years old, Seth fell asleep during the day but had no idea why he was so tired. The next day, I would recount the events of the previous night, but Seth never remembered any of them.

We scheduled a sleep study. Seth was not only exhausted but rather annoyed, convinced nothing was wrong. On the first night, shortly after midnight, Seth started with one episode after another.

In the morning, the doctor made her rounds and said, "We think there is a chance your son is having seizures. We need to transfer him to the Epilepsy Monitoring Unit."

Blindsided by the word seizure, this new development was unexpected. The length of our stay in the Epilepsy Monitoring Unit would be determined by "if" he had an episode in anywhere from three to five days and nights. The staff said it might be a week waiting to catch an episode. Sigh. I had not planned on being away from the family that long.

It seemed strange to pray for an episode, but if there was any time to have one, it would need to be now. We also prayed things would be crystal clear so the doctors could determine precisely what was happening and what to do.

Seth had dozens of probes cemented over his head. The smell of the glue was horrific.

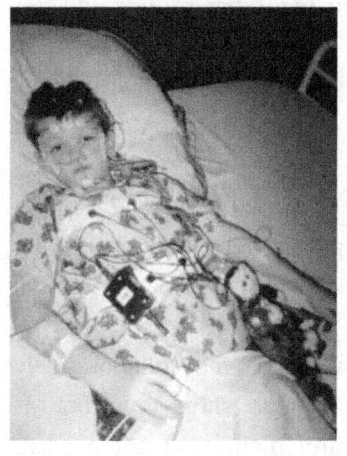

A live technician monitored the process 24/7 using probes that communicated with a machine and a live video monitor. If or when an episode began, staff instructed me to press a red button that marked the paper in the machine documenting the brain waves for later interpretation.

I settled myself in for the night under a large window on the cold, hard, green vinyl hospital bench beside Seth's hospital bed. We both drifted off to sleep.

Then, like clockwork, I awoke to Seth making a clicking noise with his tongue. He made incoherent sounds as he jerked on the right side of his body. Then his body went rigid as he abruptly sat up. I reached over to the bedrail and grabbed the corded event wand. I fumbled to hit the red episode button. Seth's right arm moved back and forth like he was treading water. Then with a blank stare, he picked at his gown. He rocked back and forth for a few seconds, then slumped over to one side (this caused him to fall out of bed at home). The unit was prepared with padded side rails and a second layer of safety with thick mats on the floor.

The door abruptly flung open, and a nurse flipped on the light. They had watched him via the monitor and saw it all unfold even before he started making inaudible sounds. The nurse called Seth's name repeatedly, but he didn't respond. She kept calling his name as other medical personnel entered.

"Seth, Seth!" they shouted until he came around. "Seth, do you know where you are? What year is it? Who is the president?"

Slowly, he attempted to answer. He looked confused. He looked around at all of the medical personnel standing over him. It was hard for me to witness that he had no recollection of what had just taken place. Seth was exhausted and eager to go back to sleep. He experienced another episode roughly three hours later.

Shortly after 7:00 a.m., the neurologist made her rounds and got right down to business.

"The spells that Seth had happened simultaneously with documented sharp waves in the brain's frontal regions. Your son's episodes are consistent with seizures."

Frontal lobe epilepsy was added to the growing list of conditions in Seth's chart. Although thankful for clear answers, this would be another painful blow in the reality of this relentless, progressive disease.

I was so grateful for the vast medical team who collaboratively helped us determine that my son's brain was short-circuiting. It explained the missing portions of time and memory. I got a crash course on epilepsy. I learned how serious it was. I also learned that anti-seizure medications are no joke. It was crucial to give him his medication precisely and on time every day. The doctor instructed me not to let my guard down–one seizure is one too many. I learned what to do to keep my son safe, and if a seizure lasted more than five minutes, call 9-1-1.

We added an emergency seizure plan to his existing IEP. Every teacher, and anyone providing care for Seth at school, was made aware that he had epilepsy. They learned what to look for and Seth's particular protocol. It was reassuring to have everyone on the same page when seconds mattered.

I needed to educate myself as well as others. I needed to be proactive and remain vigilant of possible triggers that could provoke or lessen the seizure threshold. The worst part was he was most vulnerable when we were supposed to be sleeping. The more I learned, the more there was to fear. How would I navigate sleeping with one eye open and be able to function the next day? Would I ever again "rest easy?"

CHAPTER EIGHT
THE PLOT THICKENS

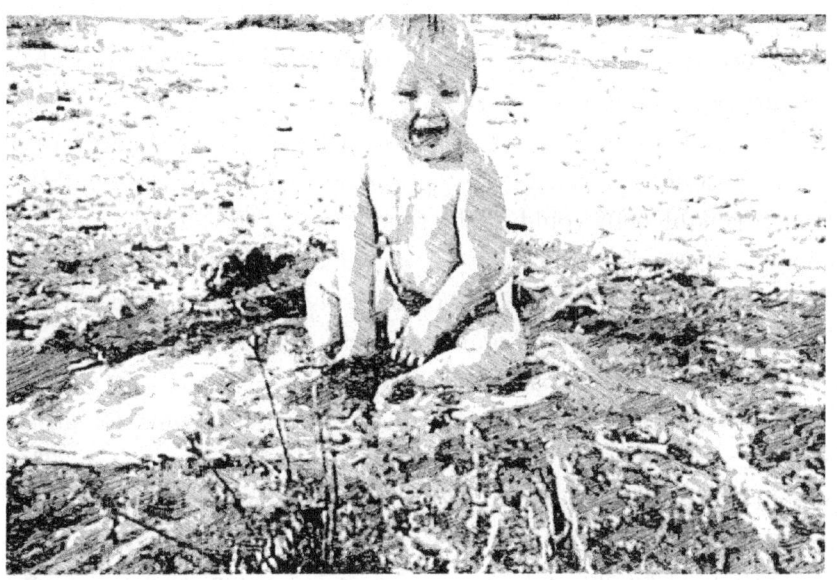

To trust God in the light is nothing, but to
trust Him in the dark–that is faith.
–C. H. Spurgeon

Seth wasn't himself. His energy dragged, weak and fatigued. Then, he began to run a fever. Although a fever is a common warning sign of childhood infection, for those who are immune-suppressed, a fever is a cause for concern.Ced warned us early on of the standard protocol for a fever–go to the Emergency Department (ED).

Our experience on numerous occasions revealed local doctors were intimidated by Seth's case. With each ED visit, I spent excessive time explaining and answering questions. After honestly admitting their lack of knowledge regarding Seth's rare conditions, they spent most of the time trying to find a doctor (including calling some at home) until they found a physician who felt comfortable being in charge of his care. Although I am glad they were trying to provide the best care for a case they had never seen before, it was challenging, especially amid a crisis and exhaustion. Therefore, we only went to the Emergency Department when absolutely necessary. I tried everything I knew to bring his fever down to no avail. Something was going on that required medical intervention.

After arriving at the hospital ED, I briefly summarized Seth's case to the front desk personnel. They promptly escorted us to a room. We were thankful Seth could avoid exposure to germs in the waiting room. The plan then shifted to . . . so, what do we do now? The staff and I exercised detective work to try and solve Seth's latest mystery.

The attending physician inquired and took notes. "Why is your son on methotrexate? What is his official diagnosis?"

"Unfortunately, there isn't an all-encompassing name for all of Seth's conditions, but I will walk you through the most serious." The more I explained, the more the doctor's body language shifted. I could tell he was uncomfortable with the complexity, and I was losing him.

Finally, he kindly said, "Look, it seems apparent that you know more about his condition than I do. I am unfamiliar with lipoatrophy or lipodystrophy, which is just one part of this. Therefore, I don't feel comfortable treating your son without consulting others. I have a doctor on call who is more educated than I am on rare diseases."

THE PLOT THICKENS   79

The two doctors agreed our best option was going straight to Mayo Clinic. At 2:00 a.m., we were no closer to controlling Seth's fever. He lay exhausted, with his face flushed, unable to sleep. I waited in the ER, concerned and frustrated. Now, I was being told to put my son, who was burning up, in the car and drive *five hours* to Minnesota to get help.

I pleaded, "You don't need to understand my son's rare disease. I just simply needed you to help me get his temperature down."

As much as I wanted to drive my son to the medical facility that knew him best, my mind was stuck calculating the risks. A spike in temperature can cause seizures in healthy children with no history of neurologic symptoms. Seth already had epilepsy. A fever plus sleep deprivation would lower Seth's seizure threshold. I was *not* about to take a chance of getting down the road and having him seize on me.

I demanded they call Mayo Clinic for advice and permission to treat. The doctor left the room to consider my request. I stood and wallowed in my frustration. *Why does everything have to be so dang hard? Why do my son's conditions have to be so rare? Why can't we just have a name that people can understand? God, please help us."*

The doctor reentered the room. "Ok, I talked with the pediatrician on call at Mayo Clinic, and he was comfortable giving detailed instructions on exactly what to do. I'm still uncomfortable about not having him at a specialty hospital. We'll treat him. We'll give it twenty-four hours. If his temperature doesn't come down, I will call Flight for Life and have him flown to Children's Hospital."

Soon, several medical professionals and medical students filled the room. They decided to give Seth an immediate high-dose antibiotic. I tried to prepare Seth for what was to come, but everything happened so quickly. Before I knew it, they had two large syringes the size of turkey basters drawn with white milky liquid in hand. Two clinicians counted to three and simultaneously jabbed both of Seth's thighs–

Poor Seth! My heart broke as he let out a wail that continued as long as it took them to push the medication. As fast as it all began, the room of white coats left. Seth refused to look at me as tears streamed down his face. I didn't blame him. No one warned him of what was to come. No one gave him a choice. I moved onto the hospital bed.

"I'm sorry, Bud. That wasn't fair to you. From now on, I promise I'll do my best to communicate every step. We're in this together."

Seth put his head onto my shoulder and drifted in and out of sleep. Nurses stepped in throughout the night to take his vitals. I experienced a roller coaster of emotions as the fever started to decrease, then spiked again. The doctors were perplexed. All of the test results were abnormal and inconclusive. Again, we didn't know what Seth was battling.

The sun crept through the hospital blinds, painting slices of light across the floor. I heard the wheels of the vitals cart rolling closer to our room. This time when the nurse appeared, Seth, fully aware and even attempting to sit up, opened his mouth for the thermometer. Finally . . . his fever had broken-hallelujah! But we had another reason to rejoice. We wouldn't find out until later that God had just orchestrated the addition of one of the most significant members of Seth's medical team.

A LITTLE CHILD WILL LEAD THEM

As the complexity of Seth's condition(s) grew, it became clear this would be a long road. Up until then, everything revolved around the clinic. We put many plans on hold. Like other families in crisis, we found ourselves putting off life "until" . . . our loved one was healed or stronger. Or until after surgery, or until they came home, or until things settled down. Until . . .

In the fall of 2009, Donnie and I decided the best way forward for our entire family was to *live life*. In-person schooling would be the first step toward normalcy. I met with the administration of a small private school. They empathized with our unique situation. Seth missed a lot of school in the year we traveled for care. Even though Seth was nine, they suggested the second-grade class as a good place for him to catch up. Seth looked out the car window for a friendly face and wondered if he would fit in. The children were lined up, ready to head into his new school.

"Mom, I don't want to go. Please. I wanna go home."

"It'll be okay, Seth. I promise you'll make new friends. The first day is always the hardest. Do you want me to walk with you?"

Seth nodded.

As we made our way indoors, Seth took a deep breath. At that moment, he was the bravest kid I knew. Despite everyone staring at him as the new kid, Seth took the Mickey Mouse medical mask Dr. Ned gave him out of his pocket. He pulled the elastic loops over each ear and adjusted the pleat over his nose. Seth was accustomed to following his doctor's orders and didn't think twice about it until now. People who knew us at church and special events expected Seth to wear his mask. These children did not.

As we made our way down the hallway, we noticed some children nudging one another and pointing to turn and look toward us. Seth's pace slowed. Uncertain he wanted to proceed, he looked up at me. I reassured him with a smile and a nod. Seth grabbed my hand and squeezed it.

We could hear kids whispering. One boy asked another, "What's that on his face?" Seth endured the snickering as we walked by, and his body language followed suit. His once brave shoulders collapsed. His head sank. His eyes stared at the ground. I didn't know how to help. I wanted to explain, but no words came. I prayed to myself, *God, help Seth feel accepted!*

Out of nowhere came a little boy. Our eyes met as he edged his way through the students. He exuded kindness as he walked toward Seth and courageously stood beside him. He confidently addressed the crowd.

"Hey, leave him alone! I feel bad for him."

Seth looked up in disbelief. Then he addressed Seth with a huge grin and the sweetest toothless smile.

"My name is Isaiah, and I'll be your friend!"

Seth's whole face turned into a smile. Even though his mask obscured his mouth, Seth's smile shone through his eyes. He now had competition for being the bravest kid I knew. The circumstances that led to meeting Isaiah would impact Seth. Seth knew how painful it was to feel like an outcast and also how good it felt to be accepted. God used those difficulties in his little life for good. Isaiah's boldness spurred Seth on to not only look for those who needed encouragement but to cheer for them.

It's no wonder Seth and Isaiah became best friends. Two little boys helped change the tone of the elementary school with kindness and compassion despite their differences.

Spring 2010

The voice on the other end of the phone spoke frantically.

"You have to turn on your television. A doctor is talking about your old neighborhood in Florida. Julie, kids are getting sick!" I stopped her.

"No offense, but Seth has the best doctors in the country helping him."

My friend insisted, "You have to see this! What if–" The call went silent for a moment. Shaken, she tried to gather her emotions. "What if this is what caused Seth's conditions?"

Although we regularly received unsolicited, sometimes crazy, medical advice from anyone and everyone, she got my attention. I grabbed the remote and flipped through the channels.

"Confirmed disease cluster in the Loxahatchee neighborhood called 'the Acreage,'" the TV reporter announced.

"I-I-I'll call you back."

I dropped the phone and sank onto the couch. My legs went numb. The stories of rare disease coming out of our old Florida neighborhood wrenched my heart. The Acreage? It felt surreal . . . The community we moved out of when Seth was two years old was making national news.

We were one of the first on our block to build there. It was our dream home away from the city. We didn't plant grass in the backyard because we thought it would be fun for the boys to leave it as it was. Seth especially loved the South Florida sand. He played in that dirt/sand mixture for hours, giggling and splashing, making mud pies to take into his "log cabin."

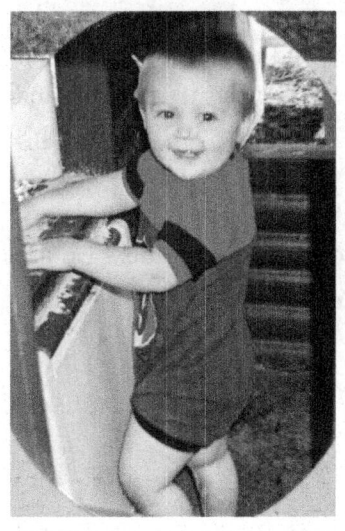

The allegations stated that soil contaminated with radioactive material was used for fill to build up the Acreage so homes could be built. Government officials had confirmed the unusual number of children who lived in the homes had developed brain and head tumors. Families were abandoning their homes in the Acreage as the cases and fear continued to rise.

My thoughts spun like crazy. I put our well water into every one of Seth's bottles every few hours to reconstitute his powdered formula! *What if—our water was tainted? What if that sand and dirt mixture that he played with daily for hours contained this radioactive material? Could there be a connection?*

I felt sick to my stomach.

For years we had racked our brains to try and figure out what could have caused this disease. I called the office of Seth's neurologist and explained what I'd heard. I coveted their professional input. They thought it was reasonable to do imaging of his brain to check for tumors. They sought to leave no stone unturned in an effort to find answers for Seth's bizarre condition.

An early hypothesis considered Seth's immune system could very well have been triggered by something. While working overtime trying to fight that something off, his immune system got stuck in overdrive. Could this be what provoked it to go awry?

Seth's neurologist told me the good news. Seth's brain was free from tumors. She also gave me wise counsel.

"Julie, you can drive yourself crazy trying to solve this great mystery. From my experience, when parents hear that their child has cancer, it's common for them to question themselves: What could I have done differently? Is there anything I could have done to prevent this? You can spend a lot of energy living in the what ifs and the land of should have, could have. Regardless of what caused your son's immune system to self-destruct, we will continue to work together, doing everything possible to give him a fighting chance."

Joshua 1:9 brought me peace. "--be strong and courageous! Do not be afraid or discouraged. For the LORD your God is with you wherever you go."

2011

Seth was born perfectly healthy without complications as a planned repeat cesarean birth. Except for a modest growth on Seth's head at birth, his early childhood health proved unremarkable. A doctor assured us early on that the growth was no reason for concern.

Seth approached his tween years. He had dealt with the unknowns of his health and changes to his appearance from head to toe. To make matters worse, the subtle growth had morphed into a thick, leathery patch that protruded from his hairline, causing alopecia (hair loss). Seth's grade school classmates began to notice, comment, and ask questions. Just as in the case of his legs, Seth found it hard to explain what was happening. He often told his peers, "It's hard to explain and understand, but God understands."

I took Seth to a specialist for a new perspective. Unlike the other doctor, this one mentioned the possibility of cancer, especially around puberty. In addition, this cluster of cells has been known to develop into secondary tumors. There was even a "syndrome" associated with all kinds of abnormalities.

In Seth's case, the doctor mentioned to Donnie and me that it was both reasonable and wise to surgically remove the growth before it evolved further. Our experience through this journey had been that if there was a slight percentage of something going wrong, Seth usually ended up being the rare statistic.

We had grown accustomed to doctors explaining that surgery was not without risks, especially in Seth's case. The doctor didn't like doing surgery on patients taking Methotrexate. He told us to expect Seth wouldn't heal as quickly as others. So, we weighed the benefits versus the risks. However, Seth's unwavering desire to remove the growth propelled us forward. Thankfully, the surgery went well, and they sent us home without incident. Phew.

To our disappointment, after a week, the wound burst open. Here we go again. Back at our local doctor's office, they sent us to the Emergency Room. The ER told us we needed to drive back to Mayo Clinic immediately.

Sigh. Like many times before, I was running on adrenaline, God's grace, and lots of coffee. I spoke with Mayo Clinic on speakerphone while I threw things into tote bags for Seth and me. Once I got off the phone with the medical team, I called a couple of friends to help with the kids the next day. Since the Ronald McDonald House almost always has a waiting list, I would likely need to book a hotel room for the night.

As I drove, my mind was racing with all the details that needed my attention. I glanced at the rearview mirror and saw a tan cruiser with blue lights flashing. Ugh. I instinctively looked down at my speedometer, which revealed my mind wasn't the only thing racing. My thoughts shifted to the speeding ticket I was about to get. So much for hotel funds!

An officer approached the car. My heart beat rapidly. He spoke in a serious yet friendly tone.

"Hello. License, registration, and proof of insurance, please. Do you know why I pulled you over?"

I scrambled to get the information he requested. "Yes, sir, I was speeding."

He leaned down to peer into the car and saw Seth with his head on a pillow. I'd put bandages around his head as a makeshift barrier to stop the blood and protect the open area from debris.

"Where are you headed?"

"Rochester, Minnesota, where my son gets treatment."

"Wait here one moment, please."

I watched him in my rearview mirror walk quickly to his patrol car. My focus now shifted to whether or not we would make our appointment to meet with the surgeon. My stomach was in knots. Thankfully, the officer kept his promise of being just a moment.

He returned my information and said, "I'm not going to give you a ticket this time, but please slow down and drive safely." I thanked him. He smiled and said, "I hope things go well for your son."

I pulled back onto the highway with great relief and gratitude.

Seth's team was waiting for us in Rochester. We were so blessed to have the gifted hands of a world-renowned reconstructive surgeon on board on such short notice. Their plan was to start an IV antibiotic drip and close the wound once and for all. I was at peace with such expertise.

After Seth and I exchanged a kiss and a smile, a man in surgical scrubs pushed Seth down a hallway to the OR. I got a cup of coffee and settled in the surgical waiting area. I looked around at the parents making small talk. I wished Donnie could be with me. Exhaustion made my eyelids droop even though I fought off sleep. I awoke disappointed in my inability to stay awake. I scanned the room, wondering if I had missed them calling me. I jumped up to check Seth's status on the surgical board. Nothing changed. Several hours passed. *It's a simple matter of re-closing the wound in a sterile environment, right? What's taking so long?* I thought as I decided to walk up to the surgical nurse's station.

"Hi. My son went in for a procedure quite a while ago. Is there a way to check his status? I'm getting worried. Here's his ID number." I handed her the slip of paper.

"One moment, please– Okay, I just called back there. Someone will come out and give you an update."

"Thank you."

I stood in front of the doors, waiting. *Why won't anyone tell me anything? What's going on with my son?* I texted my prayer warriors.

Finally, a nurse came out to walk me back to the recovery room. When I entered the room, Seth's chin was straight up, and he had a plastic mouthpiece over his lips. The post-op nurse quickly removed it and explained she was sorry for the wait but usually they don't bring parents back while a patient is still intubated.

"I was wondering what was taking so long."

This nurse promptly remarked, "I don't think you understand." The change in tone and look of concern startled me. Her eyes locked with mine and remained there. "The doctor sent me to count your son's respirations."

I didn't fully understand, but whatever complications had just happened, she was dead serious. An awkward silence was broken only by the monotone beeping of machines. Her eyes softened to reflect a demeanor of compassion. I could sense part of her wanting to reveal more, yet she hesitated. I respected that and didn't push the issue. I just wanted to be with my son. I leaned over the gurney rails and pulled him in close, my precious little boy. I looked up to thank the nurse for caring for my son so well. I had a new warmth and respect for this woman I didn't know. She smiled back at me.

"Let's try and wake him."

We tried several times. With each attempt, we got louder and moved his body. Finally, Seth's eyes opened. He scanned the room without moving his head. When his eyes met mine, he flashed that signature Seth smile. A bittersweet release filled my heart as I melted into his chest. The nurse picked up the phone and happily reported his more favorable status to the medical professionals waiting. I breathed a deep sigh. My son was back.

I decided not to share with Seth the events that happened at Saint Marys Hospital that day, and it would remain that way. His struggle to come out of general anesthesia concerned the hospital staff, but no one as much as me. As I leaned over holding him close, I thanked God for giving me back my son.

I shudder to think of how this story might have ended: Every parent's worst nightmare is hearing the devastating, life-changing news that their child didn't make it. This event shook me with that harsh reality and a wake-up call. I would no longer take life for granted. The hours of waiting etched in me a stark reminder that a routine procedure can take an unexpected turn. That afternoon taught me to appreciate the precious gift of life and realize how quickly it can end. I got a glimpse of reality that rocked me and changed my whole perspective.

My phone continued to beep with text messages from those wanting an update. Overcome with gratitude for the multitudes who prayed for Seth. I texted back, "Praise God, all is well!" I had no doubt that Seth was here safe and sound as an answer to prayers sent on his behalf.

In the meantime, removing the tumor to prevent cancer from growing and stitching up the reopened wound moved down the priority list. Hoping the scar healed discretely enough not to draw attention at school now seemed so vain, but not to a budding teenager.

Seth said, "I want to see my new battle scar. Does anyone have a mirror?"

The post-op nurse said, "Better than that, if you promise to keep that battle scar covered and protected, I will take a photo to give you. Deal?"

"Deal!"

After a quick snap of the camera, she disappeared. Soon she returned with the printed copy of the photo and an armful of supplies.

"Now you can show your friends what you were up to when you weren't at school, and they'll know what a *warrior you are*."

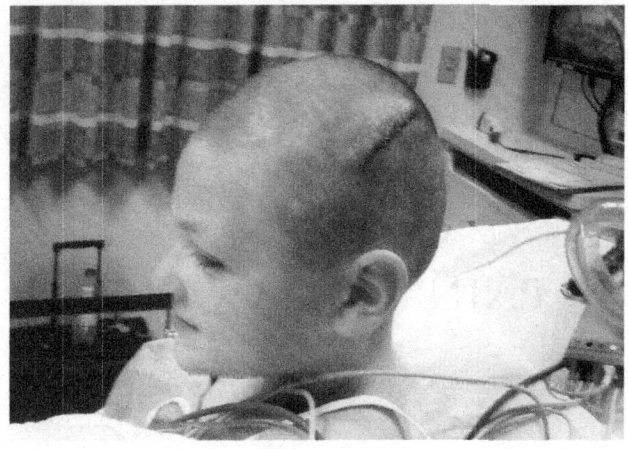

Seth smiled and stared at the photo as the nurse wrapped gauze and bandages around his head. Wound embarrassment dodged. I was thankful for a nurse who enabled Seth to share his story through photography. Seth was learning to own his battle scars.

CHAPTER NINE
PAIN IT FORWARD

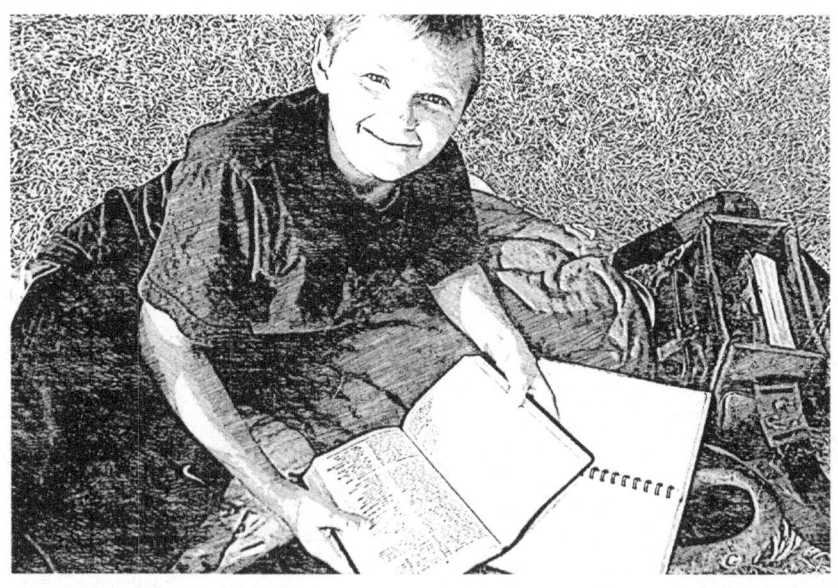

We are not entitled to a pain-free, trouble-free life. Embracing
this will ease the collision between expectation and reality.
–John Piper

At eleven years old, Seth struggled to cope with daily, consistent, unresolved pain from head to toe with no end in sight. He dealt with pain the best way he knew, but it was as rough for Seth as it was painful for us to watch. It seemed every part of his body was somehow rebelling. His organs, joints, tendons, nerves, bones, cells, and even his skin were fighting back. I wouldn't wish this on anyone. The neuropathy, the muscle spasms, and the headaches never ceased. How could he see past all this to enjoy life when he didn't have an hour free from pain? I gently rubbed pain cream on his legs. His skin hurt to be touched. All he wanted to do was to soak in hot water.

This disease seemed to be one step ahead of us. Just when the team thought they had it figured out, it changed course and attacked a new area of Seth's body. The very best doctors in the country were kept on their toes and scratching their heads.

From what we witnessed, this was progressive and degenerative. I was trying to help my son get better while fighting the possibility that he may never get better. Polyneuropathy (the malfunction of many nerves throughout the body simultaneously) was added to his chart. A lifetime of pain seemed inevitable.

Seth longed for normalcy–we all did. He never asked for pain medication. Except for a couple of hospitalizations, doctors did not prescribe narcotics (opioids). Donnie and I were on board with that, but watching Seth suffer in relentless pain wasn't the answer either. I simultaneously appreciated and despised medications. I didn't know much about pain control but knew there had to be a better way.

In researching alternative therapies and data supporting their efficacy, I found meager research statistics published in the mainstream. It was important that my son be given the opportunity to take advantage of different therapies *along with* conventional medicine. I received some pushback initiating conversations and didn't understand why. At first, I felt like this was an area that some medical professionals simply overlooked because it was unfamiliar territory. I get it–the unknowns are scary.

Whenever Seth developed a new condition, I resisted adding more medications. I questioned everything. Seth's doctor and I would have lengthy discussions to ensure that the benefits far outweighed the risks.

No doubt Seth struggled, but medications were not the long-term solution that any of us wanted for him, not even the medical team. I really struggled with the med issue. Up until this point, my husband and I were very conservative about giving our children medications, even over-the-counter ones. They were remarkably healthy and rarely got sick, so medications were unnecessary. Our children had never been on antibiotics. Now, I was being thrown into a world of prescription pills, liquids, injections, creams, light therapy, and patches, and it just kept snowballing. It kept me up at night. I wondered how we even got to this place.

For sure, Seth needed intervention. The horror of my son's body wasting away, plus the permanent disability, spotlighted the constant reminder. My son wouldn't be here if not for God's grace and modern medicine. I was grateful for access to life-saving drugs and for those who had pioneered these treatments ahead of us. But I wondered when we were ever going to be able to stop treatment. Every time we tried to wean him slightly, he relapsed. I never expected this to turn into long-term immunosuppressive therapy. A fear hovered overhead that if the active disease came back, we might not be able to keep it at bay, and we could lose him. We were not willing to take that risk.

Sometimes the weight of it all consumed me. Thankfully, I wasn't alone. We were stronger and more confident moving forward as a team. More than one pair of eyes evaluated every new symptom, test, and result. Each new condition, diagnosis, and treatment was made in collaboration with several brilliant minds. I regularly prayed that the Lord would guide and direct us all.

In the meantime, the importance of keeping Seth active was vital. His body told him he needed to rest, but we knew it was best to keep him moving. We fought for normalcy, made sure he attended school, did (modified) chores like his siblings, and encouraged him to participate in activities. Even though his body seemed to be on fire, we exercised tough love, pushing him just past his comfort zone.

When Seth experienced flare-ups, he begged for relief for his Achilles tendons. We learned this was the main tendon our bodies depended on to walk, run, squat, and jump. Seth's rheumatologist suggested administering corticosteroids directly to the affected area to minimize pain and inflammation and keep him mobile and out of a wheelchair. He couldn't inject right into the tendon because it could compromise the integrity of the fibers and increase the risk of rupture. Instead, his rheumatologist guided the injection via ultrasound to ensure the needle specifically penetrated the bursa sac, a fluid-filled sac that cushions an area of friction between tissues, such as tendons and bone. Seth felt immediate relief and was beyond grateful! It enabled him to keep going. His hinged leg braces were also a valuable support to the area.

What this disease was doing to Seth's body seemed like a never-ending battle. We were putting out fires one at a time. Understandably, Seth grew weary. The constant electricity jolts of damaged nerves got caught in a crossfire as the disease assailed through the fat layer. I learned nerves try to regenerate or attempt to repair themselves, but damaged nerves are like a downed power wire arcing wildly. We needed a drug to calm the overactive nerve pain receptors so that the pain was at least manageable. I second-guessed adding another medication, but the benefit outweighed the risk. It took weeks to see any improvement, but suddenly, it was a night-and-day difference. Seth no longer woke up in the middle of the night with leg pain and was functional during the day without fear of pain. Victory!

SEARCHING FOR ALTERNATIVES

I had a wonderful, unhurried conversation with Dr. Mirg, an anesthesiologist with a passion for children. She listened thoroughly and shared many of my concerns. She commended me for taking the more challenging, less-traveled road. We discussed ways to manage Seth's pain and help him be his best even with limited options. Familiar with the trial and error of medications we had grown accustomed to over the years, we were all learning.

Proceeding with caution, maintaining communication, and regular monitoring would be essential for implementing and balancing both natural and traditional medicine. Obviously, we weren't going to take away life-and-death medications, such as his anti-seizure medication. Yet, I hoped we could discover alternatives for lesser medications–with fewer side effects–to support his overall health. I felt like it was our only hope to (one day) wean him off some of the prescriptions.

Dr. Mirg expressed her concerns about unregulated alternatives, lack of consistency in different products, dosing, and the potential for unknown interactions with his current medications. But, she was open and willing to work through these concerns together. I presented potential options I had researched for her review, and Dr. Mirg did her own research and consulted with colleagues. In time, we moved past the "just a mom" stigma to mutual respect. It was not easy, but we pooled our resources, worked collaboratively, and refused to lose hope.

Dr. Mirg and I discussed alternatives, including a type of electrical nerve stimulation unit, physical therapy, massage therapy, including myofascial release (focuses on specific areas), and aqua therapy to help ease the pain. I looked into acupuncture and dry needling. I figured it might or might not help, but since it involved no medication, at least he'd avoid a drug interaction. However, access to alternative medicine was met with resistance by insurance, and the cost was not sustainable out-of-pocket. It was frustrating, to say the least.

Dr. Mirg encouraged my efforts and told me she appreciated my drive to find the best options for my son's unique circumstances. It inspired her to consider and push for more options in the future.

It was disappointing to hear there wasn't much room for the advancement of complementary and alternative medicine to be added in pediatrics, at least not yet. But she told us not to get discouraged. We were at the forefront of integrative medicine. She told me she would look into options in the clinic's Complementary and Alternative Medicine (CAM) department. She learned options were limited because of Seth's age. The only area of pediatrics with approved alternative therapies was Palliative Care or end-of-life "comfort" care. She shared my frustration. Seth never "fit into any box." He was treated with aggressive *adult* medications from age seven but was limited by his age for alternative, *less aggressive* treatments. Many professionals agreed it seemed backward, but their hands were tied. We determined to work together to change the current options, or lack thereof, available for young people.

To my dismay, within a year, Dr. Mirg moved to another facility. Lack of continuity is one of the frustrations of long-term care. This meant we needed to start at square one with another provider. We had gotten used to "one step forward, two steps back." It was easy to grow weary, but I needed to remember that God loved us and walked with us on this bumpy journey. I trusted that God was orchestrating just the right team, at just the right time, for all of Seth's needs.

Spiritually, Seth was ready for battle more than any warrior I had ever known. When the going got tough, he opened and studied Scripture. I often found him late at night in the dark with a book light on, reading and praying. He wrote down and highlighted passages that gave him peace and comfort. Little by little, Seth's faith grew stronger through the adversity he endured.

There were days, however, when even our tough little soldier grew weary. Seth often heard people say he was *so strong*. Others suggested yoga and meditation to "find his inner strength." Seth heard mixed messages. The truth was, many days, Seth didn't feel strong. His body was weak and getting weaker. His immune system was wreaking havoc against his healthy cells and tissues. His metabolic system was hijacked and energy depleted (inability to store energy in cells involved). He was just so tired.

On one particularly challenging day, I sensed his despair.

He cried out, "Mom! I am not strong enough. I can't do this!"

I said, "You're right!"

He looked at me wide-eyed. That was not the response he expected.

I explained. "We aren't called to be strong on our own. We are to rely on the one who is all-powerful in all circumstances–only God. Philippians 4:13 says, "I can do all things through Christ who strengthens me" (NKJV).

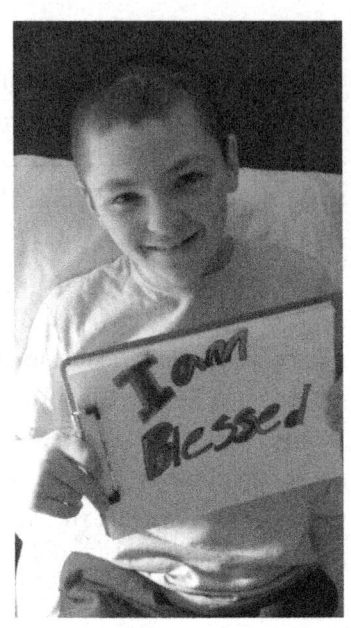

This was a pivotal moment for Seth, his aha moment. Seth realized he had the greatest truth and weapon at his disposal. He repeated Philippians 4:13 to himself over and over. Thereafter, when preparing for another test, treatment, or procedure–"I can do all things." When overwhelmed with pain–"I can do all things." He clung to *his* verse. When others asked how he endured so much suffering, he quoted, "I can do all things . . ."

For me, the preceding verses, Philippians 4:11-12, held special meaning because they highlighted the importance of finding true contentment in all circumstances. "Not that I was ever in need, for I have learned how to be content with whatever I have. I know how to live on almost nothing or with everything. I have learned the secret of living in every situation, whether it is with a full stomach or empty, with plenty or little." This journey had certainly taken us through hills and valleys and lots of needs. Over the years, I came to realize my joy, contentment, and peace didn't have to be defined by my circumstances. I had a choice.

Although at times I felt like a hot mess, and Seth was exhausted, overwhelmed, and discouraged, I saw us both as a work in progress. We were learning to find our strength and satisfaction in God through the parade of people he placed in our lives. Because of their prayers and love, our endurance to run the race of life and our faith grew stronger.

Seth didn't want to miss out and didn't want anyone to pity him.

Like most kids, he didn't want to be different from his friends. He wanted those around him to be happy. He accepted each day as a gift. He worked hard to put his best self forward, and, in turn, it seemed to bring out the best in others. People found themselves drawn to Seth. They longed to understand and engage in things that were important to him, to help him in his endeavors.

We began alternative therapies prescribed by Seth's providers. Then the fight would begin to get them covered by insurance. Even after Seth's doctor wrote letters of necessity, we had to explain, in detail, all of the things tried to no avail. I was sure that if anyone needed these benefits and services, it was my son. This was my motivation. I was prepared for denial at first but stood ready for the next steps.

I appealed and fought for the approval to go through a medical review. Oftentimes, it was apparent that those at the state level making these critical decisions were limited in their knowledge and understanding of the rare and complex. The role of advocating and educating, once again, rested on me.

Word that our requests received approval and would be paid began to trickle in. What a huge victory for Seth. I prayed that others in the future would benefit from the ripple effect. We were told our battle was paving the way.

We began to see purpose in the pain. This was especially helpful on the hard days. Seth alternated between physical therapy and aqua therapy several days a week. Seth loved aqua therapy. He told me it was the only time he didn't feel pain. We went to a special pool heated to ninety-three degrees. His therapist was shocked that Seth could kick his legs and move them without pain. His joints didn't ache like they did when he was bearing his own weight on land. It was so good for Seth in every way. However, insurance only paid for a limited number of sessions.

I had first-hand evidence of the benefits of having options available for medical treatments. In my opinion, I saw room for traditional, conventional, alternative, and complementary medicine to coincide, but access was very limited. We continued to share our journey as connections and communication continued and evolved.

During this time, I was invited and introduced as a special guest of a well-known professor of medicine, an author, and one of the world's leading experts on resilience and well-being. What a humbling honor to be a part of an intimate round table discussion at Mayo Clinic in the CAM department. We discussed caring for those with ongoing difficult medical challenges. The feedback I provided from our experience was graciously received.

As a caregiver, I was thankful for the opportunity to connect and share with other caregivers and medical personnel. We were better and stronger as we learned from each other's diverse backgrounds and experiences. After speaking with the group about my experiences with rare diseases, someone spoke up.

"I'm sorry, we didn't ask you to share your medical background."

I chuckled. "I graduated from The School of Hard Knocks!"

Meanwhile, Seth handled all of this better than anyone expected. Healthcare professionals often commented how impressed they were by Seth's positive attitude in the midst of the extraordinary circumstances. In addition, they frequently asked about the coping strategies he used.

"God. It's all God," was his unrehearsed, honest response.

He found this answer equally helpful when others asked him questions. At first, he felt uncomfortable being put on the spot. "How can you be so happy?" "How can you have such joy?" "How can you continue to show up?" Then, one day he broke the awkwardness with those three simple words he knew to be true. He boldly gave credit to whom credit was due. "It's all God!" We should have put it on a T-shirt for him to wear. Others said they were better for having crossed paths with Seth.

Aware that everyone deals with adversity in different ways, I observed that Seth benefited greatly from reading and writing Scripture. Some days, he didn't even understand what he read as he struggled cognitively (chemo brain). Nonetheless, God met him where he was and gave him comfort and peace. Seth always carried his Bible and notebook wherever he went. If we had time to kill, we'd walk out to a grassy area outside the clinic, and he'd pull out his Bible and enjoy the time decompressing. It was never by any of my promptings. It really was *all God*. God's word proved to be an anchor for us, solid and unchanging in ever-changing circumstances and unknowns. When so much of Seth's life seemed out of his control, he grew to understand the phrase, "God is in control." The concept was becoming less abstract as Seth's faith grew through reading the Bible and when he saw examples of God's help through others' love and care along our journey.

January 2012

I received a call from the head of the Pain and Rehabilitation Program (PRP) at Mayo Clinic. She informed me that someone gave her Seth's name as a good candidate for a program they hoped to implement. She asked if Seth and I would like to be part of a pilot program and, if so, be open to giving our feedback. Although the Rochester PRP is one of the first programs in the world of its kind, they wanted to implement a program geared toward younger children. They already had a three-week program for older teens and adults but wanted to develop a program for those as young as twelve (even though Seth was only eleven at the time).

We conversed for quite some time. This was a respected program that cost over $30,000 to attend. Our fee would be taken care of in full. This was an opportunity we couldn't pass up. We were so blessed to live in a country where we not only had access to such incredible care but got a front-row seat to the advancements in overall health and wellness.

Seth was shy at first but opened up to the other kids once he realized they also spent a lot of time at the hospital. Although they weren't going through the same medical challenges, they still had much in common. Living with an incurable disease, unknown prognosis, progressive degenerative disease, etcetera, is hard enough on an adult. Young people need appropriate coping skills and strategies to thrive. For us, we turned to God. He had been our strength. We had peace, purpose, and even joy in the midst of suffering. Here, we learned people process trauma in many different ways.

Staff gave each child and parent study materials. My binder was a whopping four-inches thick and crammed with information, study guides, and feedback forms to work on over the three-week program. Parent and child separated for activities, then came back together for other workshops and feedback sessions. We learned that, statistically young people who suffer from chronic pain often turn to alcohol, drugs, self-mutilation, suicidal thoughts, or other unhealthy outlets. The clinic carried a delicate balance between being informative and maintaining age-appropriate discussions for those at such a young age. Although Seth and I were pretty naive to these things, it would now be on my radar as a parent. I would be vigilant to intercept those "fiery darts" of discouragement and despair before they had a chance to take hold.

I learned that our bodies undergo changes when in "fight or flight" mode. This was the first time I heard the term. I researched and learned about two main modes of operation in our nervous system. The first is "fight or flight." The second is "rest and digest." We should optimally be in the rest and digest state eighty percent of the time. Seth and I in "rest and digest" mode eighty percent of the time? I don't think so.

One day, each patient participant was given a whiteboard. They were instructed to write down three points to share with the class, Seth willingly participated and wrote as best he could.

Name some positive traits about yourself.

"I AM A CHRISTIAN, funny, Athlete, Good frienD, a Good Brother I am COURAgous.

Name things you are thankful for.

I have God, family, fRends, Church, Mayo Clinic

Is there anything else you would like us to know?
I can do All things throo Christ."

Seth and I both found it helpful to share with others. It was amazing to find so many enduring similar struggles. We were not alone and found strength in the sweet friendships formed. Seth gained confidence. He saw the benefit of opening up as other parents shared how helpful it was to see things through Seth's lens. He was dealing with so much, yet he was not allowing it to rob him of his joy. He inspired others in faith, hope, and love to never give up.

We discussed our perspective with doctors, nurses, psychologists, physical therapists, nutritionists, and directors of the program. The theme covered coping strategies for dealing with no-quick-fix conditions and debilitating pain. Classes covered counseling, consistent sleep schedules, exercise, and meditation (for us, prayer). They also taught breathing techniques, biofeedback, and imagery. Seth favored visual and literal concepts, so "imagery," in particular, stuck with him.

In one imagery exercise, the students were told to close their eyes and imagine driving away from the hospital without appointments, testing, pokes, pain, sickness, or unknowns. They didn't have a care in the world. Seth felt empowered by that visual. No matter where he was, it taught him how to shift his focus. This would serve him well as yet another coping strategy.

Seth's classmates seemed to connect with him, and his leadership set the tone for the day. After a long day of going through the program, everyone needed encouragement. Seth's smile and quick wit provided infectious, contagious laughter. Our family had unintentionally adopted the motto, "If you don't laugh, you'll cry." Parents and staff told me that Seth's positivity made a difference in the lives of the students who attended.

Not all families were able to finish the program. We understood. Some days, Seth had to leave the program to attend medical appointments and procedures. There were nights he didn't sleep due to pain and seizure activity, but he always returned to continue with the program. Seth took it as yet another life challenge to rise above obstacles set before him.

Of all the things he could not control about his rare disease, he could control his response and whether or not he would quit. He was proud that he pushed himself to finish as best he could. The staff can attest he always had a smile and never complained. No one, not even I as his mother, could fully understand what a sacrifice it was mentally, physically, and emotionally for Seth to persevere.

Seth excelled through the program better than anyone anticipated. We were given bittersweet news by the doctors heading up this program.

"In the history of this program, which has been around for at least fifteen years, we have never graduated anyone from the program early . . . until now. Consider it a compliment. You got this!"

We were honored to hear Seth already had a lot of the fundamentals down before he entered the program. They told Seth he was thriving despite his limitations. One person joked he could probably teach the class! My first reaction was to chuckle, but as it sank in, it also saddened me. I wished my young son didn't need to be so equipped for daily suffering. So instead, we decided to focus on how God was using his suffering for good.

Seth learned a lot about himself over those three weeks. One takeaway was the power of community. Seth witnessed the tangible benefits of encouragement between peers. Although initially reluctant to join in, Seth quickly realized they were stronger as a group. It made him feel good to know this program would help countless young people in the future. All the children, who came from across the country, grew to be close friends. Seth's positive impact touched many lives. God gave Seth a glimpse of how his life was making a difference.

After several weeks of enduring brutally cold Minnesota days and nights for most of February, it was time to say goodbye to the staff and new friends we had made. Mayo Clinic staff presented Seth with a certificate validating his hard work. It acknowledged that he participated in 130+ hours in the Pediatric Pain and Rehabilitation Program. That piece of paper gave Seth tangible evidence that he *could* do all things through Christ, who strengthened him, and that all things were possible with God!

Spring of 2012

A chemotherapy shortage caused a nationwide panic. Our pharmacist delivered the difficult news that they were out of stock, and even worse, they were dealing with a rolling backorder. I knew of many like me calling various pharmacies. We all received the same response. I was certain the preservative-free version we had been prescribed for nearly four years would be especially difficult to secure. We would take any variation, and I would drive anywhere. We were desperate!

My mind replayed Seth's body's chaotic state before this wonder drug brought things under control. The thought of Seth relapsing was unfathomable. I remembered the words from Seth's doctor when he started him on this medication.

"If he isn't taken off on a very, very slow taper, this aggressive disease may come back with a vengeance, and we may not be able to stop it."

That terrified me. How could I tell my son the medicine that had saved his life was unavailable? I went into my bedroom and silently soaked my pillow case with tears. Seth would need his dose in two days. That's all the time we had.

A friend from church heard of our predicament. From her contacts in Arizona, she was able to secure one vial. Even though it was only one dose, we were beyond grateful for it. We were good for one more week. We found ourselves at the mercy of others again, having little control, waiting, trusting, and believing that God would supply all of our needs. Each week, one more vial bought us time until the manufacturer could meet the demand. We would never take this life-sustaining medication for granted again.

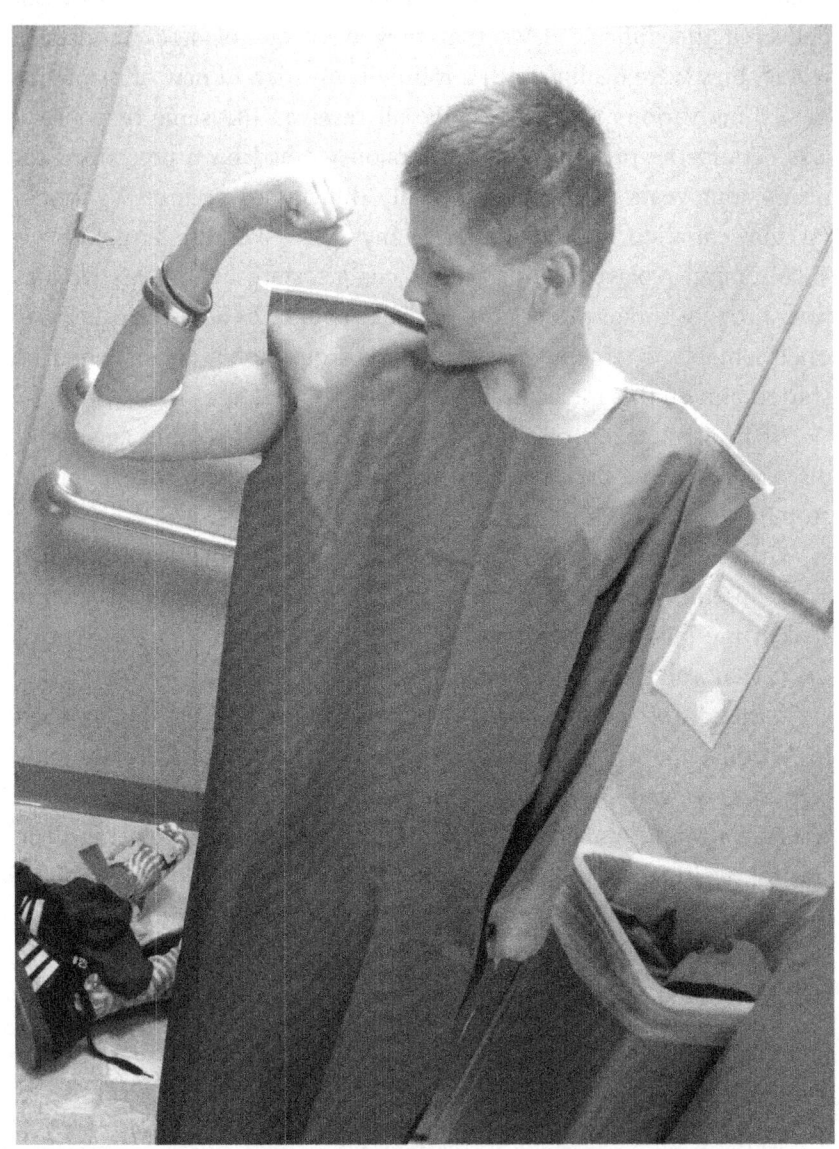

Philippians 4:13

CHAPTER TEN
A SLING AND A HANDFUL OF ROCKS

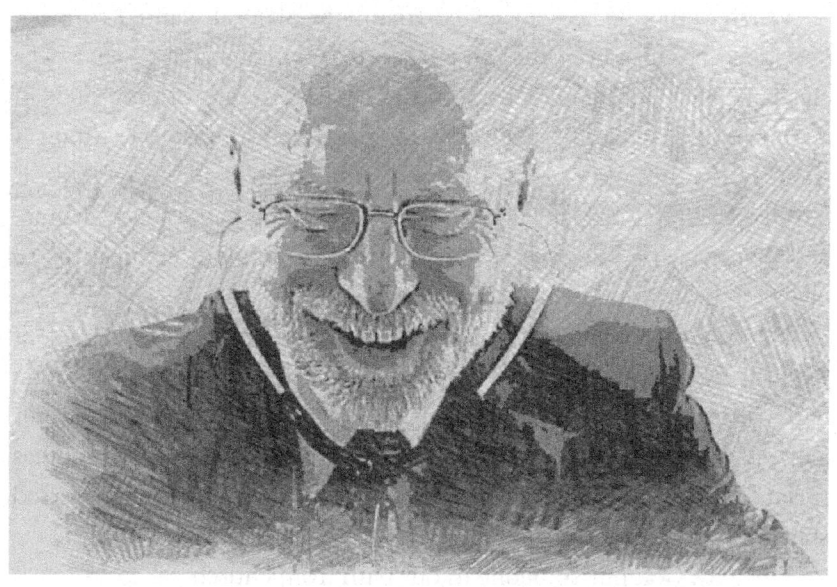

For every Goliath there is a stone.
–Author Unknown

The medical bills continued to pour in with no end in sight. There were times when I went to appointments and discreetly asked the front desk if they would be willing to hold my personal check for the co-payment until payday. The family's finances ran dry every month to pay for what Seth needed. We had to make tough choices. Donnie started selling things in the barn. His motorcycle was the first to go. Then a boat motor he'd built in which he invested a ton of time.

Donnie never complained or implied that he longed for a simpler life. After a long day, he worked on rebuilding things he purchased inexpensively or found on the side of the road. He then resold them to keep things afloat. I worked odd jobs and stayed up till the wee hours doing paperwork. No instruction manual existed for navigating the daunting healthcare system. We figured things out as we went.

When Seth's doctor suggested treatment plans, I wanted to make decisions based upon the best-projected outcome, not what was cheapest. How could anyone afford this? We were tens of thousands of dollars into this. Seth's insurance fought us on almost everything. I spent hours on hold only to be transferred to no avail. Some days, it felt like I had a phone glued to my ear. Something had to give. Donnie and I were trying our utmost, but we were maxing out credit cards to give Seth everything he needed to survive.

I didn't personally know anyone else who lived in this kind of medical crisis. I guess I lived a somewhat sheltered life. I had no one with whom to discuss our options. I felt like I was treading water alone. After trying to keep afloat for so long and making no progress toward land, the fatigue and weariness started to creep in. But God sent support.

One day, God put someone in our path from church.

She said, "I know it's hard for you to accept help, but this isn't about you. You have to think of what Seth needs long term."

She was right. Seth was already fighting what seemed most days to be a losing battle. I needed to eat some humble pie and accept assistance. Even if that meant applying for federal disability.

I had already learned to dot my i's and cross my t's by compiling documentation, logging phone calls, including names and titles of everyone I talked to, taking notes, and scheduling appointments. I saved all documentation. I felt prepared to make a strong case.

I contacted the Social Security Administration who made an appointment for me with the nearest local agency. I thought of my dad, who had suffered constant pain from debilitating cancer that affected every aspect of his life. He applied for disability at age fifty-two and was denied multiple times. He had to hire an attorney for the appeals process. Everything took a toll on him mentally, physically, and emotionally. *Four years* of denials and appeals later, it was finally approved. A few months after that long battle, my dad died.

The day had come for the preliminary hearing to see if Seth would qualify for Supplemental Security Income (SSI) benefits. I immediately felt the weight of this appointment. I knew I was facing a giant. Doubt crept in. I contemplated canceling the appointment. Seth's case was so rare and so complicated to explain. I was advised *not* to try and do this myself and that hiring an attorney was my only chance for success. But by the time I explained all of Seth's medical history to an attorney, I could already be pushing through the process. We couldn't afford an attorney anyway. I believed my son qualified, but I had to prove it on legal terms. I thought the odds were stacked against me, but I owed it to my son to fight for him. So, I made the decision to move forward. I prayed that God would guide me and help me communicate. I was nervous but confident. We needed this for the long haul.

I sat in my car in front of the federal office and tried to gain my composure. A Bible verse came to mind: "Do not be afraid! Don't be discouraged by this mighty army, for the battle is not yours, but God's" (2 Chron. 20:15).

I took a deep breath and headed into the large brick building. Inside the door, stood a uniformed, armed guard who asked my name and reason for being there. Intimidated but unshaken, I waited while he verified my information. He instructed me to sit down and wait. I noticed the vast diversity of people waiting around me. I wondered if I was the only one there for their child.

Shortly, I heard my name. A middle-aged woman wearing glasses, high heels, and a pencil skirt waited for me in the doorway. She barely cracked a smile as I followed the click of her heels with my rolling suitcase crammed full of files. She was all business. It was just as well, I thought. I was on a mission for my son and had no time for small talk.

The first order of business: sign a release for access to all of Seth's doctors and facilities to request medical records for verification. As I signed the paperwork, I joked it might tie up the fax machine for several hours. The initial question was the most challenging: What is the diagnosis? At that moment, I wished more than ever before that I had a name for my son's condition. Instead, I insisted if she would allow me the time, I would explain. I quickly opened the suitcase and presented pieces of evidence to make our case.

Medical terms, conditions, abnormal test results, treatments, complications, declines, misdiagnoses, and summaries of doctor and ER visits poured out of my mouth. I briefly read and explained the highlights shedding a glimpse of the difficult road of rare disease. The woman, who was all business, nodded and typed continuously. I showed original 8x10 color photographs that the university hospital medical photographer took of my son's body revealing the severity of his condition. I explained the progression and the long-term repercussions of this disease that affected multiple areas of his body.

She asked for evidence to substantiate each medical condition, complication, and disability I claimed. I had files of documentation at my fingertips that I quickly handed over for each inquiry. I was shaking and sweating and hoped she didn't notice. She definitely made me work through the process. Although grueling, I prayed beneath my breath to keep my composure. I understood why it needed to be a thorough process. I'm sure they'd seen their fair share of people trying to take advantage of "the system." I understood why there were systems in place.

She called a supervisor to help scan the documents. Now, two people were asking for clarification. I might not have had a name, but I had a list of medical terms of everything wreaking havoc on Seth's body for which there was no cure. They ended up taking over four hundred pages of medical records from me. They scanned every. single. page. into the governmental database accessible to the decision-makers at our state capitol.

All of a sudden, the case manager stopped me mid-sentence.

"This will do."

I was taken aback. "Do you have everything you need?"

Was there time for a closing argument? I looked at the clock on the wall. I couldn't believe my eyes. I verified that the clock matched the time on my watch–three hours and forty-one minutes advocating on my son's behalf! Part of me felt bad that I had taken so much of her time, but the other part of me was ready to continue.

My part of the process was obviously over as she shifted to doing all of the talking. To my surprise, instead of hearing about the waiting, the unknowns, and the appeal process (as I expected), the federal worker explained the process after approval. Her next words stopped me in my tracks.

"When you are approved, you will need to—"

I interrupted and repeated her words. "*When* you are approved? Don't you mean *If* you are approved?"

She put down the papers, looked me in the eyes, and said, "It doesn't happen very often, but there are times when you *know*, without a shadow of a doubt, a case *will* be approved. This is one of them." She picked up her papers and continued going over the next steps I could expect.

I tried to focus, but it was difficult. I was fighting to fully register the word "approved" in my brain while keeping my composure and processing the legalities she simultaneously explained. After finishing up the logistics, she kindly walked me out. Her demeanor had changed since we met. I sensed her empathy and compassion.

"I wish you and your son the best."

I thanked her for everything and spoke genuine words of blessing to her. Our eyes and parting smiles met as we were now connected in a new way. God answered my prayers and sent another helper along this difficult journey.

I reached my car and shut the door. Before I could turn the key, I felt a huge release. That strong, steady, unshakable patient advocate was now a hot mess melting into a puddle of emotions, overwhelmed with gratitude for how God had used her on behalf of my son.

The result of this meeting confirmed that God had equipped me for this battle. I believed Seth now had a fighting chance, even when some of the best doctors told us he didn't. I envisioned a small boy bringing a sling and a handful of rocks to fight a giant. Most would write off "just a mom" bringing a heap of papers and photos to a federal hearing as unlikely to succeed. God not only enabled me to stand before the intimidating giant of a governmental system, he also gave me the strength and clarity to explain the rare, progressive, degenerative disease with no name, no cure, and no known prognosis. This–on top of the exhaustive care of a loved one–is the battle.

So many emotions poured out of my head and heart as I drove home, both bitter and sweet. Grieved that my once perfectly healthy child was permanently disabled at ten years old, I felt anguish that I couldn't provide the thousands of dollars out-of-pocket every month for all he needed. At the same time, I felt relieved and grateful that help was on the way! This ruling would open up access to many different resources, programs, therapies, and accommodations to help Seth live his best life.

With renewed energy, I began my search, but immediately hit a wall. I found it difficult to uncover any available resources because I didn't know who or what to ask for. One of Seth's doctors encouraged me not to give up.

He said, "I don't know all the resources available in your state, but just keep digging. They're readily offered but, more or less, have to be uncovered." He thanked me for being such a great advocate and encouraged me to keep up the good work.

His words encouraged and spurred me on, but I knew already that it really was a group effort. I was learning that a big part of this journey was finding our people. We were more grateful than ever for everyone who joined Seth's team.

A whole world existed that I knew nothing of. Before this, I had never even heard of the Department of Aging and Disability. I quickly found out that even program specialists and caseworkers for the state didn't know the answers to all of my questions. I understood it was difficult, even for them, to keep up with the changing policies, challenges, programs, and resources. Budgets, grants, and other funding directly affected availability as well.

I asked if they could research the answer and get back to me or let me know how to get the information myself. I had to be proactive. Once, when Seth met with a caseworker, not a medical professional, for a program, we waited months to hear if he qualified. I found after much digging that they never filed the paperwork because they didn't feel he qualified. I had to request his file be opened in an effort to see why. There was no paper trail, therefore, no denial letter. Without a denial letter, I had no basis or leverage to appeal. Grrr.

I talked to countless individuals who said this was the way they did it, and no one had ever challenged it. I dug until I finally found out what happened. They admitted they had never met anyone with Seth's conditions. The standard paperwork didn't easily apply, nor did it have areas to record variations since he was not a textbook case. I wondered how many people who needed and legitimately qualified for programs fell between the cracks this way. I worked to change the process and hold the programs accountable to *all* individuals. I worked to be a voice for those without one.

I went to a new appointment for the same program. This time, Seth had a different screener, and instead of checking the boxes yes or no, she documented an explanation for his extenuating circumstances. Lo and behold, he was approved! It was clear that Seth was unable to navigate this system alone. The experience compelled me to get involved, ask questions, and be a voice as a patient advocate. Rather than critiquing the system, I thought my energy would be better spent sharing our journey and making a difference. Federal and state programs and advocacy groups existed because someone went before us. Now, we would do that for others to come.

Although Seth's medical conditions were rare, I learned the difficult journey affected *millions* of families. The red tape, waiting lists, and denials for treatments and access to programs were commonplace. When a child got sick, family members often had to quit their livelihood in order to care for them. Talk about dismantling the family. And that was not the primary complaint. The problem lay in the need to spend just as much time fighting for coverage as they did caring for their loved ones. This had to change.

MEETING DR. FISCHER

Our primary care pediatrician at Mayo Clinic told us of her plans to leave the clinic. We had gotten used to doctors coming and going. It's part of years of ongoing, chronic medical treatment.

I prepared myself to go into "educating" mode to bring the next doctor up to speed. Having to explain our rare journey again was exhausting. This wasn't just a regular pediatrician we needed to replace. Patients like Seth need a Complex Care Coordinator when dozens of specialists are involved. When there are questions and varying opinions, this doctor would bring it all together. This person is crucial.

I prayed about this person. I felt vulnerable at times when I wasn't sure what to do. I needed to be able to trust that this person had my son's back, that they would make decisions as if it was for their own child. I really needed to connect with this new doctor. I shared my concerns with our favorite medical secretary in charge of scheduling.

She said, "The doctor I'm going to schedule you with is my personal favorite. Trust me-you will *love* Dr. Fischer."

I never heard his name before, but she was so convincing. I trusted her opinion and left feeling much more at ease.

The day came to meet our new *quarterback* who would lead Team Seth. Seth was nervous. I will never forget that day as long as I live. The door flung open, and a very tall gentleman with a dark gray suit, blue dress shirt, and tie as bright as his smile stood in the doorway. His demeanor was warm, kind, and witty.

He said, "The one . . . the only . . . the infamous . . . Seth . . . Bayles." Seth couldn't believe his ears. Not only did he pronounce his last name correctly, but it was as if he knew him–and "infamous"? I liked his bedside manner already.

In that short introduction, Seth instantly felt known and valued just as he was.

Dr. Fischer explained, "I have been studying your case for quite some time."

An immediate weight lifted. We had never set eyes on this doctor before, yet he knew things about Seth that he could only have known after digging deeply.

He said, "I heard about a boy who was giving his local hospital a run for their money."

Seth and I looked at each other as he pulled up a seat, wondering how he knew this. Then he explained. He received a call two years prior from an Emergency Department that needed guidance, and it intrigued him. Come to find out, he had a special interest in rare diseases. In the following months, he consulted with friends and colleagues to study this little boy's complex case.

"It's nice to finally meet you."

Wait! So this was the doctor on call years ago who instructed the ER exactly what to do with Seth? I tried to wrap my mind around how God had connected the dots for this moment. I couldn't have hand-selected a better doctor for Seth. With every ounce of my being, I believe that God in his loving kindness, grace, and mercy set this up.

I thought back to that time in the ER when I was frustrated and questioning why my son had to be so rare. In hindsight, it was becoming clear. If it weren't for the rarity of his disease, and doctors in various hospitals *not* knowing what to do with Seth, we wouldn't be here. And it was exactly where we were meant to be.

CHAPTER ELEVEN
LEARNING TO COPE

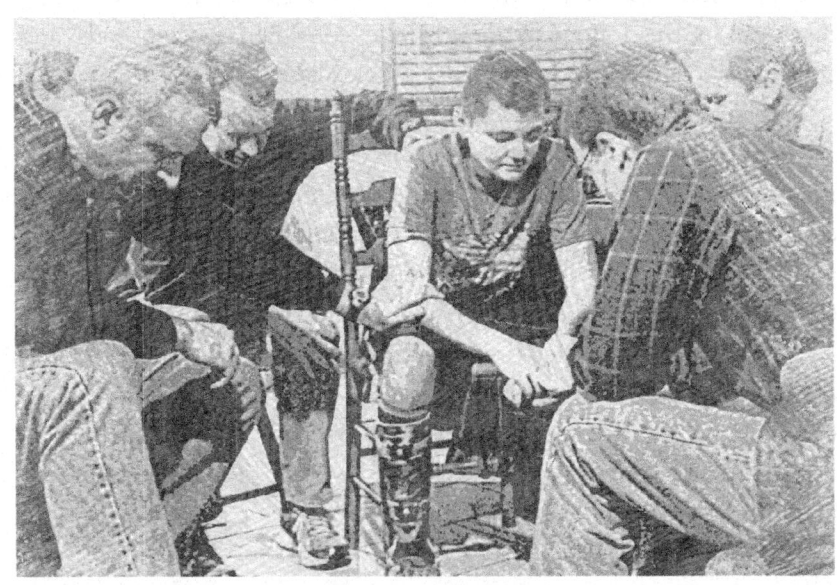

Prayer does change things, all kinds of things.
But the most important thing it changes is us.
–R. C. Sproul

I saw Seth growing exasperated, especially with his siblings. This was uncharacteristic of Seth. He went from sweet and joy-filled to having bouts of frustration and anger. His emotions were all over the place.

I got a call at work to come home. When I arrived home, I found Seth sobbing in frustration. He got angry at his siblings when they taunted him by obstructing his view of a TV show he was watching. So, he threw the remote at them. The boys thought it was funny and ducked. The remote hit the flat-screen television. Both the TV and Seth's self-control were shattered. No one was hurt, but I was concerned.

This wasn't the usual sibling rivalry. We were at a loss. Donnie and I had a dilemma on our hands. I tried not to overreact, but this could not continue.

"Seth, I know you've got a lot going on. I know it's difficult. But you cannot act out in anger like this, especially with those you love and who love you."

"I'm sorry, Mom. I love my family! It's like . . . I feel myself getting mad, and I don't want to. I don't want to do bad things. I will pay for the TV out of my allowance. It won't happen again, I promise." His head fell into my chest as he sobbed.

Was this beyond his control? Were the medications clouding his ability to think logically? Was this seizure activity? Constant pain? Is exhaustion taking over? I asked Seth questions to try and understand, but the more I asked, the more he sobbed. Our family was in crisis.

At the next visit with Seth's neurologist, she asked how he was handling things. I was honest. "He seems easily provoked, especially with his siblings."

She quickly responded, "Well, you can't blame him for getting annoyed with his brothers. They can do things he can't. It must be frustrating for him!"

Silence. I was in shock.

"That may be true, but it is unacceptable for him to hurt others because he is hurting!"

I was at a loss. We needed help. I did not intend to invalidate anyone's struggles. I'm certain what Seth was dealing with was overwhelming. This created a physical, mental, and emotional battle for him, but Seth wasn't the only one in the trenches. This was affecting the entire family.

At the time of discharge from the Pain and Rehabilitation Program, they recommended all participants find a counselor close to home as part of long-term continuing care. At that time, I called throughout Wisconsin to find someone to no avail. We had never had any dealings with mental health services, and I had no idea the process of getting into a provider would be so difficult. I was told unless he was suicidal (which he was not), a harm to himself, or others (also not the case), there weren't many options. When I found someone who seemed promising, they didn't work with kids so young or accept our insurance. For others, we had to wait nine months just to get on a waitlist.

The TV incident motivated me to press on and find alternative ways to support Seth. One arm of support came through regular visits from the leadership of our church. One day, our children's youth pastor and one of the elders from our church came to pray for Seth.

"Seth, how can we pray for you today?"

Seth hesitated, then tears started to roll down his face. Our dear pastor laid his hands on Seth's shoulders, reassuring him that it was okay to share.

"I just want the pain to stop, just for a few minutes."

We all prayed and wept together.

A friend of a friend referred us to a certified Christian family counselor. This professional was not only willing to help Seth free of charge, but he was also willing to drive forty minutes to our house. This exceeded our prayers for help. I wanted Seth to be able to regularly express his feelings and learn tangible tools to help him. Seth was receptive. He wholeheartedly wanted to press on in a positive way and prove he could do this. He really connected with this kind, compassionate gentleman. They prayed together and built trust.

Most days, Seth was more positive than one would expect for all he was going through. Most would see a strong, brave boy with no struggles. Seth put his best self forward at school, then came home and literally collapsed in his safe place. In his mind, he wanted so badly to be strong and brave, but his body couldn't follow suit.

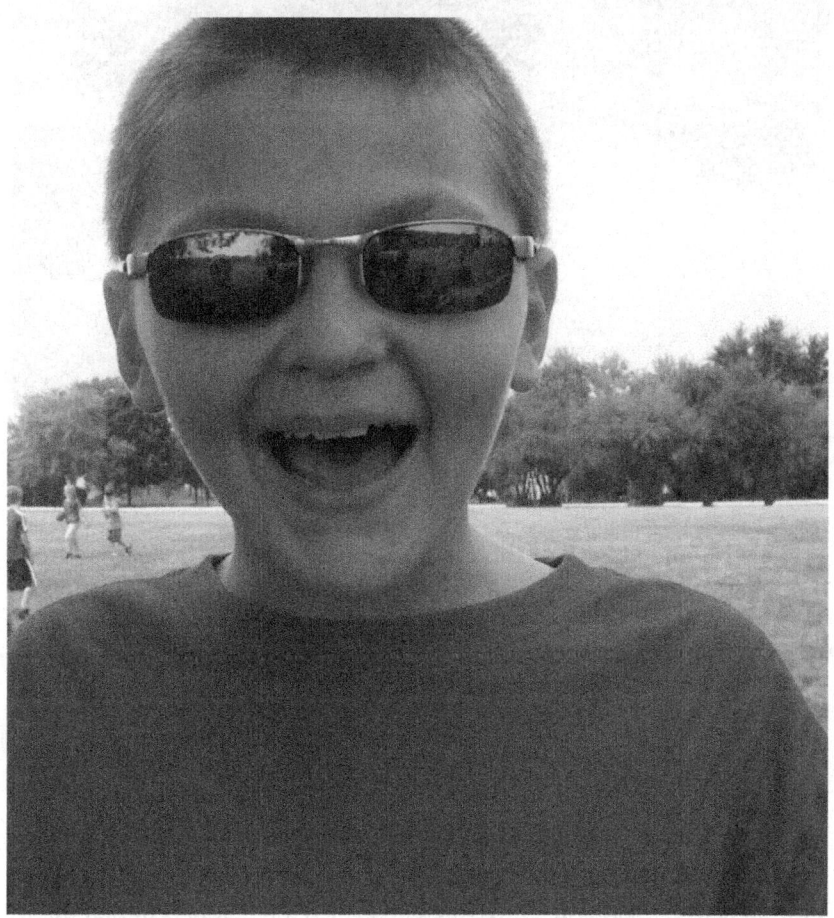

Seth at school recess

Some days his tears would flow without words. On other days when the pain got to be too much, he would lash out at those he loved most. He immediately felt remorse, but he was so tired of being sick and tired. Seth asked his counselor to help him with this particular battle. Since Seth was struggling cognitively and seemed to retain things better by picturing them in his mind, his counselor encouraged

Seth to envision a cotton ball every time he felt frustrated. It would remind him to focus on a soft response. Seth got it!

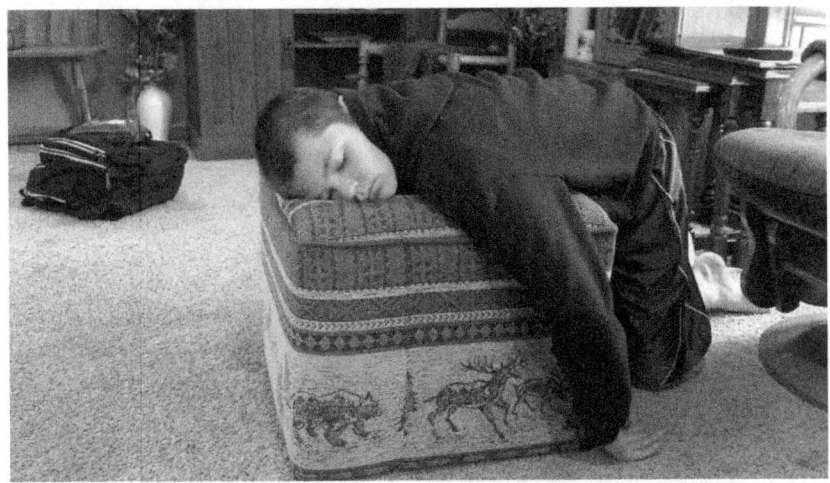

Seth upon returning home from school

This reminded Seth of the imagery coping strategy he learned from the Mayo pain clinic. Seth explained to me what he envisioned when he needed it most.

"Mom, I can see it. Dad is driving a motorhome, and you are in the passenger seat. You're smiling. Everyone is together, and we're driving away from the hospital. Everyone is happy." Seth had a detailed picture in his head as he described his sister sitting on the carpet playing with our beagle, and his brothers playing cards at the table. He grinned ear to ear as he described his vivid image. After hesitating for a bit, he asked, "Do you think this will ever really happen in real life?"

I had to turn away—I didn't want him to see the emotion that had overtaken me. I replied matter-of-factly, "You never know, maybe!" Everything in me wanted that dream to become a reality for him. Regardless, this was another tool that Seth used to cope with pain and frustration, and it was beautiful.

Being away from his loved ones made Seth appreciate them all the more. In some respects, this hardship brought our family closer to one another. Visualizing time in a motorhome with his family brought

Seth joy and peace. He thought of that motorhome whenever he was going into an MRI, having a spinal tap, heading down the hallway to surgery, or struggling with the fear of the unknown. Although it felt like the hardships would never end, Seth knew they wouldn't last forever. He had hope that the best days were yet to come. Seth was learning to trust the process and, in essence, trust the One who was in charge of it all.

When Seth turned thirteen years old, he had the opportunity to join the school band. He jumped at the chance to take up the saxophone. His great-grandfather and great-uncle played the sax. Our extended family had a tour bus that traveled the United States during the 1930s and 40s. "Bill Benson and His Orchestra" played hits from the Big Band Era during the Great Depression. I was thrilled that the saxophone would continue to be played and enjoyed by someone in our family.

I purchased a used saxophone at a thrift store and sunk a substantial amount of money into getting it fixed. Seth's infectious excitement about playing an instrument eased the financial sacrifice. I justified it by the great distraction it would offer from his pain. His band teacher was such a great role model. His love and passion for music were contagious. Seth adored him and had so much respect for his consistently positive attitude. They hit it off right away. Seth stayed after school for extra lessons whenever he could.

DRUM ROLL, PLEASE!

Seth came home from school one day and told me that Mr. Murphy had taken him off of the saxophone. I didn't understand. *Was he that bad at it? Seth loved playing the saxophone. I just sunk almost three hundred dollars (that we didn't have) into that piece of brass!* Seth wasn't phased. In fact, he was more excited than ever.

"I'm now on the drum set!"

I spoke with Mr. Murphy about the sudden change.

He explained. "I noticed Seth was struggling to catch his breath. He became winded easily, and no matter how hard he tried, he was no longer able to hold a note." Mr. Murphy was very tuned in to his students (no pun intended).

"I feel horrible," I said. "I've noticed his decreased stamina and energy. He does get winded at the simplest of tasks. I should have seen this coming."

"I am confident he will do well. I've found that kids who are going through adversity thrive on percussion because it's a great release."

I respected Mr. Murphy's insight and was thankful for his wisdom and direction. Instead of focusing on not being able to play the sax, Seth chose to focus on being able to play the drums. He never lacked the motivation to practice. Every time he sat down at the set, he came alive. Drumming became another healthy coping strategy. This was a huge step forward. Not only was playing the drums good for upper body strength and cardio, but it was also good to clear his mind. What a great outlet. When Seth struggled with pain, he would stomp out the stresses of life with each beat of the bass drum and strike of the drumstick.

Seth showed drive and focus. Mr. Murphy put him on the drums for school concerts. Seth was honored to take on that essential role. No longer was he just in the band, he was in charge of the band's overall rhythm. He had an entire team of students counting on him to keep up the beat. And Lord willing, Seth would not disappoint.

Mr. Murphy's insight highlighted my suspicions. Seth's primary doctor ordered a pulmonary function screening. When he failed one test, he was given another. The tech performing the tests was kind, but I could tell she was becoming frustrated. She called for another tech to help direct Seth in case he didn't understand the directions.

She said, "It's like, all of a sudden, everything just stops. I've never experienced this before."

Seth was trying his hardest to breathe into a measuring device. His face was flushed, but he wasn't producing the results anyone expected. The test results were abnormal but not the standard abnormal. Several medical professionals at Mayo Clinic referred us to the best pediatric pulmonologists in the country. I knew as soon as we met Dr. Miller we were in good hands. He was extremely thorough. God continued to expand Seth's team of caregivers.

A chest x-ray showed Seth's lungs had multiple pulmonary nodules in each of them. Dr. Miller spoke honestly. He had never seen anyone like Seth. He drew charts and graphs for what the projected outcome of the screening should be, then drew a line in the opposite direction, and said, "These are Seth's results."

I had never seen a doctor sit in silence, staring at a screen. I waited with bated breath to hear his thoughts but also appreciated that he did not rush a diagnosis he wasn't completely sure of. He said he needed to do more research and consult with those who regularly worked with Methotrexate and its effects on the lungs. Dr. Miller had to be certain before he recommended taking him off the medication lest Seth relapse. It was too great a risk to attempt a taper (wean off) on a hunch.

Dr. Miller mentioned several possibilities that needed further investigation to be ruled out. So much was unclear, except for one thing. The Seth factor. No matter how ineffective at getting the desired results on tests, Seth never quit. Staff asked several times if he wanted to stop, but he refused. Seth's persistence would serve him well in this long-term fight.

Dr. Miller asked me if there were any previous breathing complications.

I immediately replied, "No," but then I recalled . . .

Back in the spring of 2001, I took eight-month-old Seth to the doctor. I had a gut feeling something wasn't right. His demeanor was fine with no fever and no fussiness. However, his breathing was fast and labored. Having never seen anything like it in his three older brothers, it concerned me.

His pediatrician looked at his chest, listened to his lungs, then examined him again. He agreed baby Seth was in some kind of respiratory distress. He showed me the signs. Increased, fast, shallow breaths. Flared nostrils, chest heaving then sinking in so far you could count his ribs. He pointed at the bottom of his ribcage.

"That's called retraction." Seth's pulse oximetry measurement was extremely low. "You need to take him to the ER right away. He needs to be admitted."

I had never had a child stay in the hospital before this. It was all new to me. He had to be put on oxygen. The amount of pressure going into his tiny little nostrils was substantial yet needed. He still labored with every single breath. They said his lungs were loud and crackly but clear.

Remarkably, Seth appeared calm amidst the struggle. Baby Seth amazed the medical team by smiling the entire time. The doctors were frustrated that he wasn't a classic case. Everything they suspected and tested for came back negative. No fever, no signs of sickness. Seth's lungs were very restricted, and his pulse oximetry (a test that measures the oxygen level of the blood) continued to record alarmingly low numbers. Yet, every time they walked into the room, baby Seth was smiling and delightful. He defied logic against numbers reflecting a significant problem. He should have been cranky and miserable. They changed out several machines thinking the machine might be faulty, but they all read the same.

He truly was a medical mystery. Even as a baby, God seemed to have given Seth the ability to endure suffering with such a sweet attitude that was contagious to all those around him. Day after day in the hospital, the doctors scrambled to perform every test they could think of, yet no infection, bacteria, virus, parasites, allergens, or toxins showed up–nothing.

Seth had respiratory therapists coming in by the hour to give him nebulizer treatments. His tiny face needed to be covered with a mask and hose. He never tried to swat them away. Surprisingly, Seth wasn't bothered by the loud machine administering a medication mist to be inhaled for over half an hour. The doctors warned me that the steroids and rescue meds would make him "cranky, shaky, and jittery," but it had the opposite effect. He would smile at us the whole time.

Finally, after over a week in the hospital, God answered our prayers for Seth's pulse ox numbers to improve and remain stable enough for discharge. Doctors were still scratching their heads. They released Seth but with no answers, no reason, no diagnosis. Until Dr. Miller asked about any previous incidents, I had forgotten about this.

Here we were, nearly fourteen years later. The doctor wasn't convinced of any connection. He said that seemed to be an isolated event from infancy. I was hoping for a light bulb moment when someone, somewhere, would be able to solve these medical mysteries. Rare is frustrating. Not having clear answers and clear solutions is disheartening.

One doctor surmised that Seth had developed some kind of restrictive lung disease due to the weakening of chest wall muscles. How could a child have so much going on yet not lose his smile? Although Seth's condition continued to baffle doctors, he also continued to be remarkably happy. A self-examination of my own heart revealed a recurring battle of my own–allowing circumstances to influence my poor attitude. I knew I was in the midst of battling exhaustion, but I didn't want that to be an excuse. After all, no one I knew was more exhausted than Seth was on a daily basis. I'm so thankful for God's grace for the long haul.

I saw in my son a tangible reminder not to focus on the circumstances but to keep my focus upward. Interestingly enough, I learned the process of *inhalation* is called *inspiration*. Beyond the scientific definition, Seth's demeanor offered inspiration to many including me.

IT TAKES A VILLAGE

John Piper once wrote, "God is always doing 10,000 things in your life, and you may be aware of three of them." I used to question whether God heard my prayers. What was he doing? I only saw the suffering. I had the audacity to ask, "God, do you see him?" Then, one day, through divine providence, I understood.

Before Seth was even conceived, before we knew all the health issues that would unfold, God was working life details for his good. He loved him and had a plan. I am confident that the events the Lord orchestrated long ago in the hearts and lives of a group of missionaries in Central Africa were intended to be used decades later to save Seth's life. He couldn't find the Congo on a map, but now it was going to become very important in his medical journey.

We were beyond grateful to have Dr. Fischer at Mayo Clinic as Seth's primary physician, even though we had to drive over six hundred miles round trip to see him. Sometimes, he would be out of the clinic. We overheard bits and pieces about Dr. Fischer leading and teaching overseas, but instead of being disappointed that we couldn't see him, it increased our respect for him. We counted ourselves blessed to have a pediatrician with this kind of compassion and genuine love for others.

His administrative assistant told me that he left instructions that, even if he was out of the country, they were to always message him about Seth. He'd walk the medical team through care plans for Seth's unique case and sign off electronically. We felt a divine connection to this man. Only God knew how far back that connection went. Unbeknownst to us, God's hand in all of this was about to be revealed.

For months our insurance claims were denied. I finally got to the bottom of this when I spoke to the insurance company. They told me Seth needed a local primary care provider, and they gave me an ultimatum. Find a pediatrician in Wisconsin or they would no longer approve the out-of-state care. I couldn't believe my ears. I tried to explain that while that may be feasible for a normal situation, in our particular case, that was nearly impossible. I explained that we had traveled for ten months within our state to various doctors to find the right one, someone who could help Seth's declining health. The fact that we'd already exhausted all of our resources in Wisconsin was why we had to go out of state. They insisted this was protocol, and there were no opportunities for an exception.

Start over? I refused to believe God brought us this far only to allow my son's health to decline due to red tape. I called around desperately trying to schedule a new consultation. A lot of doctors weren't accepting new patients or didn't take my son's disability insurance. When I did reach an office that seemed probable, I felt I had to be honest upfront. I didn't want to waste my time or theirs, so I explained a bit about our predicament. That's when I lost them.

Maybe I was sharing too much. With each call, I gave a shorter explanation of our predicament. But the answer was the same, "I'm sorry we can't help you." I finally asked the next office if the doctor could call me back, so I could explain. The doctor did return my call. I was excited for a moment that this might be "the one." No such luck. Excitement turned to despair.

"Look," she said. "Technically, we have to take your son, according to our state contract, but I make a dollar and twenty cents per visit. So with such a complex case, you can understand why I simply cannot accept him."

I appreciated her honesty, but her words stung. Time was money and my son was not worth her time. Technically speaking . . . no doctor would make enough money faced with the investment of time involved in complex cases.

There had to be medical professionals somewhere within the state who genuinely desired to help regardless of compensation–right? I hung up the phone and tried to come to grips with the reality and the serious situation we faced.

We worked so hard over the last three years to get where we were. Seth was actually starting to make some headway with the team at Mayo Clinic headed by Dr. Fischer. Now, my son might not have access to that team at all. Insurance advised that for Seth's own safety, we needed a local provider so that if Seth had an emergency, someone would be willing to sign off on his care, even if that meant going out of state to receive it. Until we found someone, no claims would be approved.

I cried out, "God, you gave me this child. You created this child. You love this child even more than I do. We need you to intervene. You know our circumstances. You know what we need even before we ask. We need your guidance and direction. We trust you will provide exactly what and who Seth needs."

CONGO CONNECTION

I sent a request to my friends on social media. I didn't go into detail but asked them to "pray for the RIGHT doctor for Seth." A friend from church messaged me immediately regarding a pediatrician for Seth. I didn't put much weight into it at first.

"He probably isn't taking new patients, won't take our state insurance, wouldn't want to work with other providers or facilities or take on a complex, rare patient.

"He took care of our complex daughter. He prayed with us. He's knowledgeable, kind, and compassionate, and he's a missionary kid!"

My heart leaped, but I had been disappointed before. I didn't want to get my hopes up, only to have them crushed. I didn't care how far away his office was, I was willing to drive hours if need be. I was thrilled to learn he was only a fifteen-minute drive away. It sounded like a great match so far, and it helped to know friends were behind the scenes praying.

I called the office and asked for a consultation with Dr. Schimming.

The secretary asked, "Will this be a sick or well visit?"

"A bit of both, actually." I went on to explain some of our dilemmas.

"I am so sorry you have been through so much."

"If there is any chance that I could have just a few minutes of his time, face to face, where he could see my son so that he could see he is just a sweet little boy that needs his help—" I took a deep breath to gain my composure. "Please. Would you put me on his schedule?"

She hesitated. "I'm sure he would be willing to see you."

I thanked her profusely and hung up the phone with hope. Even though I knew there were no guarantees, we were one step closer. I was learning to trust God's timing. I once read a quote by Craig Groeschel that stuck with me, "If it's not God's time, you can't force it. If it is God's time, you can't stop it."

We were running out of time. We *needed* this doctor to agree to oversee the care of my thirteen-year-old. His medical care and coverage were counting on it. By the time our October appointment rolled around, I was sweating buckets. Part of me questioned what would happen if he said no. I didn't think I could take the news. Donnie and I and the prayer team had bathed this day in prayer. I knew I needed to trust God's plan. I was hopeful that God had led us right where we were supposed to be.

On appointment day, we made our way through a large facility and were directed to a small office painted sage green with frogs and lily pad decals on the wall. We sat down, and I reassured Seth with a smile while we waited. A man about my age walked in and greeted us. I liked the way he made eye contact and acknowledged Seth. He was soft-spoken and seemed very genuine.

"I was told you wanted to talk to me."

I took a deep breath and explained while trying not to fall apart. "We have a particularly challenging set of circumstances. We need you, and would greatly appreciate you agreeing to be Seth's primary doctor. We don't need you to do much. We just need a doctor within the state for insurance purposes."

"That is a relief because just looking at his med list, I would have to go back to school just to be able to prescribe one of these meds." We chuckled, and it lightened the mood.

I said, "We would be willing to sign anything to release you from liability if that would make you more comfortable. We are not trying to replace Seth's primary physician who knows him best. I mean, we have come to love Dr. Fischer—"

"That wouldn't happen to be Phil Fischer, would it?"

"To be quite honest, I'm not sure."

"Is he really tall?"

"As a matter of fact, yes, he is."

The tone in the room changed. He took a moment to compose himself. I got chills from head to toe. This was so much bigger than us.

Dr. Schimming began. "Growing up, my parents were missionaries in the Congo along with the Fischers. Our parents were good friends, and, as a teen, I followed this doctor [Fischer] around through the villages. I wanted to be just like him."

Although it seemed unbelievable that we were talking about the same person, I was convinced it had to be. Dr. Fischer fits the profile of often being out of the country for medical service to others. Oh my–both of us were taken aback by how these journeys played out. He sat back in his chair. Silence. I could tell by the emotion on the doctor's face that Dr. Fischer was just as important, if not more, to Dr. Schimming than he was to us. I tried to piece it together in my mind.

Dr. Schimming continued. "Over the years, I've thought about him often. I wondered where he went and if he was still practicing medicine. My family lost touch with him."

Then he asked if I would give a message to Dr. Fischer for him. What he said next overwhelmed me.

"I am a doctor today because of him."

With tears in my eyes, I told him, "I would be honored."

He smiled and said, "It would be my pleasure to share Seth's care with Dr. Phil Fischer."

I could hardly wrap my brain around what I had just heard. As Seth and I left the office, I looked up at the beautiful sunset, and it hit me how big our God was. The God who created all things and flung the planets and stars into place loved us so intimately and cared for us so deeply that he placed a doctor–inspired to be a doctor by our Dr. Fischer–fifteen minutes from our home!

CHAPTER TWELVE
THE NEED FOR SPEED!

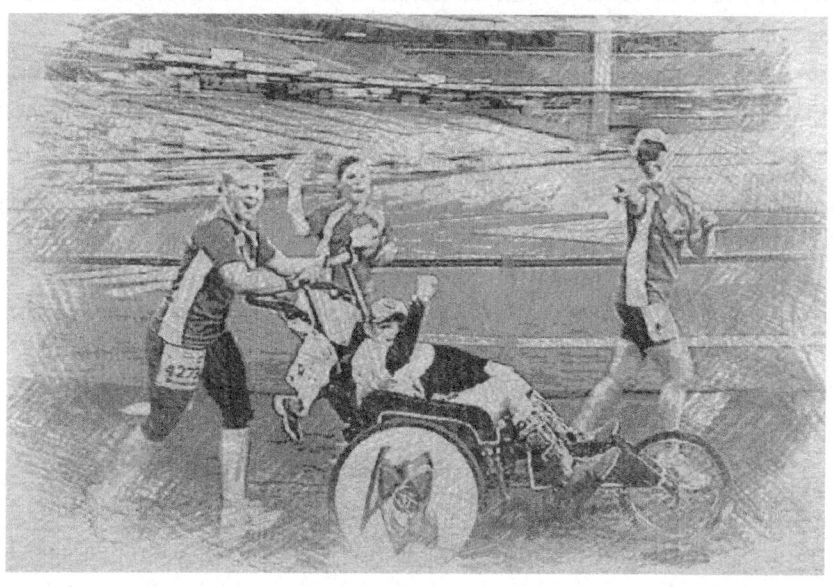

Hardships often prepare ordinary people for an extraordinary destiny.
–C. S. Lewis

FEAR OF THE UNKNOWN

For several years, when the Ronald McDonald House was full, we stayed at the same hotel. We routinely parked on the same ramp and took the same elevator to the same floor. During this particular stay of several nights, we settled into the room. Seth mentioned he forgot something in the car. When he asked if he could go grab it, I offered to go with him, but he immediately contested. He wanted to go by himself. Even when walking was painful, twelve-year-old Seth was determined. I nodded in agreement just as Mayo Clinic called to discuss our appointments for the next day.

I finished the call and thought it was odd that Seth wasn't back yet. I didn't want to overreact thinking he would return shortly. Maybe he stopped at the gift shop in the lobby or needed to use the restroom. Maybe he was talking with someone. After all, Rochester was our second home.

I waited another few minutes, but I couldn't fight my gut reaction that I shouldn't have let him go alone. But we felt safe here, and he knew this place like the back of his hand. I opened the door expecting to hear the clicking of his cane down the hallway. Silence. Seth was nowhere in sight. Maybe he forgot which room we were in. I noticed he had been getting more and more forgetful lately. He had lost two brand-new cell phones at the hospital. No one turned them in, so to teach him the value of money and to be more mindful, I told him we were not buying him another. I now regretted that decision.

I searched the entire floor, the elevators, and the lobby. My heart started to race. I went back to the room in case I missed him. I retraced his steps. I eventually made my way to the parking garage. I opened the door to find Seth standing in the middle of the garage. With the small bag he went to retrieve in his hand, he was shivering in only a white undershirt in the middle of a frigid winter in Minnesota.

"Seth! What are you doing?" He gasped and made his way toward me as fast as his legs would carry him. "Let's get inside and warm up." I took off my sweater and put it on his goosebump-filled arms, "Why were you just standing there?"

"I-I forgot the room card– I-I couldn't get back in." He started to cry.

"Why didn't you go in with other people coming in and out?"

"People asked me if I needed help, but they were strangers. I didn't know what to do!"

Seth's former confidence and self-sufficiency had dwindled, and it scared both of us. My voice quickly changed with empathy as I felt responsible.

Once we got to the room, I said, "Let's go over some ways you could have handled this differently. When the door opened, you could have gone inside the door. You could have gone back to the car to get warm; you had the car keys in your hand. You could have gone around the building to the front door." I realized the more options I gave, the more it overwhelmed him. With a blank stare, Seth was clearly at a loss, scared, and confused. His head dropped.

"I couldn't think of all that."

My eyes were filled with tears, not only in relief that he was back with me but heartbroken at the reality that my son no longer possessed the problem-solving skills he once had to keep himself safe. His older siblings babysat, cooked, and increasingly took on more responsibility when they were Seth's age. When Seth should have been gaining skills, it seemed he was declining cognitively. I wanted to cry with him. Instead, I diverted the conversation quickly to a more positive inquiry.

"Well, did you get what you needed? Let's go get some hot chocolate."

Triumph! Seth Is Fourteen

It was Friday afternoon on a brisk fall day in 2014. A friend from school asked Seth if he wanted to be in the Kenosha Marathon the next day. Seth was puzzled. He chuckled.

"Marathon, like running? I can't run a marathon!"

"You would be in a cart, and people would push you."

Seth's ears perked up. She went on to tell him that her mom would be there, taking turns with others, pushing him the whole way. The person her mom was going to push had to cancel at the last minute.

"The only thing is. . . you would have to be able to sit for like five hours. Can you do that?"

Seth listened intently and pictured it in his mind. Seth wanted to do anything asked of him and loved a challenge to do hard things.

Without hesitation, Seth replied, "Sure!"

Seth came home eager to tell me about the conversation. I asked questions making sure I heard him right. He had already set his mind to do this. We were to show up at Lake Michigan by the lighthouse by 5:00 a.m. I had only watched bits of the Boston Marathon on television, so I had no idea what to expect in person.

Although I didn't know what Seth was committing to, I was thrilled someone was willing to invite him. Seth had gotten used to not being included in friends' parties, gatherings, or sleepovers. I don't think they meant anything mean or intentional. They probably just assumed he wouldn't be able to participate in things and didn't want to make him feel bad. We've found that others sometimes avoid things and people they don't fully understand. Often, if people didn't know what to say, they didn't say anything.

We arrived within a block of the Kenosha lakefront before we hit roadblocks. Thousands of people flooded the streets. We asked for directions, then walked toward the myTEAM TRIUMPH box truck and a large red, white, and black tent. Despite the cool wind blowing off the Great Lake before sunrise, a cheerful group had gathered.

Several ladies in red volunteer shirts made eye contact with smiles and introductions. The entire group was super welcoming, kind, and sincere. They made Seth feel like a superstar for just being him! They brought Seth to a state-of-the-art race chair with a sign displaying the words "Captain Seth." The air was filled with excitement, cheering, and high-fives. We wanted to know more about this organization.

We were thrilled with the values of an organization that paired able-bodied athletes called "Angels" with those differently abled, referred to as "Captains." This fostered inclusion, friendships, teamwork, and experiences that would not be possible otherwise. God had placed Seth in a group of selfless Angels. Wow!

Countless volunteers offered behind-the-scenes support: planners, set up, tear down, pit crews, and more. They planned months in advance for marathon day. The intense training commitment of the runners was nothing short of unbelievable.

Organizers explained that Seth could participate in marathons, half-marathons, triathlons, and even one day an "Ironman" in a team with myTEAM TRIUMPH - Wisconsin Chapter. Opportunities abounded throughout the state and all over the country.

"Triathlon? What's that?" Seth asked.

Christian Jensen, the executive director, explained, "It's a run, a swim, and a bike ride."

Seth's eyes lit up. He loved the water. With the help of an Angel, Seth could experience the two-mile swim. A swimmer would pull him across a lake in a raft tethered to their waist. What a thrill to experience gliding across the water. This was far greater than Seth could have ever imagined. As he prepared to settle into his race chair, he started to laugh.

"This is so much cooler than I thought. When they said I would be riding in a *cart*, I pictured being in a shopping cart for five hours!"

We all chuckled. Seth seemed relieved. The aerodynamic chair was built for comfort, with pads, footrests, seat belts, headrest, the whole nine yards. It was quite impressive, especially for a teenage boy with a "need for speed."

Seth would be accompanied by three Angels for this race. One of them pinned on his race bib. After he was strapped in, everyone gathered around. Fifteen race chairs with captains were placed beside each other. Christian stood in front announcing each captain by name. As he did, the crowd roared. The smiles on those captains' faces were priceless. They were all feeling the opposite of isolated and alone. And then, hats came off and heads bowed as he led everyone in prayer. This was our favorite part. To hear his words of blessing and see the

Angels laying their hands on my son in one accord gave me goosebumps.

Seth got to know his crew over the course of the run. Seth learned a lot about his Angel companions seeing them stretched to their limit mentally and physically for five grueling hours. Their commitment never waned. Seth told me they were so kind, constantly making sure *he* was good. These were women that we had never met before that day. They immediately seemed like they had known each other forever and treated him like family.

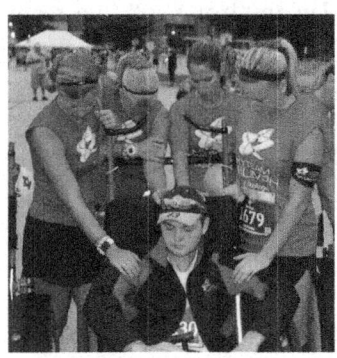

Little did we know that the Angel relationships were the beginning of changing his life and the lives around him forever. The connections, this organization, and their mission for these deserving humans came as a gift from God. And it came at a time when Seth had begun to feel the weight of his declining health.

Because of this event and organization, Seth's focus shifted. He no longer focused on what he *couldn't do*. He looked forward to what he *could* do.

Seth told me how amazing the marathon was. When he was out along the lakefront with the wind blowing as they pushed him, listening to the crashing waves, he said he felt God's peace. For the first time in a long time, he actually forgot about his medical conditions.

To see Team Seth cross the finish line together brought tears to my eyes. Team members collected their medals. Seth couldn't believe how heavy it was and stared at it in disbelief. The ladies told me Seth smiled the entire five hours.

One Angel joked, "His face may hurt in the morning!"

When asked if he wanted to do this again sometime, he immediately shouted, "YES, please!"

Seth brought his medal to school and told everyone about his life-changing experience. His peers and the staff thought it was so cool that he completed a marathon. This gave Seth new motivation to press through treatment, get out of the hospital, and get better in order to get back to the training runs and races with his new best friends.

Soon, many Angels joined Team Seth. I told these awesome gals they had become like second moms to Seth.

"We like to think of ourselves more like the cool aunts," one replied.

I knew it was going to be one adventure after another. Seth and I chose from a list of marathons across the state. Seth eagerly anticipated the next race, city, and adventure. The selfless Angels trained all year. I drove Seth to training runs, and eventually, they picked Seth up at the house. After they trained together, they treated themselves to popsicles or ice cream. They were, for sure, the cool aunts. They trained without Seth in the winter but impressed me with their commitment to running at 4:00 or 5:00 a.m. before work. They showed such dedication through all types of weather, any day of the week, even on holidays.

When Seth rode in the chair, people came out of their houses to cheer Seth's name. Oftentimes, they held up bags of pop tabs and offered words of encouragement. Seth passed that encouragement on to the ladies when they struggled with fatigue. He made them laugh and cheered them on, and they reciprocated whenever Seth had a bad day of pain. They were all stronger together!

Seth's go-to verse, Philippians 4:13, became the Team Seth motto and central theme.

"I can do all things through Christ who strengthens me." Those words were written on their hearts, wristbands, and plastered on posters cheering him on in the community. That verse became a lifeline for many.

Over time, Seth grew taller and taller until he outgrew the adult race chair. Medically, his growth was not expected. Back when Seth was eight years old, he started aggressive treatments which he is still on today. We were warned of the side effects, such as stunted growth. Understanding this, we decided to proceed because the benefits outweighed the risks. Seth's case continues to prove doctors can make educated predictions, but God . . . He stepped in with the final word and unexpected results.

Seth was now bigger and taller than most of his Angels. With his head well above the back of the chair, it became more difficult for the cool aunt Angels to push him, make turns, and stop. Seth couldn't move his legs which made his arthritis and neuropathy worse. Without our knowledge, Seth's Angels fundraised to purchase a customized chair built and adapted for Seth's special needs.

Countless individuals got involved, including schools, churches, local businesses, and nonprofit organizations in Seth's honor. His measurements were taken to customize a new race chair specifically for him complete with colorful decor: Team Seth, Philippians 4:13, the Pittsburgh Steelers logo, and others were displayed on the wheel covers.

As an old African proverb says, "If you want to go fast, go alone, if you want to go far, go together." It's one thing to run twenty-six miles for yourself. It's a whole different mission to run twenty-six miles while pushing, pulling, and steering the extra weight of another person plus a steel vehicle up and down through various terrain while tending to *their* needs. Not for the faint-hearted. God bless his Angels!

It was incredible to see the number of sacrificial people who signed up to join his team. There was even a waiting list! A few guys joined the team. Seth had five hours to talk sports and share his faith and life's journey. We were humbled by the outpouring of so many who lined up to help get Seth across the finish line. Races were filled with new adventures, occasional costumes, and hilarious selfies.

Seth felt a connection with people who accepted him and celebrated his uniqueness. He met outstanding people along the way and learned from other captains fighting their own battles. How beneficial to share and hear the stories that made us who we were. Event leaders asked Seth to attend various talks with other captains at public events and schools. One event was at his previous elementary and middle school.

"We have a celebrity in the house!" the principal announced to the packed gymnasium. The crowd erupted as Seth grabbed the mic. Then the gym grew silent as the kids from kindergarten to eighth grade and staff listened. His words were few but powerful. It was healing for him. Once bullied for his disability, he now had a platform to turn that around and make a positive difference.

Knowing there might be someone in that gym who felt they were in a hopeless situation and tempted to give up, Seth went down the bleachers and gave high fives as the students lunged to reach out their hands. Life had come full circle.

It was neat to see the ripple effect. Soon, the younger generation asked to be a part of what he was doing. Several of Seth's Angel's children went from cheering on the sidelines holding Team Seth signs to training and eventually becoming Angels themselves. Seth's younger siblings did the same by taking turns pushing Seth in our hometown Progress Days Run. What a beautiful thing to watch Seth and his siblings together. No limitations, just love.

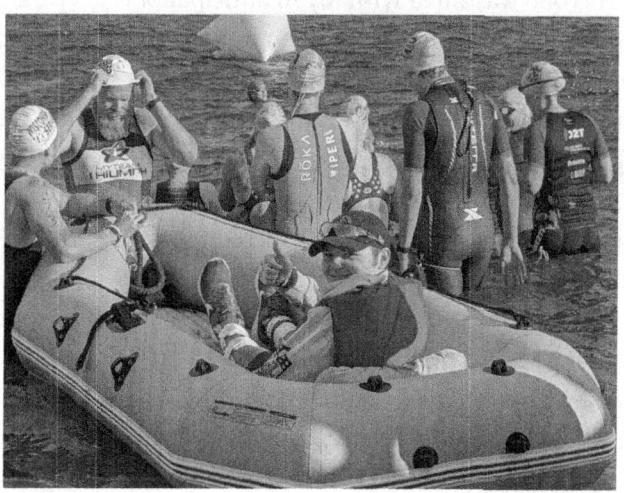

Team Seth prepares for the swim portion of the triathlon. Ah-mazing

Christian Jensen said this about Seth, "Every once in a while you come across someone you know God is using for big things, someone who demonstrates grace and strength through indescribable challenges. From the moment I met Seth, I knew this was a special man with a heart for God. He constantly puts on a smile and positive attitude for others despite all that he faces on a regular basis. His faith and servant's heart is an inspiration and example for everyone looking to make a difference in this world,"

YOU WISH!

Several adults familiar with Seth's case suggested that now would be a great time for a referral to Make-A-Wish®. When the battle is long, and there seems to be no end in sight, it's helpful to be able to step away, gain a new perspective, and renew strength for the fight ahead.

In the spring of 2014, Seth received a letter stating he had been approved to receive one wish. Shortly thereafter, Janet and Sharlene, two wish granters from Make-A-Wish Wisconsin came to our home. They showed up with balloons, treats, and a large gift bag for Seth. They gave him a token good for one wish. Seth's siblings received gifts as well. Everyone was filled with joy in anticipation.

These lovely ladies had done their research. They already knew many details about Seth, his family dynamics, interests, and passions. They knew he loved the Pittsburgh Steelers. When they mentioned Make-A-Wish had worked with the Steelers before, Seth's eyes lit up. In fact, they said the Pittsburgh Steelers and the Green Bay Packers might have been two of the most incredible teams they'd worked with.

Janet and Sharlene got down to business. "Seth, this is your time to choose one wish. I wish to meet...I wish to be...I wish to go...I wish to have...Anything you want."

We all thought Seth would say he would like to meet the Steelers or go to a game. But without a shadow of a doubt or hesitation, Seth said, "I have this dream about a motorhome with my family all together."

Sharlene said, "I'm not sure the rules would allow us to give you a motorhome, but we can check for sure. We can give you a camper, like one that you pull behind a truck."

"Oh, I didn't mean one to keep. My dream is to *ride* with my family *all together* in the motorhome going down the road. My dream is that my dad is driving, and my mom is in the passenger seat, and my family is in the back while we're going down the road. I have dreamed of this for so long."

"Ohhh, you want a motorhome *experience*. I'm sure we can make that happen. So where are you going in the motorhome with your family, Seth?"

"I don't know, around the block?"

Janet and Sharlene chuckled. These sweet volunteers encouraged Seth to think on a bigger scale and dream big. They gave him a suggestion.

"The farther away you go, the more time you get to spend with your family."

Seth grinned ear to ear. They discussed different destinations he would like. One stopped Seth in his tracks.

"The Grand Canyon? I've read about that in history books!" Seth squealed with delight. That was it! His one wish was to go with his family in a motorhome to the Grand Canyon.

Since Seth is one of seven children, a family excursion is not a typical one. Make-A-Wish Wisconsin went on a mission to find a motorhome with nine seat belts. Donnie and I took on the daunting task of finding a time when all nine of us could take off work, school, finals, sports, and prior commitments.

When Make-A-Wish finally found a motorhome large enough to accommodate our family, only two weeks (back-to-back) in the whole season were available. If we couldn't make it work, we would have to postpone it until the following year. Not wanting to disappoint Seth, it was a no-brainer.

Without hesitation, I said, "We'll make it work." I called a family meeting.

"Countless people have been working behind the scenes to make Seth's wish a reality. I know all of your commitments are important, but we will need to do this during the third week of August."

I knew we'd have conflicts and hard decisions to make, but I was prepared.

Seth said, "Mom, do you know what falls in between those dates?"

"I'm sorry, these are the dates, they are set in stone."

"It's my BIRTHDAY!"

We all laughed and shared his excitement. How perfect! With all the focus on choosing dates that worked for everyone, that special date was overlooked. What greater gift than to celebrate his fourteenth birthday with his wish of a lifetime. We felt God's hand guiding and directing the details.

Finally, the last detail we had to work out was securing coverage for the family business. We had run a not-for-profit thrift store for the past six years. We needed to keep the store open and operating smoothly. Because we had missionaries and various ministries that counted on the income the store generated, closing it was not an option.

As soon as we let our church know, they jumped into action. Their love for God and our family showed as they stepped up. Before we knew it, they had coordinated over fifty volunteers to run Christian Mission over the thirteen-day trip. *Oh. My. Lanta!*

Do I need to say Seth enjoyed every mile of the trip? Even though many of us were carsick, we made sure the trip was everything Seth dreamed of. He played cards at the table with his siblings just as he had envisioned. He loved the comfort of the loft over the driver and passenger seat. Most impressive to Seth was not having to stop to use the restroom, he was able to use it as we drove down the road. The simple joys!

Even though all of Seth's doctors supported the trip, they expressed concern about Seth staying deep in the forest without immediate access to emergency medical attention. Also, his doctor expressed concern about the hot August temperatures in Arizona. Seth had developed a heat intolerance. Also of concern, Seth wore a heat-activated patch that lowered his blood pressure. Excessive temperatures, causing Seth's body temperature to rise, could release too much medicine too quickly. This would cause a dangerous drop in his blood pressure.

As we entered Grand Canyon National Park, we sensed God's presence working out details large and small. I breathed a sigh of relief when I saw a large red cross/medic building near our campsite. How like God to provide perfect and consistent temperatures in the 70s for the entire trip. Our praise and thanks focused on Him.

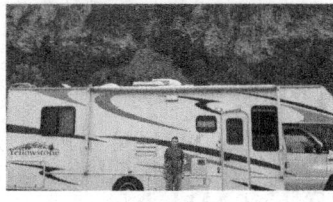

Seth was in awe of God's magnificent creation as he took in the breathtaking scenery, especially the majestic canyon. It was far greater than he ever imagined. So, we celebrated Seth's fourteenth birthday in Grand Canyon National Park. It was filled with wildlife like elk and mule deer that wandered right up to our campsite. But most importantly, we experienced it all together.

We could not be more grateful to Make-A-Wish Wisconsin, and all those who give to this organization, for making this dream come true. Our family continues to reflect on that cherished time together. It helps to recall the good on the hard days. We give thanks to God for the precious gifts of life, family, and memories. We pray we never take them for granted.

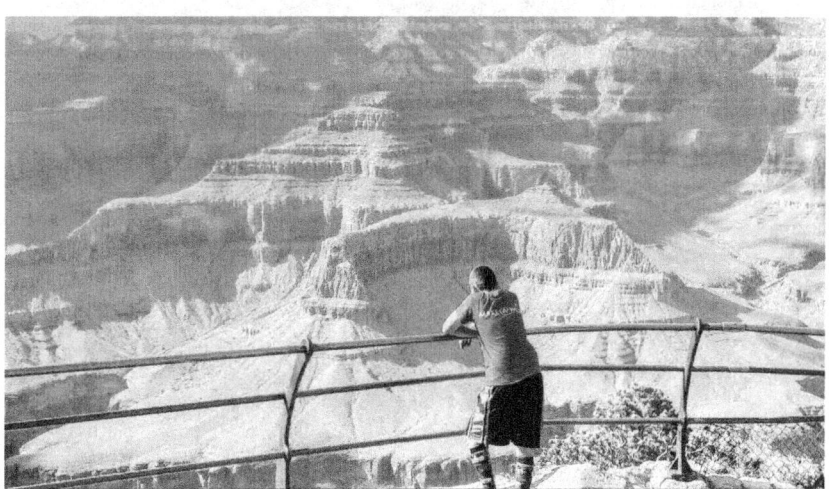

CHAPTER THIRTEEN
WHEN ONE DOOR CLOSES, ANOTHER BURSTS OPEN

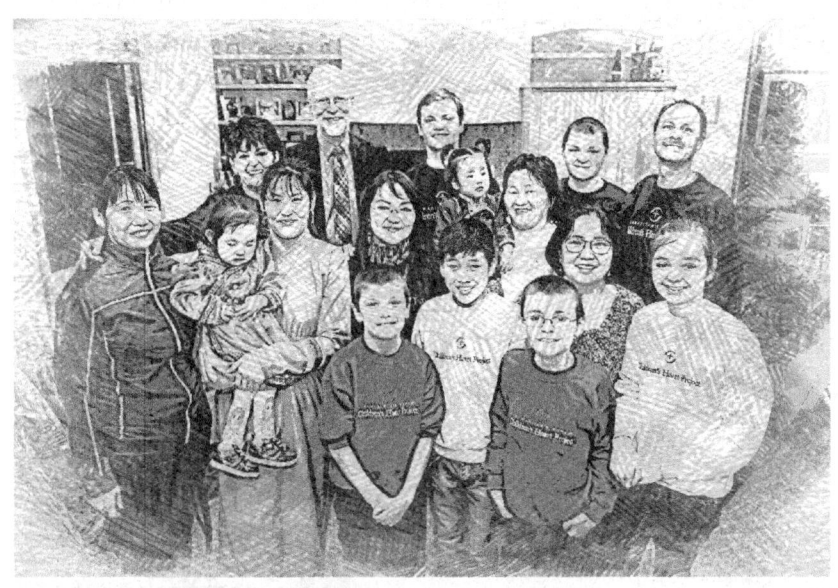

You can give without loving, but you cannot love without giving.
–Amy Carmichael, missionary to India

UNEXPECTED VISITOR

Juggling home life, being a mom, and volunteering full-time at our non-profit, took a toll. Overseeing the full-time care and advocating for a medically complex child added to the load. My schedule involved frequent ten-hour commutes to Mayo Clinic. After a long day of appointments, I drove home with Seth late into the night. Once home, extra responsibilities awaited. Running the 6,500-square-foot thrift store six days a week took hard work, yet I loved it. It was gratifying to support mission work this way. However, committed to the day-to-day operations, my health teetered on the brink of burnout. Sleep was sparse. I was livin' on a prayer and a pot of coffee.

One morning, I opened the store and greeted the customers waiting at the door. A gentleman dressed in a brown suit jacket entered. He spoke with a heavy accent.

"May I speak with the person in charge, please?"

I reached out for a handshake. "You're speaking to her. How can I help you?"

The man smiled and nodded. "Oh, nice to meet you. My name is Titus from The Gideons International. I want to thank you for the substantial donation that Christian Mission made to our work this past month." He went on to tell several stories of lives impacted and, again, extended his wholehearted gratitude. Just as our small talk wrapped up, he asked, "I don't mean to impose, but are you alright?"

His inquiry took me aback since I had just met the man.

"Why do you ask?" I was obviously not doing a good job of hiding that I was not okay.

"I just sensed something and wanted to know how I could pray for you."

I barely succumbed to tears in those days–no time for that. But I sensed his sincerity. Then he did something I rarely saw after one asks how someone feels. He took the time to stick around and listen.

"Quite frankly, I'm exhausted and a bit overwhelmed. I just got back early this morning from being out of town with one of my sons. You could pray for healing for my son."

His dark eyes were so kind and comforting. He listened as if he were pondering what I said. Afterwards, he said something that I would never have anticipated.

"Have you thanked God lately?" Awkward silence. I stood there puzzled. Then he asked, "May I tell you a story?"

I nodded in agreement and with great curiosity. Then, he opened up about his own family's painful journey.

I, too, had a son that was in need of healing. My baby boy was not well, very sickly. No one could figure it out. He would cry out in anguish. Eventually, he developed sores that covered his entire body. When we would see improvements, we thanked God. When things didn't change, we thanked God. In the waiting, we thanked God. In the midst of suffering, we thanked God. We tried all kinds of doctors and treatments, but we got no answers.

When he was about two years old, things took a turn for the worse. His breathing became shallow, and I felt like death seemed imminent. My wife and I rushed in the middle of the night to the house of an elderly Christian pastor who was visiting us from India. I gave my son into the hands of that pastor to die in his hands.

I will never forget how Titus described that pastor holding his son's limp body and crying out to God. His story pierced my heart as I wiped tears flowing down both cheeks. I felt the anguish as I pictured it in my mind. I was relating in my own way to his suffering and surrendering.

"The pastor prayed something like this, 'Lord, take this child if it is your will. But Lord, if it is your will, give him a new life so he may lead many to you. In Jesus name, I pray. Amen.'"

Adrenaline replaced my fatigue. I was on the edge of my seat, listening to every word. Miraculously, that baby boy did not die that night.

When Titus shared, "He went on to be a thriving young man who is serving the Lord today," it so moved me and strengthened my faith.

I thanked him for sharing and asked if he was visiting the area. He said he had moved his family to Wisconsin years ago. In fact, he was a member of a church in the neighboring town. I eagerly said I was born and raised in that town. I knew exactly where his church was. It was only a few blocks from my childhood home. He asked what church I attended, and I told him.

"That's where my son is a pastor!"

I was shocked. I struggled to contain my composure when I asked his name, and he revealed who his son was. Pastor Josh was that baby boy on the verge of death? How was this possible? Our family loved him–he was instrumental in the young adult ministry and poured into my own adult sons' lives! I was astounded to think I had the honor of seeing the prayer from *decades* ago, come to fruition. Now, I understood what he meant about thanking God in and for adversity.

God's loving-kindness and mercy had poured out over a baby in the middle of the night just like it was pouring over me decades later–over a weary mama in a thrift store amidst strangers. I didn't know what God was doing through our suffering, but I was learning to trust Him and thank Him. I was stronger that day because God sent me an unexpected messenger.

It had been seven years since we felt called to start Christian Mission. The thrift store work was difficult but good. I loved working side by side with our seven children. They learned valuable lessons in business, work ethic, and service to others. The best part of it all? The joy of giving funds away.

But having a child with critical health conditions who needed extra attention had taken its toll. Never knowing when I had to leave everything and drive ten hours (round trip) for medical emergencies made it more difficult. Our church's business administrator, was our secretary, treasurer, board member, accountant, and friend. We had two wonderful part-time employees, and several faithful volunteers. Still, it was a huge undertaking and juggling act to make it all work. We needed all hands on deck, especially while Seth and I had to be away at the hospital.

I often felt guilty, but the kids never complained. Since we lived next door to the store, the children were able to come and go, but most of the time, they wanted to be right in the center of the activity. Even though we set up a special playroom for the three youngest in the back room, complete with a slide and foam jumping area, they had more fun sorting. The children mastered the role of donation sorter. They helped separate clothing into two different piles, sellable and unsellable. They could see a spot or hole a mile away. It was a constant "treasure hunt" going through bags. What excitement when they came across a game or toy. It was like Christmas morning every day! Their favorite "job" was making sure every donated game had all the piece parts, as I instructed them.

They told me, "Mom, we have to *play* the games to make sure they work!"

Ahh, such dedication. Come Saturday, did they long for play dates with their friends? And miss a Christmas morning? Not a chance.

The stairs in the sorting area led to the gas station and pizza shop directly above us. On Fridays, the kids could turn in the *Bayles Bucks* they earned for cash. With money burning a hole in their pockets, they couldn't wait to shop upstairs. Drawn to the sports cards, candy, brownies, and orange drinks, they plunked down their well-earned cash. Playing games, eating treats, and trading cards with family wasn't as bad a gig as my *mom guilt* led me to believe. It was a good life.

The work was never caught up, especially after being away. I often put in extra hours just to make a dent. My sister Donna often volunteered her time after work. After store hours, Donnie took the children home. Donna and I locked up and worked into the night.

We were blessed with more donations than a small army could handle. The community was incredibly generous. A third of the store was the sorting area which often piled up over our heads. Although the work was non-stop, we saw God's provision as a huge blessing and avenue to give. The sales supported many missions that made an impact in our community and around the world.

To keep to our homeschool schedule, we set up a video classroom in the store. In addition, the children learned business skills by pitching in. Our oldest programmed the computer and cash register, created our logo, and ran the register. Once our second oldest secured a driver's license, he picked up donations. The middle children, including Seth, helped sort donations, and everyone helped with the younger ones. They loved it. To this day, all seven children possess a strong work ethic and live with purpose.

Our non-profit helped us build relationships with all kinds of people in the community. It offered jobs for people working off jail time, fines, and community service hours. I led a Bible study for women after hours at the store. We received thank you notes, letters, and photos from our community and many countries around the world. We posted pins on a world map for notes we received. It hung behind our front counter as people entered the store. Our children saw first-hand the ripple effect of where God was working through their efforts.

Our older boys took several mission trips to gain new perspectives and build relationships with others in different cultures. Being able to provide resources and meet needs blessed us. I marveled to see how God used a family with seven kids from a small rural town to impact others across the US and the world.

But, for everything there is a season, a time, and a purpose, and seasons don't last forever. Although we felt called to this ministry, and it was thriving, something had to give. Our family dynamics became more complex as Seth's conditions grew more complicated. Life became increasingly difficult as we tried to teach school, run a business, and raise a family.

After much prayer and consideration, the time came to close the doors of Christian Mission, a very tough decision. Both pain and peace tugged at our hearts as we let this part of our lives go. No regrets. We trusted God's plan. The "Going Out of Business" sale and selling everything we had acquired was difficult. But, in the end, the total sales were beyond anything we could have imagined.

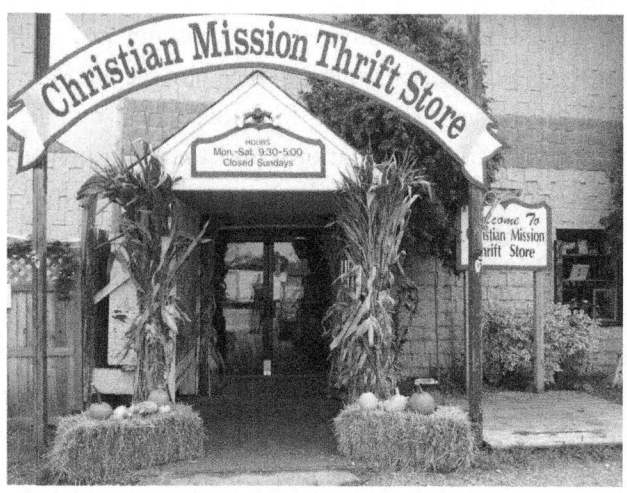

The entrance to our family's store and mission

CHILDREN'S HEART PROJECT, A NEW DOOR BURSTS OPEN

It was time to close the chapter and the books on the Christian Mission Bank account. A substantial amount of money remained for our family to choose what we felt led to do. We always included the children in our donation decisions. I remembered a conversation Seth and I had with Dr. Fischer months prior. During one of our routine visits to Mayo, Dr. Fischer told us about an event he attended to celebrate the one-thousandth heart surgery through Children's Heart Project (CHP). His excitement was contagious. How wonderful that CHP did this right where Seth received all his medical care. We were especially intrigued because we had so much love and respect for Dr. Fischer. Anything he was a part of was something about which we wanted to know more. We went home and researched the Children's Heart Project and learned it was a division of Samaritan's Purse. When we watched film clips about it, I cried.

The more we learned, the more our hearts were drawn to be a part of the project. This, we decided, was what we would do with the money leftover from Christian Mission. We learned three children were waiting to come to Mayo Clinic from Mongolia. We had enough money to sponsor all three and give to the churches that hosted the children. We were so excited to have the opportunity! It's out of the overflow of what we've been given that we joyfully give.

The long-standing relationship between Dr. Fischer and us made being a part of this project feel like we had come full circle. Enabling other children and families to experience the care we had been blessed to receive helped us see purpose in pain. Maybe we were called to this.

To be honest, we weren't exactly sure where Mongolia was. We searched the Internet and studied this vast land of mountains, plateaus, and high altitudes. Our children eagerly researched more about the fascinating culture of the nomads. They learned the portable dwellings (circular tents) they had lived in for thousands of years were called a yurt or a ger. This opened up a whole new world we never knew existed. Seth's medical crisis might have been the deciding factor in closing our doors at Christian Mission, but we found ourselves here because of his medical conditions. Doors were opening at Mayo Clinic for our family to continue to give, serve, and reach others around the world who were also hurting. As someone once said, "God often uses our deepest pain as the launching pad for our greatest calling."

The Ronald McDonald House asked if Seth would like to be the featured houseguest for the annual Hearts and Diamonds Spectacular. What a huge honor. It filled us with excitement, but I was a nervous wreck. That meant I would act as the keynote speaker. Speak in public? I would rather have another c-section without an epidural. To add to the mounting pressure, the Hearts and Diamonds Gala was the largest and the most anticipated fundraiser of the year. At $250 a plate, I was clearly out of my element. Seth was adamant he didn't want to speak but was thrilled to be the guest of honor. I couldn't disappoint him, so I had a speech to write.

At the same time, Cindy, the director of the Children's Heart Project called. She heard about our donation and wanted to thank us. We had a lovely conversation. She took time to listen as I shared our connection with Seth's beloved physician, Dr. Fischer, and how we wanted the sponsorships to be in his honor. We knew of his enthusiasm for the project, but we didn't know he was also a huge friend to the project. So humble, he never spoke of what he did continuously for children around the world. We had even more love and respect for him, and our desire to be a part of this project intensified. God was connecting the dots far beyond what any of us could have orchestrated. Then Cindy said something that took my breath away.

"We would like to invite your family to meet the children you sponsored."

I never expected this opportunity. Overwhelmed and overjoyed, I couldn't wait to tell the rest of the family. To be able to provide for these families meant so much, but to actually meet the recipients would be life-changing.

Cindy went on to say, "The story of Seth and Dr. Fischer is too incredible not to share. Would you mind if we documented this journey?"

I politely declined. I didn't want the attention. But she convinced me it really wasn't about us. It was a testimony to how God brought all this together for good through Seth's treatment, connection with his doctor, Mayo Clinic, and heart patients from all over the world. She said sharing the story would inspire others and give God the glory, not us. Cindy was a wise woman. This was God's story, not ours. And God was not finished writing it.

"Julie!" I heard an excited voice when I answered my phone. "Jeff, from the Ronald McDonald House." Since I am horrible with names, I tried to visualize him at the house by connecting the voice. "You, Seth, and the family are going to be staying with Allison and me as our houseguests!"

We talked for over an hour. Jeff was hilarious. We had an undeniable connection in God, Mayo Clinic, the Ronald McDonald House, and the Children's Heart Project.

"And I hear you're going to be the guest speaker for the Hearts and Diamonds Gala!"

"Well, I submitted my speech. I am not a speechwriter, so we'll see."

"Aah, yeah, I was in that meeting when it was read. It was perfect. It was a unanimous yes! I will be the emcee for the event. You will be at the head table with me, so Seth and I can hang out while you speak."

My jaw dropped, and my shoulders relaxed as a huge weight lifted. God had answered several prayers. He knew I was terrified and sent Jeff to put me at ease. We wouldn't have to worry about getting a hotel for several days. God had gone before us and worked out every detail. I felt peace, had great joy, and a newfound anticipation for the upcoming gala. I couldn't wait for Seth to meet Jeff. This connection became the gift that kept on giving in our lives. What a timely blessing.

We spent the next few days getting to know the people who opened their homes to complete strangers. We didn't know it at the time, but God was setting up one of the most important relationships in Seth's life. The new friendship with Jeff and Dr. Allison reaffirmed God's goodness to us. Their hospitality was an over-the-top blessing as they welcomed our large family into their home and hearts. Jeff and Seth bonded like two peas in a pod. I have no doubt God brought them together.

BEHIND THE SCENES

The next day, a crew from Children's Heart Project arrived at Jeff and Dr. Allison's. They were some of the most down-to-earth, compassionate people I'd ever met. I was thrilled to meet those behind the scenes who made the magic happen. Cindy and Theresa, someone everyone lovingly referred to as Mama T, ran the project like a well-oiled machine. To see them in action and witness their hearts and the way they served families was inspiring. Seth was intrigued by the film crew. Arthur, Justin, and David, the director, videographer, and photographer, unloaded the equipment, including a stellar drone they used to follow our car in one scene. They worked around our appointments and preparations for the Ronald McDonald House Gala. They jumped in our car and followed us on our busy schedule taking raw footage along the way. They shared their talents and love for God and people by creating a marvelous compilation of our journey. We were so grateful for Cindy's vision for sharing our story and assigning a dedicated top-notch crew who worked tirelessly. From the combined strength of the film crew and everyone involved, God unfolded a beautiful story.

We met the host families, the host church, and volunteers who supported the families coming from overseas. I quickly realized writing a check was the easy part. These dedicated servants were the essential boots on the ground. They spurred us on to want to give, serve, and love others more.

We found out Justin had recently returned from a film project in the Congo. Upon further discussion, we learned that he stayed in the exact house in the remote village where Dr. Fischer spent so many years as a missionary practicing medicine! I teared up, unable to wrap my brain around this global connection. We couldn't make this up if we tried. It regularly amazed me how God intertwined people's paths down to the smallest of details.

Meeting the group from Mongolia with Dr. Fischer by our side marked a highlight of our lives. Two remarkable Samaritan's Purse interpreters handled the communication between us and our new Mongolian friends. Nothing was spoken that did not go through the tireless effort of the interpreters. They were on call twenty-four hours a day for four to six weeks as companions to the mothers who traveled with their children.

One of the heart surgery recipients, a boy a little older than Seth, was substantially smaller and quite weak because of the years his heart had not functioned properly. Yet, his face shone with the sweetest smile and demeanor. The two other children were adorably dressed in Mongolian attire, colorful and decorative, complete with traditional headwear. I soaked in and celebrated our differences as well as our many similarities.

I stood back and watched God work miracles right before my eyes. Seth's suffering would not be in vain. He sat down with his new friends and, through the interpreter, shared the purpose he found through his own pain. He recited his favorite verse. They prayed together. This precious Mongolian boy committed to pray for Seth. Such a beautiful connection in shared suffering.

We knew that God brought eight people from the other side of the world in his perfect timing. I marveled at all the people he networked to make this happen. As we spent time with the families and the interpreters, I had to hold back tears from the wonder of it all. Even though the clinic didn't have a specific surgery to give Seth a chance at a normal life, these families would. We could not have been happier. The children would return to Mongolia with their physical hearts transformed, but we never expected our hearts to be transformed as well. We prayed, applauded, cried, and grieved with them like they were our own. They were family to us now.

View the short film project here

Seth, Fifteen Years Old

It was time. The Ronald McDonald House made sure every detail for the Hearts and Diamonds Gala was memorable for their guest of honor.

Because Donnie and the kids had gone home for work and school, I felt especially nervous. The House went all out to give us the royal treatment leading up to the event: a clothing allowance, hair, makeup, and a mani-pedi for me. That evening, a sleek, black limousine picked us up. Dressed in our best, we experienced a pinch-me moment as we admired the leather interior. We felt like celebrities as we stepped out onto a red carpet. Even though I felt as far out of my comfort zone as possible at such a sophisticated event, I committed to seeing the goodness of God and being thankful. I didn't want to take anything away from Seth's night.

Seth looked like a million bucks. His snazzy tuxedo, complete with his signature smile, lit up the room. Since Seth's favorite color was royal blue, Jeff decided to honor him by wearing a royal blue vest and bow tie. I was so grateful he was there with us. And me? Talk about a hot mess. I tried to gather my thoughts. I was nervous about what people would think of my speech. Would I lose my place? Could I pull this off?

Nearly faint and sick to my stomach, I had to focus on the task at hand. I wanted to be transparent and honest about the way diseases strike families and how the Ronald McDonald House made the challenges easier to bear. I thought I was ready, but the more I soaked in the ambiance of the wealth represented in that room, the more inadequate I felt. Who was I to speak before a sold-out crowd of medical professionals, CEOs, philanthropists, and dignitaries? My worst enemy was my own inner critic. I could feel beads of sweat slowly dripping down my sides. So much for my sequined elegance.

Thankfully, the staff from the Ronald McDonald House were wonderful and supportive. They told me to be myself and not try to be anyone else. A mom with a real, raw, inspiring story only needed to speak from the heart and from personal experience. Their advice eased my self-induced inferiority complex. Seth was counting on me. *Mama, pull it together.*

Seth and I were seated at the head table. I had never eaten like this. I didn't recognize half the food. It was so fancy, I didn't know where to begin. My Grandma Benson taught us the importance of proper etiquette early on. She used to say, "Emily Post would say—"

But at this table, I forgot everything. I couldn't think straight. I couldn't eat. I discreetly looked around to follow everyone's lead. The wait staff served one course after another of exquisite food. My stomach twisted into knots, so I picked at pieces to be polite.

I had never spoken in public before, and here I was expected to give a speech for the elite of Rochester. I felt the blood drain from my face.

Jeff leaned over Seth and whispered, "Julie, you don't look so good."

"I don't feel so good. I don't belong here."

He immediately started listing all the reasons why God called me to this place for this time. He reassured me that God would equip me. "Can I pray for you?"

"Yes. Please."

Right there at the table, the three of us huddled up and prayed. I immediately felt the "peace that surpasses all understanding." I felt empowered–with God's strength. Jeff looked me in the eye.

"You good?"

I nodded and smiled. Jeff jumped up and stepped behind the podium to officially kick off the evening.

Jeff made sure he announced Seth as the star of the evening. He invited Seth to sit in a chair he placed beside the podium. Jeff was in his element as he worked the crowd.

"Seth asked me if I was going to wear my Ronald McDonald socks tonight. Well, yeah!"

Seth pulled up one of his pant legs to proudly display the famous red and white socks showing from beneath his leg braces. With that, Jeff stepped out from behind the podium, propped his leg up next to Seth's and pulled his pant leg up to display a matching pair. Everyone cheered.

As Jeff introduced me, I prayed a last-ditch plea. *God, speak through me. Not my words but yours.* They were definitely his words because mine seemed so inadequate. It was almost impossible for me to fully express the amount of gratitude we had for this organization. When we were in desperate need of help, the Ronald McDonald House opened its heart and doors to us.

With God's help, I blocked out all distractions. I spoke from my heart. I shared our journey of faith and hope through adversity. I saw people nod in agreement.

"This could be anyone's story. Sickness is no respecter of persons," I said. "One day, my son was perfectly healthy, and the next, we were in a race to find appropriate medical care to save my son's life . . . . We all want the best for our children. We all want a life free from suffering, disease, and pain for them."

At times, I hesitated in an effort to maintain my composure. I looked up to see several people wiping their eyes. I realized the people in that room were more like me than different. Regardless of the vast differences in backgrounds, cultures, economic, educational, or professional statuses, we shared a common bond through Seth's journey. God used our medical struggle to touch hearts with empathy, compassion, and love.

I was startled when the room erupted with a standing ovation. Overcome with emotion, Seth could only look out at the audience cheering for him.

As Jeff returned to the stage, he gave Seth a "you're a rockstar" hug as the crowd continued to applaud and cheer on their feet. Seth grinned from ear to ear. God was able to use whomever, wherever, whenever, and however He chooses. He is not limited by our limitations.

I am reminded from Scripture, that God, through His mighty power at work within us, is able to accomplish infinitely more than we might ask or think.

People made their way through the crowd and lined up to speak to me. One by one, they encouraged me. Many of these well-known people said God used the words I spoke to stir something in them. Some said they were struggling with their own health challenges, and this gave them hope and strength for the battle. Countless medical professionals said their zeal for what they were called to do was renewed. Corporate executives expressed they wanted to give more and do more because of hearing our story. Dignitaries tearfully shared that our message penetrated their hearts and spirits. Philanthropists said they were compelled to invest their resources into the Ronald McDonald House and Mayo Clinic on our behalf. That night affirmed our stories are a source of connection and are often intertwined. So much can be accomplished when we recognize the power of community.

I will be the first to admit I was the most unlikely, unequipped, unexpected person to write or speak at this or any event.

But God.

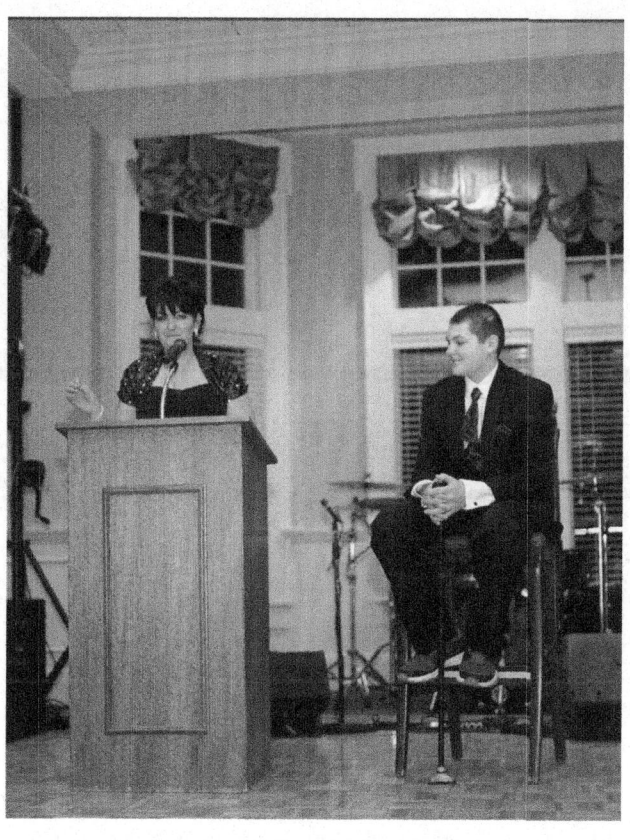

CHAPTER FOURTEEN
IRON SHARPENS IRON

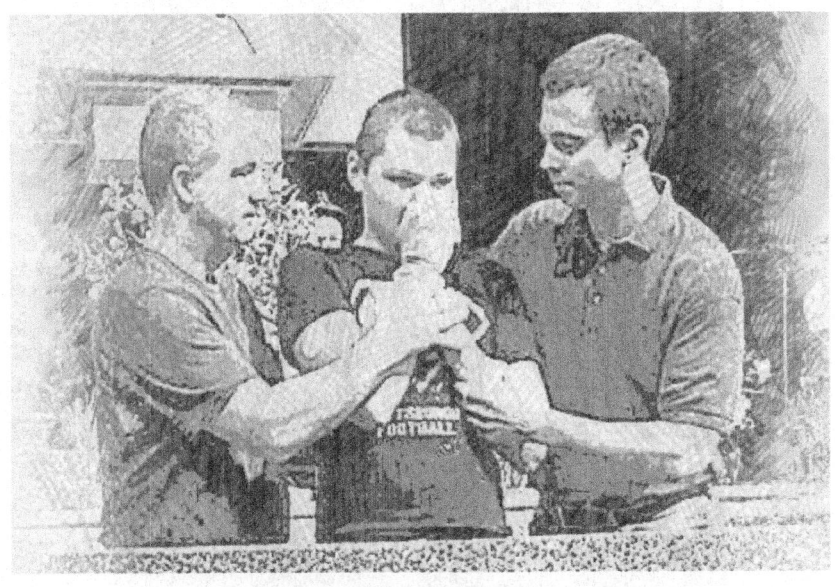

God deliberately chooses weak, suffering and unlikely
candidates to get His work done, so that in the end, the glory
goes to God and not to the person.
–Joni Eareckson Tada

Fall 2014

The Bristol grade school administrator, Mr. Gale Ryczek, and Seth had developed a close relationship. Seth looked forward to seeing him daily. They talked about sports and always kept tabs on each other. They both faced daily health challenges and encouraged one another to stay strong. They spurred one another on with projects and excitement for doing good. I would often hear them mention each other.

Even though it was difficult for Seth to get up and get going each day, he knew it was a gift. When, occasionally, talk about staying home was mentioned, I would say, "Think of someone that wouldn't be encouraged today if you didn't show up." Seth had a zest for life, and it was contagious.

Mr. Ryczek called with excitement he couldn't contain.

"Hello. Gale Ryczek here. I've got some pop tabs I want to give Seth. You might want to bring an empty vehicle–with the seats down."

When I got there, he was more excited than a kid in a candy store. He beckoned me to follow him as he giggled and talked a mile a minute about how he acquired the tabs for Seth. He brought me to the storage room inside the service entrance. I could hardly believe my eyes. A drum sat filled with hundreds of pounds of tabs! He said they had to use a forklift to transport it. He could hardly wait to get Seth out of class and show him.

Seth's reaction brought tears to Mr. Ryczek's eyes. Seth squealed with delight as he worked to bail the tabs into transferable containers. The moments discussing how incredible this was and how grateful he was to Mr. Ryczek were priceless.

Mr. Ryczek said of Seth,

"There are kids that come along, that bring everybody else together and make it a better place for everyone. That's Seth."

Seth no longer dreaded the next trip to the clinic. Instead, his mind was set on transporting those little pieces of metal to the Ronald McDonald House.

Kindred spirits, Seth and Jeff, were inseparable, even more so since our time together at the gala. When we made the trip to Rochester, Seth couldn't wait to see Jeff. Whether hanging out at the Ronald McDonald House, church, Children's Heart Project missions, outings around town, or killing time between appointments, the time Jeff and Seth shared together was always time well spent. Jeff was a kid at heart and had a gift for making everyone around him laugh.

I never saw laughter as a gift from God up until this point, but meeting Jeff changed my perspective. After a long, stressful day, what a stress buster to release the weight we carried with a good chuckle. I had almost forgotten what it was like to laugh to the point of tears. Missing loved ones at home and being in survival mode for so long, that intense laughter reminded me good existed even in the hard places.

Jeff gave us a precious gift–his time. He spent hours sitting in the waiting room with us and made a point to pray with Seth in pre-op before his many surgeries. When Jeff wasn't traveling the world on medical missions with his wife, mentoring kids at the local schools, or volunteering for countless organizations, he could be found executing one of his shenanigans. And, for a moment, Seth would forget about life's troubles.

The best part of this sweet friendship was their faith connection. It's just like I read in Proverbs 27:17, "As iron sharpens iron, so a friend sharpens a friend." They fed off one another, encouraged one another, strengthened one another, and prayed for one another. God knew Seth would need this dynamic brotherhood for the road ahead.

May 2015

Our family attended a church youth group ceremony one summer night called "Moving Up and Moving On." It was a celebration of gratitude for what God had done and in anticipation of what God would do in the future in the students' lives. Seth graduated from the elementary program and moved up into our church's middle school program. As was customary, each graduate received a leatherbound Bible and a book. Seth received *Don't Waste Your Life* by John Piper.

I had never witnessed Seth immerse himself in any book as he did this one. It was as if a lightbulb went off.

He said, "Everything makes sense now."

He knew why God had spared his life and sustained him thus far. Because of Piper's book, Seth now wanted to serve, love, give, and live life with purpose and passion more than ever.

Since this book had such an impact on Seth, I did some digging. I listened to the original message from John Piper from the year 2000, which inspired the book. I was six months pregnant with Seth when this message was presented to a crowd of forty thousand youth. As God was knitting Seth together in my womb, he prepared a message through Piper that would not only change Seth's life in one of his darkest hours but change hearts and lives for generations to come.

As Seth read this book, each chapter renewed and strengthened his faith like never before. Up until that point, "chemo brain" fog and seizure activity pushed Seth to discouragement. He had trouble retaining information and remembering scriptures. Through the words in that book, God met Seth.

Seth often came to me and said, "Mom! Listen to this," and read me parts that spoke to him. He highlighted and underlined and dog-eared pages devouring the message. He loved Scripture in a new way and began to more fully understand his purpose in life and suffering. Seth was determined to *not* waste his life.

Dr. Fischer continued to be a special part of Seth's overall well-being. Instead of primarily focusing on abnormal test results, he paid equal attention to Seth's mind, body, and spirit. Wisely, Dr. Fischer understood how they all connected. We had gotten used to new doctors not knowing or taking the time to get to know the person behind the chart. Dr.

Fischer, however, wanted to challenge Seth to live his best life. He achieved this by engaging with Seth about his interests and life goals. Seth was excited to share that he just started reading *Don't Waste Your Life*.

"So, you aren't going to waste your life by living it solely to pick up seashells on the seashore?"

Dr. Fischer had obviously read one of the examples in the book. He encouraged Seth to press into being intentional and purposeful.

Seth said, "I feel like it's hard for me to concentrate. I thought I would always be a pastor, but I don't think I could go to seminary. I can't picture myself standing at a pulpit. I can't even stand for long periods without my legs hurting." He hung his head as though his dreams were crushed.

Dr. Fischer spoke words of encouragement and life into him. He said, "There are many avenues that God calls us to minister. You could be a hospital chaplain, for example."

He encouraged Seth to be open to God's calling for his life, whatever that might look like. This was a huge encouragement to Seth. At the same time, Seth's pediatrician, Dr. Schimming, and his rheumatologist also spoke life into him. This tag team that God put together strengthened Seth for the road ahead. Although Seth's physical conditions weren't improving, Seth embraced hope, joy, and peace. That made all the difference. His extraordinary medical team gave top priority to Seth's overall well-being: mind, body, and spirit.

Seth began to experience increased episodes at night. They appeared to be breakthrough seizures but were more aggravated. He would gasp in his sleep. Getting a full night's rest became a rare luxury. We were both exhausted. I learned that managing epilepsy is a constant work in progress. The many and ever-changing variables create a lot of trial and error. We learned how crucial it was to keep in constant contact with Seth's neurologist, so I called him and discussed what was going on.

He ordered another sleep study with an electroencephalogram (EEG). We prayed for results that were clear and wisdom to know how to help Seth.

After a twelve-hour observation, medical professionals told us the news. Not only was Seth having what appeared to be seizure activity, but he had also stopped breathing several times per hour during the night. His doctors and I were disheartened and frustrated. We didn't expect this. Obstructive sleep apnea was common for someone born with abnormalities, in the older population, in someone with a heavier build, a wider neck, who was overweight, or for those who snored. Seth met none of those conditions, and was, again, the rare exception. Seth didn't show sleep apnea in previous sleep studies, so it could only be explained as one more unfortunate sign of progressing deterioration. Seth was assigned a pediatric sleep medicine doctor to treat his sleep apnea. Now he needed a Continuous Positive Airway Pressure (CPAP) machine every time he slept.

The team explained the complexity of the situation. Both epilepsy and sleep apnea have their own concerns individually, but together they could lead to serious complications and increased risk of death. They told us it was *imperative* that Seth's seizures were controlled and that Seth wear the CPAP mask any time he slept, even for a nap. This became part of Seth's new normal.

Upon doing my own research, I found out about another danger lurking, something known as SUDEP Sudden, Unexpected Death of someone with epilepsy, who is *otherwise healthy*. My heart sank as I read those words. Since Seth was *not* otherwise healthy, I could only assume he was at an increased risk.

Learning how serious uncontrolled seizures were and the prevalence of SUDEP was a valid concern and startling reality. Each year, more than 1 in 1,000 people with epilepsy die from SUDEP. I shuddered to think of going in to wake Seth only to find his body lifeless. I was no longer the same mother or caregiver. I could no longer plead blissful ignorance to the possibility of one of these horrific health conditions taking my son's life. What a heavy load for any parent to bear. I wouldn't say I lived in fear, but I had to actively fight when fear crept in.

I found out it's not uncommon for doctors to avoid a conversation about SUDEP. I suppose because no one wants to invoke fear. How does one tell a parent who is dealing with the initial shock of having their child newly diagnosed with epilepsy that their child has a higher chance of dying unexpectedly? But I beg the question - *how could you not?* We tell our new parents about Sudden Infant Death Syndrome (SIDS) and what puts their babies at higher risk. It seemed to me that parents of children with epilepsy needed to be equipped with as much information as possible so they could be proactive in lowering risk factors for SUDEP. I found the following quote by Jim Abrahams, founder of The Charlie Foundation to Cure Pediatric Epilepsy helpful.

The medical destiny of each of us and our children is largely up to us. To think otherwise can be damaging. There is a tendency when we walk into a doctor's office to want to hand over our problems to the doctor and say, 'Here it is, please fix it.' It's comfortable, it's easy, and more often than not, it works. Just as we take comfort in deferring to them, many doctors are unwilling to confide in us that we may have stepped into one of Western medicine's black holes. There are many black holes, and they are deep . . .

So what does that mean? It means that our medical problems and our children's medical problems are precisely that—OURS. At first, that's a pretty intimidating and perhaps a seemingly foolish concept, both to us and to some physicians. After all, they went through years of education. They've seen countless patients in their practices. And then we walk into their offices with a disease we probably don't even know how to spell. How presumptuous and perhaps foolish of us, the patients, to ask and then pursue the hard questions, learn the side effects, get the second opinions, do the research, and participate in the cure— in short, to become proactive.

Ironically, the 'side effect' of participating in our medical destinies may not only lead to getting better sooner. It is empowering.

I researched and learned how all of this may play into Seth's particular situation. I needed to be precise and timely with his medications, make sure he got adequate sleep (sleep deprivation lowers the seizure threshold), and make sure he was compliant with his CPAP. I needed to maintain regular communication with his doctors, reporting any changes or breakthrough seizure activity. His neurologist warned Seth of the major implications of drinking alcohol and other risk factors that he could control. We understood and were more than willing to do our part. But the reality staring me in the face was—no guarantees.

My natural instinct was to worry. I struggled with the fear of not being there in the middle of the night. We rarely left Seth alone, but no one could be there at every moment, especially while we slept. I knew worry and fear didn't help. God was teaching me to trust him. I prayed for wisdom as I educated myself on how to give Seth the best chance for living as normal a life as possible.

We all needed rest. Rest–a gift from God, vital for mind and body. I needed to trust that God was in control and that he loved my son even more than his dad and I did. I had to come to grips with the fact that God didn't guarantee a life without hardships, but He would be with us. And no one offered peace and crushed fear like God.

SETH'S PUBLIC PROFESSION OF FAITH

For many reasons, Seth often couldn't attend his high school youth group. That didn't stop Pastor Ortiz from meeting Seth where he was. Pastor Ortiz cared deeply about the outcome of his students' faith. He regularly asked to pick up Seth and take him to a fast food place where they hashed out life, struggles, victories, and God's goodness. God worked through this man to show Seth that God had not abandoned him.

Seth had expressed a desire to follow Jesus' example and be baptized. He met with the pastoral team from our church to study Scriptures on the significance of baptism. Seth made the decision to follow Jesus when he was quite young, but now that he was fifteen, he felt compelled to make his profession of faith public.

This day was a momentous occasion. The scheduled baptism service fell on Easter Sunday. On March 27, 2016, Seth proclaimed publicly and boldly in front of family, friends, and the congregation his faith in Jesus as his Lord and Savior. We embraced the symbolism of Seth submerged under water to represent leaving his old life behind. What joy to watch our son come up out of the water as a symbol of rising to a new life of faith in Jesus Christ. With this outward expression, Seth was declaring the transformation that had taken place in his heart—not a religious facade but evidence of a personal relationship with God.

Following Jesus didn't mean the absence of struggles. This progressive disease was no joke. There was no quick fix. Our weaknesses were a daily reminder of our desperate need for God. Yet, through it all, God was good to us. He never left us. We sensed his peace and presence in difficult times. Amazing grace . . . how sweet the sound!

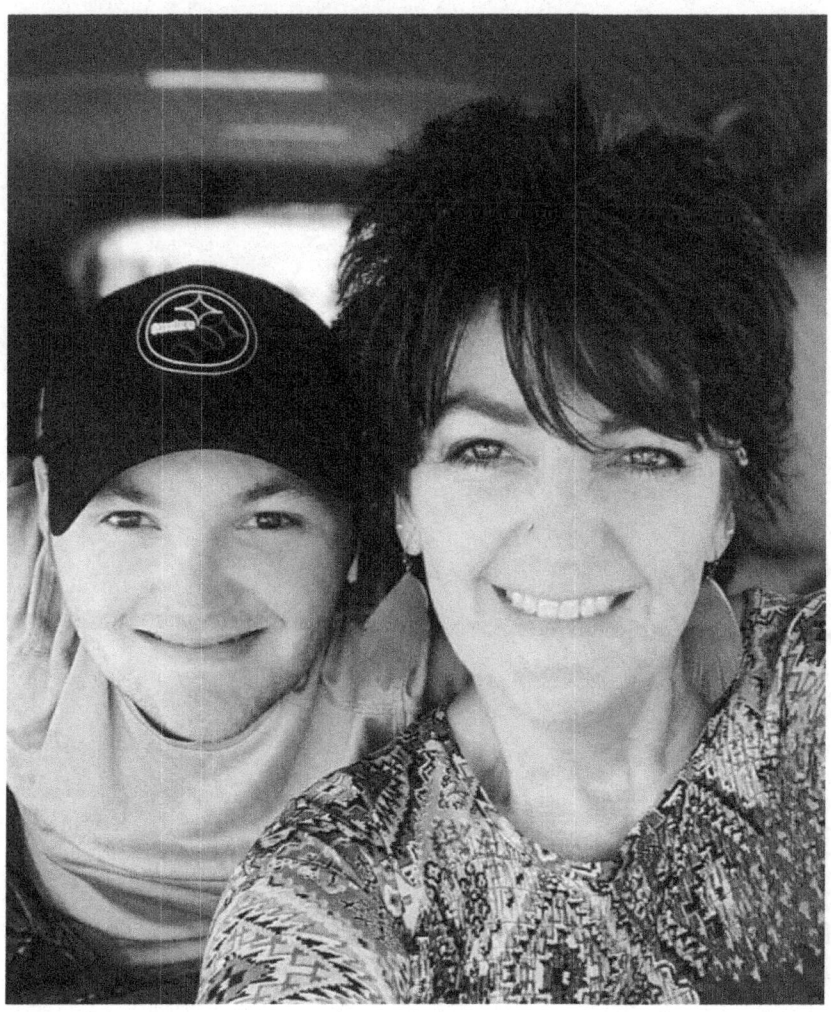

On the road again

CHAPTER FIFTEEN
THE POP TAB KID

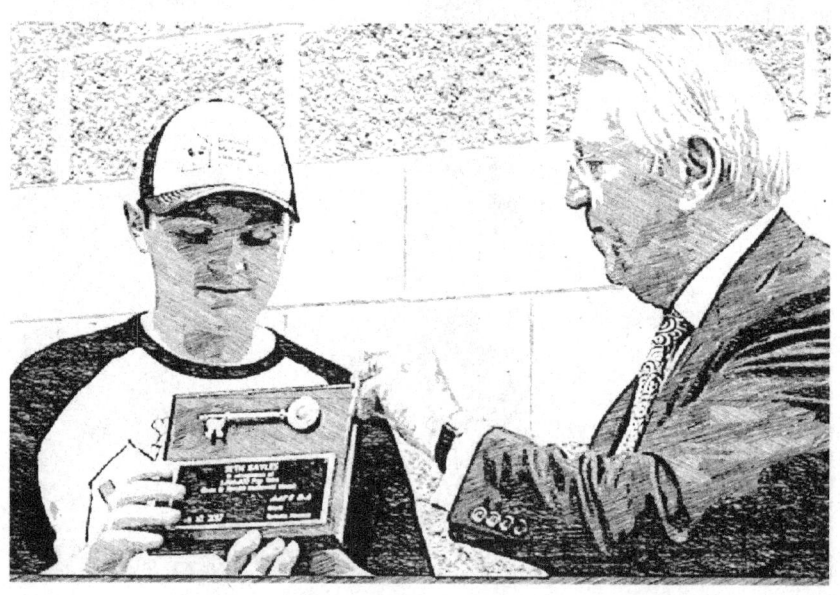

I alone cannot change the world, but I can cast a
stone across the waters to create many ripples.
–Mother Teresa

Spring 2016

Seth came home super excited. After four eighth-grade classes watched videos of various charities, the eighth-graders unanimously voted for Children's Heart Project as their class service project! Seth said everyone had been talking about it. The kids were as thrilled to be a part of it as much as Seth. They set a goal to raise enough funds to sponsor one child to come to the United States for life-saving heart surgery.

The students planned a bake sale and dodgeball tournament. They ordered red wristbands with hearts on them. Inside were the words, "In honor of Seth Bayles." A classmate and his mom ordered team shirts printed with "For Seth." The bake sale donation jar collected a record-setting amount. Someone saw Mr. Ryczek take a cookie off the sale table, drop a hundred-dollar bill in the jar, and walk away.

Another classmate of Seth's had a death in the family, and the funeral was the same day as the event. The family decided all memorials in honor of their grandfather would be made to Children's Heart Project. We felt overwhelmed with love.

On tournament Saturday, many of the school staff, board, and community members volunteered alongside our family. Our tribe, once again, rallied around Seth. More importantly, they rallied around children in need of life-saving medical care. Because of our family's connection to the project, the school asked me to accept a check for the project from the four eighth-grade classes. When I arrived at school, Mr. Ryczek stopped me as I entered the building and asked if I would come into his office.

When he told me to have a seat, I knew this was about more than money. I will never forget the honor of him sharing his heart with me that day. He explained the details of his own health struggles. I had no idea that he was going through aggressive medical treatment. He told me Seth changed his outlook on life. Obviously moved by what he was trying to put into words, tears flowed down his face. His brief silence pierced my heart. I had always known this man to be a strong leader whom I respected. His long-standing dedication to the community was undeniable. I was humbled and moved to hear how personally Seth affected him.

He said, "On the worst days, when I feel like I can't do this, I am reminded of Seth. He's going through many of the same health challenges, yet the other day he asked me how I was doing and told me he had been praying for me. He was praying for *me*! He shows up, with the biggest smile, never feeling sorry for himself. He walks down the hallway and high-fives kids the whole way. He makes everyone feel important, that their life matters."

Both of us were struggling to contain our emotions. I never knew any of this.

He said, "This school needed this project. It was extra special for all of us." Then, he wiped his face, took a deep breath, and said, "Now, let's go get that check."

The students and staff of Bristol School made Seth's exit from middle school meaningful and memorable. Together, they were able to give a priceless gift, the gift of life and hope. I saw the heart of what was most important at that school: care for one another, character building, and celebrating life. The class of 2016 united for the greater good! To me, those life lessons were even more valuable than the academics.

SETH'S SIXTEENTH BIRTHDAY WISH

Rites of passage: Sixteenth and eighteenth birthdays, *quinceaneras*, gaining the freedom (and responsibility of) a driver's license, applying for jobs, and registering to vote all mark milestones in life. For various reasons, including epilepsy/seizure activity, completing driver's education would not be on Seth's check-off list.

Seth and I discussed other kids, often friends from the Ronald McDonald House, who never made it to such a milestone. He recalled sitting beside a friend in the hospital weeks before she went to heaven. The Ronald McDonald House gave us so much more than just a roof over our heads. We built relationships and realized many others, especially in other countries, were worse off than us. This kept

Seth grounded and helped keep his conditions in perspective. Because of that, Seth rarely felt sorry for himself.

His sixteenth birthday especially had him thinking of others. Kids he knew were spending their birthdays at the hospital, the Ronald McDonald House, or whose parents were spending their child's birthday without them. He recalled a time, several years prior, when we were staying at the Ronald McDonald House for several weeks. That day, we walked past the room of a girl he had gotten to know well. Her door was decorated with crepe paper, balloons, and a big number "16." Seth felt so bad that she had to spend her special day away from her friends, family, and school.

"Mom, can we buy some presents to cheer her up?"

Elated at the initiative Seth took, and with time to spare before we had to be back at the clinic, we ran to the store. Seth joyfully picked out several gifts of art/coloring books, make-up, nail polish, and candy. The empathy he felt for this girl was replaced with the thoughts of what joy this would bring her.

We talked on the way back about the beauty of giving anonymously. We took everything to our room, and Seth wrapped them with great care. He was so excited. He put everything in his coat and scoped out the situation to ensure we avoided any witnesses. I waited at the elevator, and he knew what to do. He dropped the gifts at her door and scampered back to the elevator out of breath with a huge grin–mission accomplished. We giggled all the way back to the clinic.

Seth's own sixteenth birthday arrived with great anticipation. He felt the depth of the gift of life and all he had been given.

"I know what I want to do for my birthday. I want to give gifts to the Ronald McDonald House. I have so much; I don't need anything, but the Ronald McDonald House always needs stuff."

Seth and I made a short video explaining his desire. Donnie secured a U-Haul trailer and Grandma Sue made a banner for the side that read, "Seth's Ronald McDonald House Supply Drive." His siblings supported him all the way. They made posters and set up a tent at the intersection of two highways near our home.

On his big day, Seth sat by the intersection to greet a steady line of people who drove from two states with groceries, supplies, and pop tabs for The House. Some stayed for several hours to show their support. Strangers stopped and asked what was going on. It gave Seth an opportunity to talk about the Ronald McDonald House. He was so in his element sharing about things that mattered.

Seth's friend asked his mom if her company could help Seth's cause. His mom was not only honored to be a part, but planned a shopping spree. Myself, Seth, his friend and mother walked up and down each aisle, tossing in items they thought could bless families. In the end, we filled five shopping carts. Seth couldn't wait to deliver all of this. This birthday turned out greater and more memorable than Seth could have imagined.

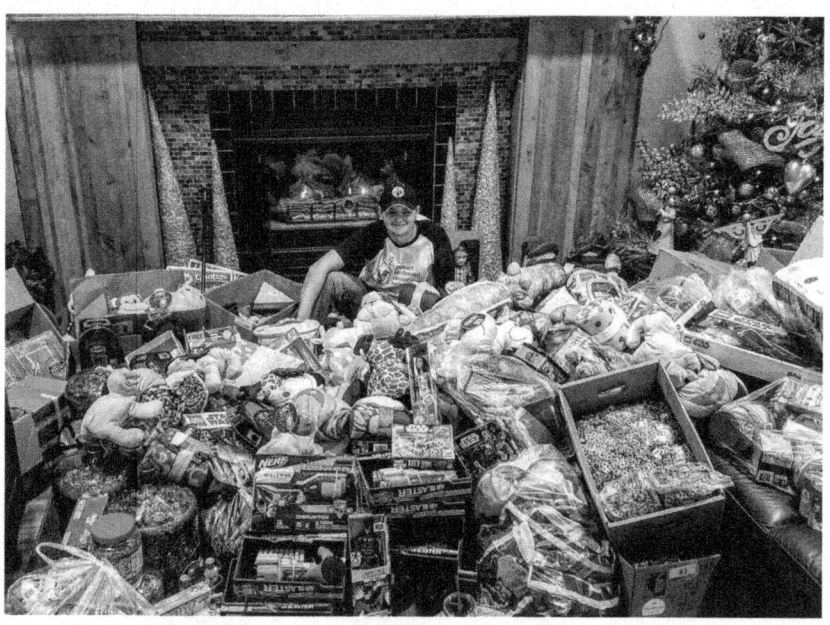

Thanks to community support, Seth is surrounded by items he donated to the Ronald McDonald House.

PUSHING THE DRUMMER TO SUCCEED

The 2016-2017 school year was Seth's freshman year. The band teacher, Mr. Scheele, offered Seth all of the opportunities and accommodations needed to continue his love of drumming. Seth loved the thought of being in the band for his high school years. What he didn't expect was to also join the Pep Band and Marching Band.

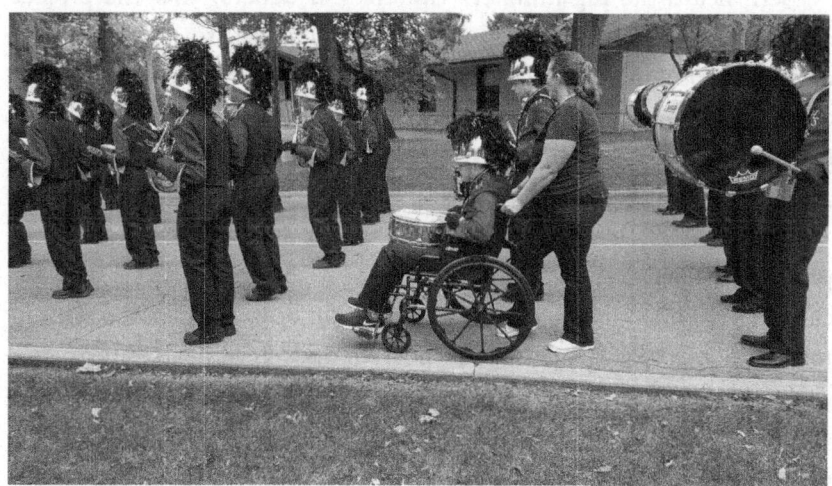

Seth was uncomfortable, at first, thinking he'd be a burden for people who had to push his wheelchair outside around the grassy football field and around campus. He was assured, however, that a number of people were eager to help. Parents and students took turns pushing him *for four years*. The selfless labor of others enabled Seth to play the snare drum and partake in parades around the community. A highlight for him that fall was a day trip to Chicago where he participated in the nationally televised Columbus Day Parade. Seth experienced miles of spectators who enjoyed the Westosha Central Band and festivities. What a memory!

MAY 2017, MORE THAN A TINY PIECE OF METAL

The Ronald McDonald House officially announced its plans for expansion. It launched a historic campaign known as "Love Tremendously, Hope Exceedingly." The expansion was desperately needed and many years overdue. The project would bring the current forty-two rooms (that consistently logged a waiting list) to seventy rooms, along with many needed improvements and amenities to better serve families. Because the house meant the world to us, Seth wanted others to be able to experience it rather than go to a hotel.

Seth heard the big numbers (millions of dollars) that the project cost, but he wasn't intimidated. He felt compelled to make a difference. He committed to more fundraising and announced he would collect ONE MILLION pop tabs. Seth knew we served a big God and learned to ask big. He had seen time and time again that nothing was impossible with God.

Seth's sister, Janae, wanted to help her brother. She asked the principal of her grade and middle school if she could start a pop-tab campaign in his honor. The principal was all for it. Excited and willing to put in the work, Janae made posters and created a contest. The class that collected the most tabs received a cupcake party. She committed to buying the cupcakes with her own money. She never expected the outpouring. Seth and I spoke to the winning classroom. The kids were so excited to meet him and commit to helping other kids. They also made blankets and cards for the children staying at the Ronald McDonald House. Kids helping kids–what a beautiful thing.

Seth talked pop tabs with anyone who would listen. Our wonderful Bristol Fire and Rescue station became a major, long-term drop-off location for tabs from the community. The captain and lieutenant put out the word to other firehouses to collect tabs. "Firefighters 4 Charity" multiplied Seth's efforts in a big way. Seth traveled to firehouses, businesses, local pubs and restaurants, our local county fair, outreach events, and more to talk and receive tabs. He gained notoriety as "The Pop Tab Kid." No one who met Seth looked at those little pieces of metal the same way again.

Our village hosts its annual Bristol Progress Days celebration one weekend in July. It's the biggest event of the year for our neck of the woods. Generations ago, our family was proud to have our very own "Pop" Benson as the grand marshal of the very first Bristol Progress Days Parade. It has been a highlight for our family ever since. The annual celebration offered a perfect opportunity to move Seth toward his pop tab goal. He came up with the idea of creating a float of pop tabs to enter in the parade. It would be quite the undertaking.

We borrowed a trailer and worked nights in our barn decorating it. Firefighters 4 Charity created and donated two giant personalized banners. The entire perimeter of the float was made up of clear totes roughly half-filled with tabs. Reporters wrote articles about the purpose of the float and word spread. The entire community was all abuzz. Word-of-mouth spread like wildfire.

The celebration kicked off Friday night with softball tournaments. Bristol Firefighters had taken the liberty to purchase five hundred pairs of red and white Ronald McDonald socks, better known locally as "Seth Socks." It was pretty cool to see the players and umpires, along with adults and children in the stands, wearing knee-high red and white cotton socks in Seth's honor.

By noon on Sunday, thousands of people had lined the streets. Seth waved from the passenger seat of his dad's truck that pulled the float. His younger brothers were on either side throwing candy and receiving tabs. We never expected people to run up to both sides of the float to dump their pop tabs in the bins. It was so much fun!

After the parade, Seth continued to collect into the night. The bins overflowed! We added buckets, cans, and various containers from our house. More important were the fascinating, powerful, and touching stories of how people connected with Seth and his heart to give back.

One teenage girl and her mom came to meet Seth and share how he inspired them. She showed us the polypropylene back brace she wore for scoliosis. She told us she had always been ashamed of it. She never wanted anyone to know she wore it underneath her clothes. She said she saw Seth in the newspaper in shorts with leg braces made of the same material. She was surprised that he wasn't ashamed and thought that was amazing. She was determined to be like Seth and embrace her physical challenges.

We heard another powerful story when a woman brought her load of pop tabs. As Seth thanked her for the huge donation, she started to cry. She explained that she and her husband collected tabs for years for various charities. It was something they enjoyed doing together.

Although he had passed away over a decade ago, she kept them in her office as a reminder of him.

She said, "I just couldn't bear to part with them. They're the last thing I had left. Then, I read about you and your goal in the newspaper, and I knew this was where these tabs were supposed to go."

Seth was so moved. He expressed his gratitude and said, "I'm honored to receive them to give to the Ronald McDonald House." They embraced with tears.

I watched in awe as strangers came together in the midst of challenges and helped one another ease the pain by doing good. At the end of the long yet sublime weekend, we dismantled the float in the dark, in the rain, and loaded the tabs in a waiting U-Haul truck parked in our driveway. Our entire family planned to head to Rochester first thing in the morning wondering and hoping if Seth made his goal. It had only been eight weeks to the day since Seth announced his goal publicly. Even if there weren't a million tabs in that truck, the support from the community was nothing short of miraculous. This quantity in such a short period of time was beyond imagination!

When we arrived early the next morning at the Ronald McDonald House in Rochester, Minnesota, we were shocked to have the House staff, volunteers, the Rochester Fire Department, Mayor Ardell Brede, and local camera crews waiting for us. The tabs were received, weighed, and the individual count was calculated.

The grand total, ladies and gentlemen, . . . drum roll, please . . . 1.7 million tabs! Holy Hamburglar! God honored Seth's desire to give, big time. We saw Psalm 37:4 all over this effort. "Take delight in the LORD, and he will give you your heart's desires."

At a local press conference, Mayor Brede took to the podium and asked Seth to come up. He was taken aback by all of the attention. All Seth wanted was to do what he could to help with the expansion project. He never expected recognition. Collecting tabs felt like a small token of giving back for all the support he had received over the years.

Because of Seth's efforts, Mayor Brede announced and officially proclaimed the week of July 10 to July 16, "Pop Tab Week." He presented Seth with the official proclamation. Seth was beyond excited that every year the city of Rochester would bring awareness to collecting and donating pop tabs to the Ronald McDonald House. His hope that more people would get involved and offset the cost of running each house came true. And it really did "take a village."

What happened next was even more remarkable. The mayor presented Seth with "The Key to the City." This sobering moment brought silence except for the clicking of press cameras. Then, cheers and applause erupted from the crowd. I don't think Seth had the ability to fully comprehend the magnitude of such an achievement. It took time for this extraordinary recognition to truly sink in. Someone told us it was only the second of two keys that the good mayor had handed out in his fourteen years in office. Seth's jaw dropped, but words didn't come. He was truly speechless by this humbling, once-in-a-lifetime honor.

JULY 2017, A FLOOD OF PURPOSE

Having accomplished the pop tab mission, Donnie and the kids headed home from Rochester. Seth and I stayed behind for appointments. After a long day at the clinic, we settled in and I turned on the evening news. The local Minnesota station showed aerial footage of Burlington, Wisconsin, underwater due to flash flooding. Burlington, our neighboring town? I was in shock! I called home. Donnie told me we had a flooded lower level, and the water was rising. Oh, no!

"Julie, I can't talk. Me and the kids are bailing water. Stuff is floating. The water's coming in faster than the sump can pump it out. Gotta go." Click.

I recalled it was raining the evening we loaded the U-Haul. We tried to dismantle the float full of pop tabs in the rain. It had not let up the entire time we were gone. *Stuff is floating?* Then I remembered. Before we left, I asked the kids to get every bin from the basement they could find for the tabs. In their haste, they must have dumped the contents on the floor. That must be the "stuff" Donnie was referring to.

Donnie later called and explained he and the children were cutting up pieces of soggy basement carpet and hauling them up the stairs and outside to the road for bulk trash pick up. The clean-up went on for days. He had to stop to go to work, but then came home and continued where the kids left off. I felt so helpless and distanced from being able to help.

Seth and I arrived home to a growing problem–mold. What a mess. Who knew how fast mold could spread up the drywall? Seth went downstairs devastated to see how much mold had already grown inside his wooden bass drum. He immediately got a nosebleed. I got him upstairs, as he struggled to breathe. It was obvious the restricted and reduced capacity of his chest wall muscles put him at extra risk. A friend called after seeing the devastation on the news and encouraged me and Seth to "get outta there." She even made hotel reservations for us.

Donnie wasn't able to take time off work, so he couldn't stay ahead of the mold. It was now twelve inches up the walls and into the inner drywall. Our church reached out to check on families in the area. I rarely asked for help, but since they asked, I described our dilemma. They thanked me for sharing and reassured me help was on the way. They sent an email to the leaders and immediately received replies from many who wanted to help.

The church ordered a grasshopper green thirty-yard dumpster to be dropped in our driveway. The Samaritan's Purse Disaster Response Team called me. I had no idea they were already deployed with a command center set up in our area. *Thank you, God!* He supplied a mighty army!

I will never forget the sea of vehicles that steadily streamed into our driveway backing up all the way onto the highway in front of our farm that Saturday morning in mid-July. A sea of orange shirts representing Samaritan's Purse volunteers joined our church members.

The first thing they said was, "It was obvious from the moment we talked to your church, how much they love you and wanted to serve you . . . . We don't usually have this many people working together at one site, but we thought it was important to link arms and serve you together. It's an honor to come alongside them."

Soon, two of the Billy Graham Rapid Response Team chaplains made their way over. Seth told them that he wanted to be a chaplain one day and asked if he could pray for them. They were quite moved that someone asked to pray for them. Afterwards, everyone scattered like ants and promptly set to work. Yard cleanup, gutting the lower level, carpet, linoleum, drywall removal, and chopping up furniture all happened at the same time. They sprayed everything down with a non-toxic, anti-mold solution. Everyone was so efficient and positive. Surely, "many hands make light work." The group accomplished everything from start to finish in only four hours.

I can't say enough about the volunteers, including three who were well into their seventies. They drove their own vehicles all the way from Kentucky and Connecticut at their own expense. I couldn't believe that they slept in sleeping bags on the command center floor to come and clean mold off our basement walls. I had to ask about their stories and their motivations for being there. Their selfless service and why they chose to do this changed me. I wanted to hug the snot out of them.

We didn't grieve the loss of stuff–we had all that truly mattered. We filled that green dumpster with a household of stuff, and the only tears shed were those of gratitude for those who helped fill it! We gathered as a large group. Samaritan's Purse volunteers handed me a special Bible inscribed with words of encouragement from everyone who helped us bear this heavy burden. We bowed our heads and gave thanks to God for it all: faith, family, and friends, new and old. I witnessed that sometimes it was the hardest things in life that made the biggest impact and the strongest bonds.

The Ronald McDonald House staff asked if they could tell Seth's story as their next short film project. Honored yet hesitant, I agreed. A professional film crew come to my house? After a flood? Oh, my. They made plans to send a professional photographer, videographer, and film crew from Encore Public Relations to our home in Wisconsin.

BEHIND THE SCENES

Director/Producer Laura and business partner, videographer/photographer Shawn, put our fears to rest. They embraced our small town and our journey, and we became fast friends. It was chaotic packing two weeks' worth of events into two days. Laura and Shawn made it seem easy. Filming continued in Rochester as they documented a day of our life at the clinic. Seth was exhausted but knew it was important to share his journey to help others. They also filmed a pop tab commercial featuring Seth and his three younger siblings. Epic! At first we felt reluctant to be put in the spotlight, but when all was said and done, the opportunity to share our story was a blessing, and I could only thank God.

View short film project here.

RIPPLE EFFECT

The Communications Director of the Ronald McDonald House said this about Seth, "He's so focused on the positives. He's going through things that most kids couldn't imagine going through, most adults couldn't imagine going through, and he does it with a mindset of 'how can I help others?' I think that just speaks to him and his family . . . They have really become part of our story."

A local radio station named Seth's donation to the Ronald McDonald House the number one "most tissue-worthy, heartwarming Rochester story of 2017." It was humbling to witness the impact one boy had through the beautiful collaboration of countless individuals. And the ripple effect of Seth's desire to make his life count continued to expand, beyond what he could have imagined. The worldwide headquarters of a Fortune 100 company got involved. Since it was so close to our home, we knew many individuals who worked there, but one employee and friend, in particular, took the liberty of sharing Seth's story internally. She showed the Ronald McDonald House film project, based upon Seth's desire to give back, during a charitable giving drive. Employees were inspired to collect pop tabs in Seth's honor for every trip to Rochester. Many of their employees took advantage of their employee match program and signed up to give monthly to the Ronald McDonald House in Minnesota, their charity of choice.

We developed partnerships with several local businesses. Seth's school, Westosha Central High School, led fundraising events. They designated all the proceeds from the sale of socks, wristbands, and ice cream at lunchtime for the Ronald McDonald House. School clubs got involved. Classes held penny wars, a pop-tab drive, and the week concluded with an assembly. The entire school and community packed into the gym where Seth's Ronald McDonald film project was shown, and we talked about overcoming adversity. The school surprised Seth when they presented him with a check for the Ronald McDonald House.

The Association of Business Students took it upon themselves to create Seth's Journey shirts with Philippians 4:13, his signature Bible verse, on the back and sold them in the school store. Several "Miracle Minute" collections were done at various high school events. With the stands filled with spectators, we watched in awe as buckets were passed up and down the aisles for only sixty seconds. Unprecedented amounts were raised! One time, nine hundred dollars broke the record for a one-minute collection. Business owners regularly jumped on board to match the funds.

The school staff was behind Seth every step of the way. The Sheriff's Department and Fire and Rescue partnered with the school to join his efforts. The school hosted a "Color Run" with all proceeds going to the Ronald McDonald House.

Seth and I spoke at a student-run Fashion and Art Show with all proceeds going to the cause. Seth even modeled a pop tab vest he created in the car during the commute to and from Mayo Clinic. Many said they felt Seth brought out the very best in our community.

We were beyond thankful for the part people played in helping him in countless ways. Ironically, people regularly expressed their gratitude to Seth for allowing them to be a part of something bigger than themselves. We realized through this journey that the majority of people wanted to give. They just didn't know how or what. Seth was simply an instrument orchestrating a much bigger plan and purpose. And we can't mention all those who wished to remain anonymous. We loved them all.

What a blessing to be a blessing!

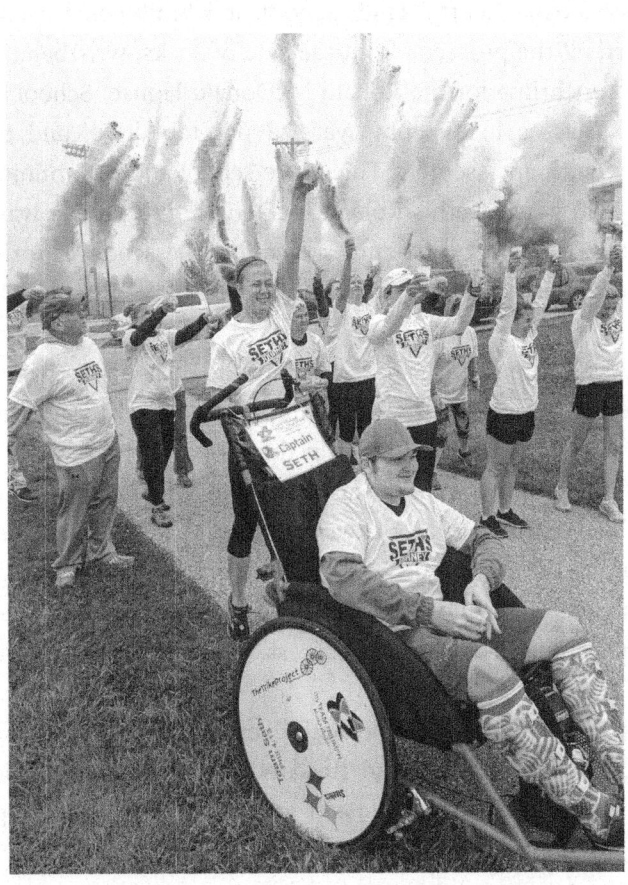

CHAPTER SIXTEEN
NOT REJECTION . . . REDIRECTION

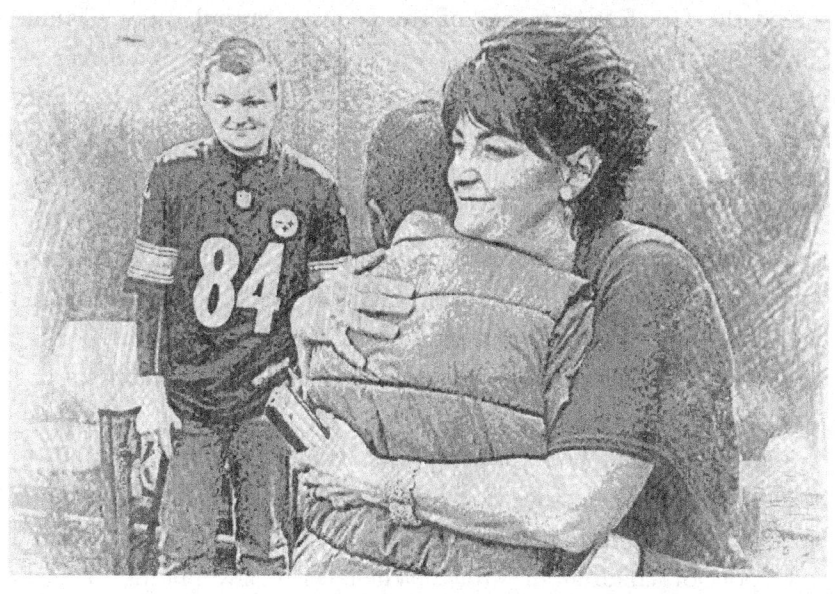

Instead of dwelling on the pain within,
reach out to someone else's pain.
–Nick Vujicic, *Life Without Limits*

My heart leaped out of my chest as I heard the pulpit announcement. Our church was sending a group to Kenya. I perked up wide-eyed.

"If you feel a calling to minister to those in Africa, come see me after service in the foyer for more information."

I leaned over and nudged Donnie making eye contact. I couldn't contain my excitement. I pointed to my chest and mouthed, "Me! Me! I'm going." He tried to focus on the message, but I could not. My mind was traveling a mile a minute. Everything said from that point on was a blur.

We loved running the Christian Mission. God blessed us with a great crew of like-minded servants who helped with that calling. We had the privilege of seeing the fruit of our labor every month as we supported ministries all over the world. Donnie and the older boys served the less fortunate out of the country several times. Donnie taught the boys how to weld, which they used several times to improve living conditions at an orphanage. The boys felt led to return to Mexico to finish the welding project when the opportunity arose.

I always stood in awe at how they returned with a new perspective. I envisioned one day going on a mission trip as well. I dreamed about what an African village would look like, what the kids' voices sounded like, and ways I could bond with the children. Already supporting these ministries motivated us to work hard and send resources, but I longed to be more personally connected.

Our family had been packing Operation Christmas Child shoeboxes for nearly a decade. Every year we looked forward to sending boxes to the impoverished and unreached all over the world. I had a soft spot for children in Africa. Whenever I saw photos of them receiving shoeboxes, my heart melted. It felt incredible to be a tiny part of what God was doing on the other side of the globe.

As the church service ended, I cornered Donnie. I poured out my heart like a volcano with all the reasons I should do it. Since we closed the doors of Christian Mission, I no longer had to be there all day, six days a week. Donnie gave me all the reasons it would be difficult. I am the dreamer, and he is the realist.

He said, "We'll need to get a full-time nurse for Seth. Plus, who would care for the other children while I work? How are we going to come up with the money to get you there?" Realizing how determined I was, he finally sighed and said, "If it means that much to you, we'll figure it out."

I bolted out of the sanctuary to find my contact. With heart pounding, I spotted him across a sea of people and made a beeline for him.

I blurted out, "I want to go to Kenya! I want to go so bad I can taste it!"

The chatter in the foyer faded into the background. His response caught me off guard.

"Julie, that's so far for you to be away from Seth."

What? He's declining my help for the mission trip? My heart was crushed on the spot.

He continued in a kind, gentle tone, "I don't think it's wise, Julie. If anything happened to Seth, and you couldn't make it back in time you would never forgive yourself."

The hard reality of his words sucker-punched me. He spoke the truth, and we both knew it. This wise word of counsel came from someone I respected, a long-standing elder of our church and a friend. He prayed with us many times, visited us at Christian Mission and our home. He wept with Seth. He spoke life into Seth. I knew he was right, but I was heartbroken. I didn't understand. My desire was for something good and godly. Why would God plant this desire, yet derail the details from coming to fruition?

A photo of a boy and a story on social media grabbed my attention. I stared at the photo as sadness and empathy overwhelmed me–he looked so sad. I shared the story of this boy named Albert with our family, and we prayed for him. Seth felt his pain and cried out in prayer. We prayed Albert would be able to get help medically and emotionally and that he would find friends who loved him unconditionally.

I started to feel guilty that we had access to some of the best doctors in the world. It made us appreciate God's goodness even more. My mama heart couldn't get the image of Albert out of my head and heart. When I learned he had no parents to care for him, my heart shattered.

As the world followed Albert's story, we saw God move mountains. His story reached a well-known journalist who contacted her friend, the president of an international Christian relief organization. They began to work behind the scenes. People around the world began to contribute financially and pray for all of the details.

Soon, I learned of the most exciting news–Albert was not only coming to the United States, he was coming to the Mayo Clinic in Rochester. My heart leapt! Praise God, he would get the same world-renowned medical care that Seth had been getting. Who but God could have seen this coming? Who but God could have orchestrated the details? From a remote jungle in Africa to Minnesota, God was on the move.

We contacted our prayer warriors and asked them to pray that we would, somehow, get the opportunity to meet Albert. We knew it would be a long shot . . .

What I had earlier perceived as rejection (going to Africa), God redirected to something far greater than I would have asked or even imagined. While in my car running errands, my phone rang. It was William who had become a friend through the charitable projects we had done together at the hospital. After small talk, he got right to the point.

"There is this boy, Albert—"

"Wait! I know Albert. We've been praying for him!" Astounded, I pulled over to the side of the road to listen to every word he said.

"Yes, I thought Seth could be an encouragement to him. Would you be willing to come on Wednesday? I will be there with him at the clinic downtown for his initial testing."

I could barely believe my ears. I looked at my calendar and realized we would already be there. Albert and Seth's appointments were on the same day.

"It would be an honor," I said as I squealed with delight. Prayers answered!

I needed to stuff my excitement and tread lightly. We needed to consider things like this little guy being homesick and in culture shock. I couldn't imagine all that this precious boy had to deal with. I felt sure he must be scared about all of the unknowns. Even though unknowns were commonplace to Seth, he still got anxious about new medical procedures. I thought about the promise I made to Seth early on in his treatment. "You will never have to do this alone. I will be with you every step of the way." I recalled what a great comfort that was to him. We were called to do this for Albert–to be there for him.

January 18, 2017

Unlike our usual trips, the five-hour drive to Mayo Clinic was filled with excitement, hope, and anticipation. Seth asked many questions about Albert. We didn't know much. We just wanted to show him unconditional love. We stopped at a store to pick up a few gifts for Albert. They "happened" (God wink) to be having a huge sale. Ninety percent off of certain gift items. The only items left were Star Wars-themed. I personally didn't know much about Star Wars, but I am all about a good deal. I grabbed all the Star Wars things left: a blanket, robe, action figure, etcetera, and smiled that the only action figure they had left was African-American.

We arrived at the radiology waiting area while Albert was still in testing. We met with William, who was escorting the group on Albert's behalf. We were so honored and excited to be there at that moment. At the same time, Jeff and his wife, Dr. Allison, came to see Seth. William was also a friend of theirs, so we all chatted before Jeff, and Dr. Allison had to leave for a flight across the ocean for medical mission work. I hugged them extra closely in our goodbyes. I prayed God would keep them safe. My heart overflowed with a growing adoration for friends who sacrificed their own comforts to serve others in Jesus' name. I wanted to live like that.

William introduced me to Kim who volunteered as Albert's host mom. Kim and her husband, Frank, were members of the host church, Autumn Ridge. We got better acquainted while waiting for Albert to come out of his procedure. It was good to be together, but I was obviously distracted. Unable to contain my excitement about meeting the boy for whom we prayed, they cautioned me not to have high expectations. Albert wasn't making eye contact with anyone, and he would probably be exhausted after extensive testing. I understood and prepared my heart for whatever time God allowed. To see him, smile, and introduce him to Seth, so he knew he wasn't alone, would be enough.

After two hours, Albert finally came out to the waiting area. I knew he was only at the start of what would be a long road ahead. I met a man, whom I assumed to be his interpreter, wearing a dark-colored plaid beret and a bright smile. When I first laid eyes on Albert, I tried to stifle my excitement. The darling boy standing in front of me was our answer to prayer in the flesh. As Seth and Albert stood beside each other, my heart overflowed with gratitude. Not a doubt lingered that we were meant to cross paths.

I felt the weight of people's stares in the waiting room. Albert's head hung low. It took me back to Seth's initial battle struggling with what others thought. The stares and whispers, people moving away like he was contagious. He was self-conscious about the look of his diseased legs and leg braces. Many commented that Seth handled the weight of it well, but it was still heavy.

One day, Seth came home from school after being mocked, laughed at, and called *robot legs* by some classmates. Those words cut as he told me he "felt like a freak."

"Mom, why would God allow this to happen to my legs?"

I said, "It must be tough, hurtful, and frustrating to have others stare and make fun of you. I'm sorry this has happened to you. You know how awful it made you feel?" Tears welled up in Seth's eyes as he nodded. "Maybe the lesson is never to treat people that way and be there for others that need a friend."

Seth paused, deep in thought. "Yeah!"

Looking back, this marked a shift in Seth's thinking. The heartache he experienced when bullied became a springboard to empathize and encourage others. As a result, Seth became hypersensitive to those who needed extra support at school, at the hospital, and in his community.

Seth now had an opportunity to befriend Albert. What a match made in heaven. Roughly the same age, both boys had endured more suffering in their young lives than most could fathom. Yet, regardless of countless differences, they found they were more alike than different, and suffering had brought them together.

As Albert stared at the floor, I instinctively sat at his feet. I hoped my presence would take some fear and anxiety away. I prayed for the right words. I spoke a few words, then paused to let the interpreter translate. Silence. I spoke again and waited—I was a little distracted, wondering why the interpreter, who was sitting right there, wasn't interpreting what I was saying to Albert. I was puzzled.

I continued praying, asking for something, anything, even one word that would make a difference and be an encouragement. I wasn't sure if he understood as he continued to stare at his lap. I decided to break the ice and grabbed the gifts we had brought. Our younger boys had sent along matchbox cars they had gotten for Christmas. They wanted to connect with Albert, too. We bought a small dry-erase board. To show him how it worked, I wrote the names "Seth" and "Albert" on it.

I was thrilled to see him smile. I learned that he *loved* Star Wars! Of all American movies, this was one he knew and enjoyed at his host home. Chalk one up for another confirmation that God planned the details. Albert immediately picked up the action figure.

He looked me in the eye and said, "Thank You!"

My heart overflowed. I thought, *Wow, that was excellent English. He must have practiced conversational sayings before he came.*

Later, William graciously pulled me aside to explain that they speak English in Liberia. I had no idea. He smiled and continued, "Albert has a temporary guardian escorting him, not an interpreter." I felt foolish for not knowing this, but he made me feel better. This was only the beginning of what I would learn about the beautiful people of Liberia.

I shared things about Seth, hoping it might spark a connection. When I told him he loved to play the drums, Albert didn't know what they were. I showed him a video, and his face lit up. Seth said he would bring his drumset the next time we came, and they could play together. A smile appeared as he nodded. Things seemed to be turning around.

We were already planning our next get-together with drums when we had to get going to Seth's appointments. Without warning, Albert put out his bandaged arm and leaned in for a hug. I pulled him close and melted. I don't know what that hug meant to him, but it meant the world to me.

Our visits were encouraged by Albert's presence and friendship. Someone asked me for suggestions to connect with others despite barriers. As a mom of seven, six of them boys, video games came to mind. Albert caught on quickly, and before we knew it, he was squealing, high-fiving, and celebrating victories, and we witnessed the power of community.

As Seth and I traveled back and forth, we sometimes brought Seth's younger siblings as extra playmates for Albert. He thought it was neat that Seth had a big family. This would not have been possible without Albert's host parents, Frank and Kim, opening their home to us. They generously offered our entire clan an open invitation to come and stay in their home with Albert anytime we wanted. We accepted without hesitation. We commuted almost every weekend, plus days Seth had appointments. It showcased another beautiful example of God's purpose and plan through Seth's journey.

It didn't surprise me to learn that Seth's beloved doctor, Doctor Phil Fischer, was a huge part of pulling all of this together. He and his wife hosted Albert in their home for a while and helped him through some complications. We saw in them such selfless, caring, compassionate individuals. They opened their home countless times over the years to people they'd never met. They inspired our family in countless ways.

About eight of us sat in the waiting room during Albert's surgery. Someone from the church brought a wonderful spread of food to pass the time. After about twelve hours, the surgeon came to give a report. This unbelievably gifted, world-renowned surgeon was the same one who performed surgery on Seth's head in 2011.

This humble doctor spoke words of encouragement to *us*. He said it was a beautiful thing to care so deeply for someone you've just met, which was exactly what he just spent the last twelve hours doing in surgery. I knew Albert was in the very best hands.

Over the next four months, we witnessed Rochester's incredible hospitality of faith, hope, love, and service to its patients. We continued driving back and forth with some of our children to make memories, pray together, laugh till our stomachs hurt, and become family in Christ.

We brought Seth's drum set and watched Albert enjoy playing. We dyed Easter eggs, rode bikes through the neighborhood, ate new foods, and so much more. Kim and Frank threw a huge celebration for Albert's sixteenth birthday (now Seth and Albert were both sixteen years old). Their large home overflowed with laughter, hugs, memories and so much love.

Just as Seth had experienced, a community of (once) strangers rallied to love and serve unconditionally. In hindsight, I saw God shut the door for me to travel to Africa because God had something better. God didn't reject my plan, he simply re-directed it. He brought the mission trip to us. Seth wasn't the reason I couldn't be a part of missions, he was the reason for it! I didn't have to raise funds to go out of the country. I didn't have to leave my other children or find a nurse to care for Seth. God understood the situation better than I did. God not only gave me the desire of my heart to love on these beautiful Africans, but many of our family members got to have a direct part also. Seth was able to continue his medical care. Albert and Seth were able to hang out at the clinic at the same time together. It was a win-

win all around without even a language barrier. Also, we weren't limited to the ten-day, short-term mission trip. Instead, we had sweet fellowship with one another for nearly five months! During this time, Albert was able to build many special friendships and lifetime memories.

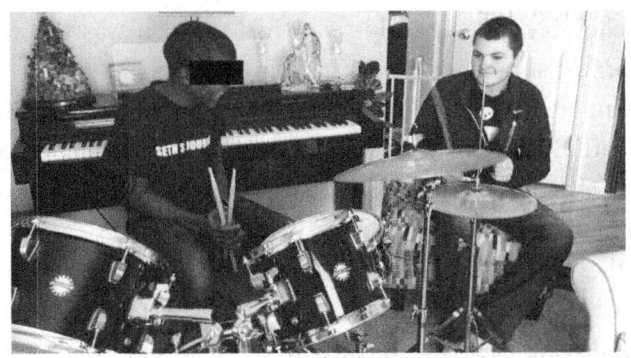

Albert shrieks with delight as Seth shows him how to play drums for the first time.

Couldn't have orchestrated the details if I tried. Only God could write this. These two boys from vastly different places on the globe were so similar. Not only were they close in age but in countless other ways. Academically, they were both years behind, but between the two of them, they felt no judgment, and it brought them closer. Once outcasts, God formed a friendship that changed and grew their lives forever. Emotionally and socially, I watched two boys connect over LEGO video games, food, and drums. Their shortcomings weren't on display. They finished each other's sentences. They were just two guys having a great time together.

For me, I realized, with God anything was possible. I loved learning about Albert's culture, his likes and dislikes, and I enjoyed his sweet giggle. I realized the enormous obstacles both Albert and Seth had overcome without bitterness. It was an attitude check for me.

The day arrived to say our final goodbyes. A caravan of vehicles drove to the airport for a send-off. The mood was solemn and heart-wrenching. At the airport, Albert remained quiet. He took off one of the cross necklaces from around his neck and gave it to Seth.

Seth was quite moved and said, "You are my best friend. I will never forget you!"

Until then, I didn't know if Albert even had a best friend. It was an emotional moment for us all. I snapped a photo of the two of them, although I already had an imprint in my mind that would last far longer.

The thought of Albert leaving was painful, yet we attempted to be happy for his homegoing. We fought back tears as our dear friends who loved Albert gathered with us around him. Jeff and our friend Pastor Woody led a group of us in prayer huddled in the middle of the terminal. Hearts and lives had connected. And then, he was gone.

Two days later, our friend Justin, the Samaritan's Purse videographer, sent me a video clip he knew Seth would love. It showed Albert on the ground in his remote African village after the helicopter landed.

"Hi buddy! Hi! . . . . Seth, I hope we'll see you again. Bye!"

I bawled like a baby. Knowing we will see him again one day in Heaven was worth giving away a piece of my heart. God showed me tangible evidence of how He could use our suffering in this life for eternal good. Forever intertwined. I knew, for I had seen and lived it first-hand, we were better together.

CHAPTER SEVENTEEN
THE PILLS ARE GONE!

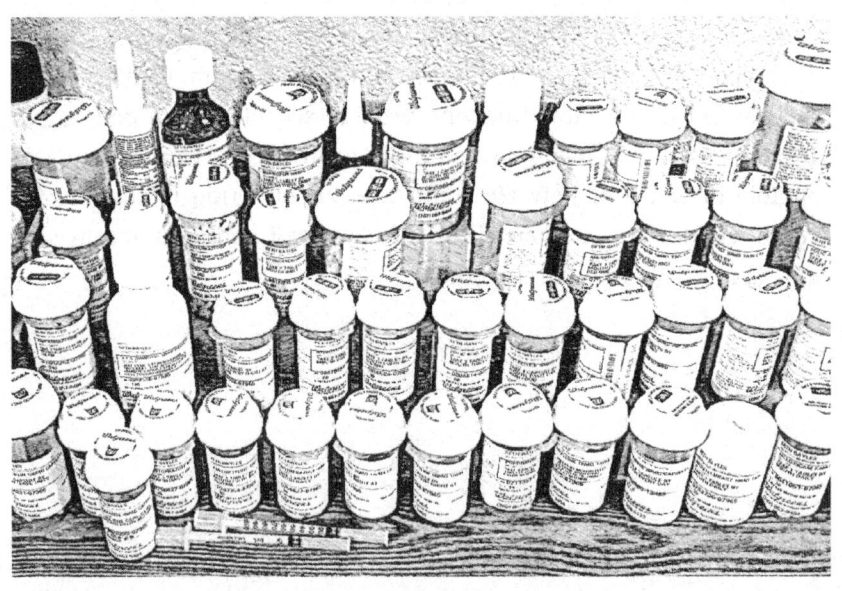

We don't meet people by accident. They are
meant to cross our path for a reason.
–Author Unknown

July 2017

Everyone who knows Seth, knows what a *huge* Pittsburgh Steelers fan he is. I used to be concerned about how much emphasis he put on following this football team until I saw it from a different angle. I was grateful for the distraction from the hardships he faced on a daily basis. When he watched football, he enjoyed the thrill of connecting with people on a different level. Seth shared his love of football with everyone he met.

Only God knew, over the years, how many countless individuals would come together to give Seth the opportunity and the thrill of cheering for the black and yellow in person. On our next trip to Rochester, we were invited to Fagan Studios for an event filled with surprises. A private concert awaited with Seth's favorite local band, Light 45. Seth met the drummer, Critter, who asked him to sit in and play. What a huge honor for Seth to play percussion as Justin sang "I'll Fly Away" for a packed house.

Our director friend Laura, shared Seth's journey with her friend Elaine. Elaine wanted to do something special for Seth and invited others to join her. Unbeknownst to us, the people in that room, and from all over the US, collaborated to bless Seth. That night Elaine presented Seth with two tickets to see the black and gold in Pittsburgh! The crowd cheered as he was, once again, speechless. The airline tickets, also included with the gift, were presented in a gift bag covered in black and gold stickers with the names of those who donated to make this happen, including the states they were from: Pennsylvania, Minnesota, New York, Alabama, North Carolina, and Wisconsin. Love in a gift bag. The date of the game tickets fell in August during the week of Seth's seventeenth birthday. He and his dad would soon be off to Pittsburgh for Seth's first-ever plane ride.

I was so excited for them yet anxious about making sure all of his medical equipment and abundance of medications arrived intact. Few realize the full weight of traveling with a medically complex child. I decided the safest way to pack over two hundred pills he takes weekly was to put the seven-day pill container in the large outside pocket of

Seth's CPAP machine. Donnie would take it as his carry-on bag to be kept with him at all times.

I knew Donnie was capable of caring for his son, but mentally planning for all the "what if" scenarios was a full-time job. It had become second nature to me in our travels, yet I never got used to it. Nor could I prepare for what was about to unfold.

Donnie and Seth made their way to the O'Hare airport security checkpoint. Security made Donnie open Seth's CPAP machine case and take the motor out to place it separately on the x-ray belt. He then asked Donnie to take off his belt and empty his pockets; everyone knows the routine. Seth was wanded, then asked to step out of his wheelchair. Donnie helped Seth up and explained Seth's tube feeding machine. They also checked the chair. By this time, they had to rush to make their connection. When they arrived at the gate, Donnie realized the pill container was not in the CPAP bag.

Donnie called just as their flight was about to take off.

When I answered the phone, I heard his frantic voice. "The pills are gone!"

"Yeah, right." I thought he was joking.

"I'm serious. The last I had them was at the security checkpoint. The doors are closing. I have to go. Can you call security and figure it out? Thanks. Love you, bye."

I felt gut-punched. The very thing I feared had, in fact, become a reality. Seth was without his life-saving pills. My mind raced as I tried to figure out where to start. The most logical conclusion was the pill container had been taken out at security and not put back in the bag. I just happened to be talking with Laura and Elaine at the time and asked them to pray. Not much is scarier than Seth not having his medications. Laura offered to contact the corporate office.

I called airport security and waited through transfer after transfer. Valuable time was being lost. My brain was multitasking to the max. I thought maybe I should just get in the car and drive back to Chicago. If the pills were there, I would have to get them anyway. But even if I got them in my possession, and even if I made it to the post office before closing and overnighted them to the hotel, Seth wouldn't have his evening pills. Those included five (of his ten daily) anti-seizure pills that he *had* to have that evening along with the other major meds. So many unanswered questions. Since I couldn't communicate with Donnie while he was in flight, I didn't know where to start to try and remedy the situation. I felt helpless at home.

I spent the next four hours on the phone. I spoke with countless people from the airport, from security level one to head security and video monitoring. I asked if they would pull the tape to see what could have happened.

I called our local pharmacist and explained. I had just seen her the night before getting his prescriptions filled and telling her about the big weekend trip. She said she wouldn't waste time going to the airport because the pills were probably long gone. She heard of meds being picked up or confiscated because they weren't in the original prescription bottles. She was gracious but explained the insurance couldn't be run because it was too soon to order a refill, and we needed an abundance of pills. She said I could file a report with the airport, but it would take days and wouldn't help now. She suggested I call the Pittsburgh pharmacy, inform them of the life-threatening complications, and ask for an emergency supply.

He needed like forty anti-seizure pills to get him through the four-day weekend. This is not the normal quantity dispensed for most emergencies. One of the meds wasn't carried in stock. It was becoming more and more complicated and heart-wrenching. I had pills at home I could ship to the hotel, but overnight shipping could cost up to fifty dollars. He wouldn't have his night pills in time, and there was a chance *that package* might not make it there either. Then, we'd be back to square one.

The corporate director of the nationwide pharmacy called me. A calm voice assured me that help was on the way. She even gave me her private cell number to work more efficiently as the plan of action unfolded. In the meantime, their Pittsburgh pharmacies had already been contacted regarding an emergency supply of all of his pills. She told me I didn't have to do anything and was not to worry about the cost. I was ill with relief and on the verge of tears of gratitude.

Meanwhile, back at the airport, the director of security reviewed the footage of Donnie and Seth going through security. He didn't see a pill container. Donnie was racking his brain. What could have happened? He just didn't understand how the pill container disappeared into thin air. I told him as we spoke, others were working behind the scenes to help. We praised God for His provision and for favor with people that didn't have to go out of their way to remedy this, but did.

No matter how well-intentioned a planned getaway is, complex medical conditions and medications don't take a day off. Nagging hardships, complications, and limitations are reminders, but so are things like kindness, hope, and unity. Donnie rented a car and drove to two Pittsburgh pharmacies that had scrambled to get Seth's replacement pills. When Donnie and Seth finally received the envelope of pills at the pharmacy, they saw a highlighted, handwritten message, "Welcome to Pittsburgh!" Donnie and Seth were one step closer to game time and enjoying much-needed father-son time. But there was another piece to the story.

Donnie received a message from the airport. A gentleman from Ohio found thousands of dollars of pills in his CPAP machine bag. He called the airport with this concern, and the airport knew immediately to whom those pills belonged. The man must have been going through security at the same time with the same CPAP machine. It finally all made sense, mystery solved-phew!

The airport shared contact info connecting Donnie and the gentleman. Realizing neither could use the other's CPAP machine or masks, they needed to meet up as soon as possible to exchange bags. Since Donnie had already rented a car, he and Seth took off from Pittsburgh, Pennsylvania to Ohio.

Donnie never had one negative thing to say about this mix-up. He said, "Everything happens for a reason. We don't always know what that reason is, but God is always in control!" Donnie's response to things often helped me put life's curveballs in perspective.

I've always known Donnie to be a people person. He talked for quite a while with this gentleman and found out they had a lot in common. Donnie found out he was flying back from Wisconsin after attending a Make-A-Wish™ Wisconsin golf outing fundraiser. Donnie was excited to share that Seth was a "Wish Kid" via Make-A-Wish™ Wisconsin. All agreed it was a blessing that the challenging circumstances led their paths to cross.

We learned a lot through this experience, especially me. This mama bear was trying so hard to figure out what happened, who was responsible, and how the problem would get resolved. I often viewed things gone wrong as frustrating injustices and inconveniences. Instead, I felt convicted to put my focus on the blessings, the people God placed in our paths, and the opportunities to extend grace and love. Sigh. I was a work in progress.

Fall 2017

Seth's regular abdominal pain increased after he returned from Pittsburgh. Some days it was almost unbearable. He was reluctant to eat because he knew it would cause pain or vomiting. We went to the gastroenterologist countless times. Seth was growing weak and weary. We had tried everything: elimination diets, natural methods, and homeopathic means.

A team of multiple doctors at Mayo Clinic planned a surgical procedure to get answers. The doctors instructed Seth to follow a strict clear liquid diet in preparation for surgery. We settled into a hotel near the clinic for his two days of a digestive cleanse. Seth's abdominal pain increased with no results.

The day before his surgery, I looked over to see Seth with his knees up to his chest in pain. Silently, he soaked the sheets with his tears. Going to the ER had always been a last resort, but it being after hours, we were out of options. When I tried to help Seth get up, he cried out in pain. He started to vomit profusely out of his nose and mouth. I grabbed an ice bucket and pushed him in his wheelchair to the parking garage.

The gal behind the front desk in the ER asked why we were there. I tried to explain, but she interrupted.

"--So, he probably ate something wrong."

I told her he hadn't eaten in several days per doctor's orders. She told us to have a seat. The triage experience with a physician's assistant gave us more of the same remarks.

"He probably has some sort of a stomach bug."

"Can you page Dr. Fornago? She'll be performing surgery on my son tomorrow."

"We don't routinely page doctors after hours unless it's an emergency."

I insisted, with more emotion and passion than all of the encounters combined, that they *look* into my son's abdomen. Seth had been strong, but we needed answers. Reluctantly, they agreed to do imaging and wheeled him to radiology.

The weight of it all consumed me. I sat alone in the room and sobbed in frustration. I prayed and pleaded with God to reveal what was wrong. Exhausted and overwhelmed, I could only imagine what Seth was going through. We didn't feel heard and felt no one but God understood. I began to question everything. What if we can never get to the bottom of this? How can he live like this?

A new doctor entered the room with the results. "Your son has complete bowel obstruction, possible ileus, needs NG decompression, and possibly emergency surgery. We are consulting with a pediatric surgeon right now and keeping Dr. Fornago informed."

"What's NG decompression?" I was trying to process what was happening while trying to understand the medical terminology.

"We insert a tube through the nose and into the stomach and attach it to a mechanism to pull out the contents of his stomach. Right now, there's nowhere for the contents of his stomach to go. The scans reveal your son's colon is severely dilated. We need you to step back, please."

The nurses scurried to gather supplies, ripping packaging open and connecting tubes into devices on the wall.

They have to pump his stomach? Without any pain meds administered, the nurse inserted and quickly fed a hose through Seth's nose without warning. It was hard for me to watch as the team fed more and more tubing while they shouted, "Swallow, swallow, swallow!" Seth coughed and gagged before it finally reached his stomach.

Seth was admitted and stabilized in preparation for exploratory surgery with an endoscopy and colonoscopy that had been planned for the next day. The surgeon covering for Dr. Fornago talked with me after the procedures.

"I had trouble navigating the scope due to redundant colon (extra loops). I found *recognizable food* in his stomach as well as air and liquid lodged in his intestines. Quite honestly, I've never seen anything like it before."

He was shocked when I told him Seth hadn't eaten solid food days before this procedure.

"I am sending you to our Nuclear Medicine Department to test for delayed gastric emptying."

The results revealed what the doctor had suspected, Seth had gastroparesis. They told Seth to avoid eating even more foods like popcorn, corn, grain, nuts, seeds, anything with peels, raw fruits, or veggies, etc. Seth had already suffered from malabsorption (even supplements weren't getting absorbed), was anemic, and now he wasn't supposed to eat these good, fiber-rich foods.

I was growing more frustrated. *What was happening? Why now? How can anyone deal with this long-term?* I asked a ton of questions and asked to meet with a dietician. We avoided what we thought were trigger foods. We tried a gluten-free diet even though biopsies and blood work confirmed he did *not* have Celiac Disease. Seth grew hesitant about eating because he knew the painful after-effects. One day Seth said at a time of weakness, "I can't take it anymore."

Dr. Fornago, one of the best gastroenterologists in the country, told us we needed to "reset" Seth's digestive system. This was a last-ditch effort. Complete stomach rest for the next six weeks, at the very least, then we would reassess. Seth would be 100 percent tube-fed with formula–no exceptions. Dr. Fornago had a straightforward conversation with her seventeen-year-old patient.

"I'm not going to sugarcoat it, Seth. This will be very difficult to get used to. Everyone around you is going to be eating. You are going to physically feel hungry, but you need to convince yourself you are okay. Your body is getting everything it needs just in a different way. You are one of the strongest, most positive patients I know. You can do this!"

JANUARY 2018, A NEW WAY OF LIFE

A nasogastric feeding tube was placed down his nose and throat into his stomach. It was like the one he had in the ER but much thinner and it would be left in. It wasn't traumatic this time, and Seth was hopeful things would improve. Just as the doctor warned, however, it was a big adjustment. Overnight, the entire family felt guilty for eating solid foods.

The week after Seth's tube was placed was his younger brothers' birthdays. Gabe and Luke agreed it would be too difficult for Seth to have a birthday cake as part of their celebration. They graciously chose to forgo that tradition this year. Once again, I was touched to witness the selfless, sacrificial attitude of Seth's siblings.

Seth soon started to feel like himself again. His color returned. Seth's labs came back showing he was no longer anemic. No infusions to schedule! We didn't realize how much the limitations of his diet, due to horrific stomach issues, affected his overall health. The formula he was able to digest was a God-send. I personally couldn't imagine not being able to eat, but by God's grace, Seth, again, persevered and conquered.

The biggest worry for him was how being attached to a continuous feed formula pump would limit his day-to-day activities. Thankfully, he was pleasantly surprised. Few realized the subtle backpack he wore to school held his lifeline. For the most part, he made the most of it, staying active and enjoying life. Sometimes, he even forgot about it. He still had some days of nausea and stomach pain, but when we turned down the administered rate of the feed to dispense more slowly over hours, things went much better.

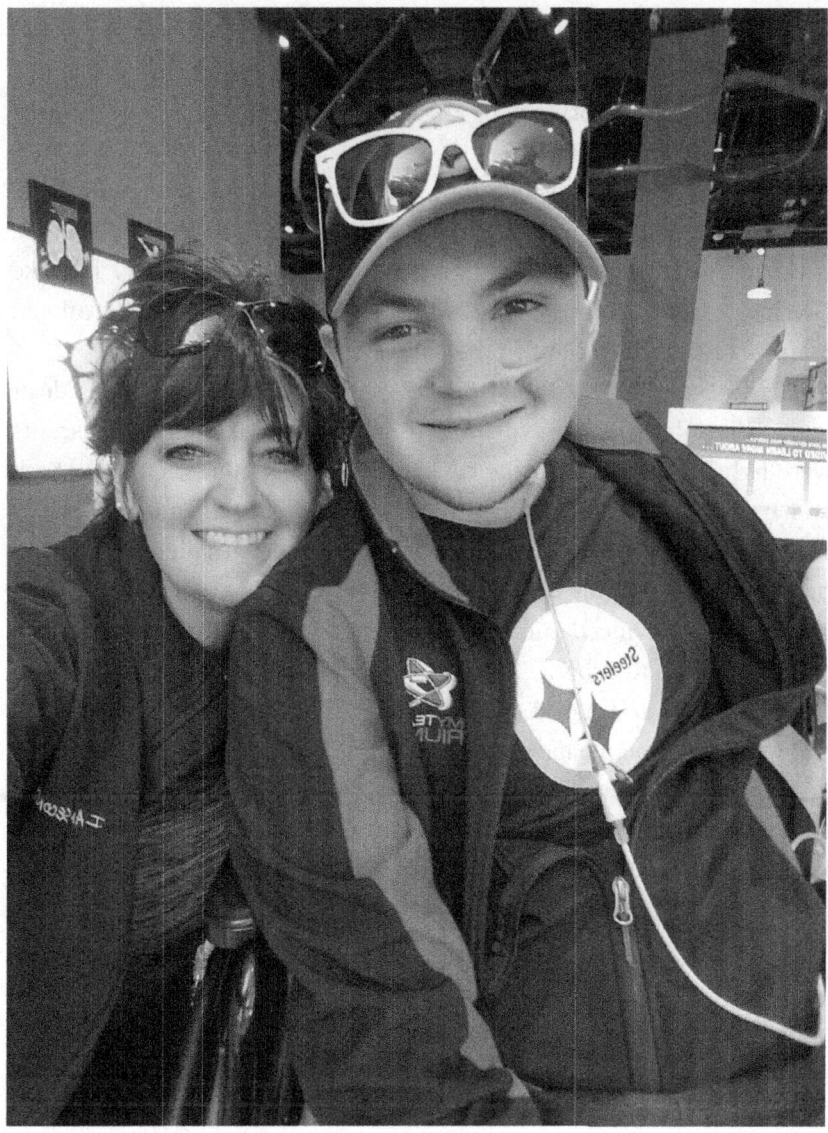

Seth never let things stop him. He was happy in school every day he wasn't at the hospital. However, it was challenging for him to be in the cafeteria watching everyone eat. The smells really got to him. One day, he went into the hallway to get away from it all. Seth found himself in the midst of the students walking by and loved it. He talked to everyone who passed. He developed quite a warm relationship with the janitor who told me Seth was one of the few who engaged her in conversation. He decided this was where he would spend his lunch period. He looked forward to the high fives, bro hugs, and mutual shouts of encouragement.

Everyone seemed to love him. Others told me his joy, kindness, and intentionally taking the time to engage with others was rare. He truly appreciated people and life. Both were a gift to him. I felt like God placed him in a unique position to understand and help others. Seth was a beacon of light in the hallway.

Seth began to hear the struggles his high school classmates dealt with. When he tried to explain it to me, I realized many adolescents were fighting enemies in silence, battles in their minds. One day Seth and I ran into one of his classmates. He shared with me the impact Seth had on him. He explained his struggles with depression and health challenges that no one could figure out. Contemplating taking his life, he convinced himself that no one would even notice if he didn't show up to school. That very day, Seth came up to him, greeted him by name, and asked how he was doing. At that moment, Seth showed him someone *did* care and *would* notice.

A popular saying circulating at the time said, "In a world where you can be anything, *be kind*." I had just witnessed how a simple act of kindness changed–and even saved–a young person's life.

Seth needed orthopedic surgery. It included the breaking of a bone, resetting, and the placement of screws. Arthritis was wreaking havoc and causing this shift along with relentless pain. Seth's rheumatologist told us he was "maxed out" on the amount of corticosteroid injections one could have. After an evaluation, the orthopedic surgeon recommended surgery as the most optimal long-term solution, but he was hesitant. As always, the immunosuppressive drugs Seth was on meant surgery would not be without difficulties, risks, and a longer healing time than most. Seth always opted for the best chance to remain mobile.

On the day of the surgery, Seth was hopeful but nervous. Wanda, the certified nurse practitioner, noticed his anxiety. She already knew Seth from years before, and she was aware of his feelings that morning. She asked him about the activities that were important to him, so they could help him get back to life at its fullest. She found out he couldn't play football but loved the game, especially watching the Pittsburgh Steelers. I loved watching them interact and thanked God for her.

Soon, they wheeled Seth down the hallway to the OR as they had countless times before. My spirit felt heavy that morning for all the challenges Seth dealt with, especially over the last few months. Major life changes, unable to eat solid food, a tube taped to his face 24/7, emergency room visits, as well as surgeries from head to toe.

THE POWER OF MUSIC

In March 2018, I found myself in a familiar place again–alone in the surgical waiting room. Wall monitors displayed patient numbers and statuses. I spent some time in prayer. As I grabbed a cup of coffee, I tried to shut out the sights and sounds of the busy clinic. I received a notification on social media that someone shared a video with me. It was titled "Mayo Clinic Doctors Sing." When I clicked on it, my heart skipped a beat.

Two men, dressed in scrubs and still wearing their surgical hats, sat at a baby grand piano in the foyer of one of the buildings. One played the piano; the other was singing his heart out. The voice that poured out of the singing doctor's lungs was unlike anything I had heard before. Soothing rhythms filled my soul with peace as if he was singing directly to me. Tears filled my eyes as the doctor sang words I needed to hear. "It'll be alright . . . " God's peace poured over me through these two doctors. My heart overflowed with gratitude for all of the people God worked through to bring comfort to me and my family.

It may have been a simple song to some, but to me, it placed a soothing balm on my wounded, weary heart. I found out they were orthopedic surgery residents. Upon looking closer, I realized they were playing the piano at the Saint Marys Campus in the building where Seth was having surgery at that very moment. Who knows, maybe they had learned of Seth's rare case as residents. God had, again, used the staff of Mayo Clinic as vessels to encourage us. And the day wasn't over yet . . .

"CAST" AND CREW

A post-op nurse emerged and called my name. I grabbed my things and rushed to meet her as she took me back to the recovery room. When I entered, Seth was resting peacefully under several warm blankets. The nurse checked his vitals and initiated small talk.

"Steelers fan, huh?" I was a little puzzled as Seth was not wearing his usual Steelers hat.

I asked with a smile, "How did you know?"

"Well, the cast kind of gave it away!"

Curiosity got the best of me. I pulled back the blanket covering his leg. I was shocked and delighted. I could never have anticipated what I saw–a cast all decked out in true Steelers style! What doctor team would do such an incredibly thoughtful thing? Someone crafted cutouts and decoupaged a coating. I stifled tears. I couldn't wait for Seth to wake up out of anesthesia to this most wonderful surprise. God supplies all of our needs–and throws in some wants–just because He can.

Wanda came in to check on Seth who was still fast asleep. I knew she had to be behind this special work of art. I impulsively reached out to hug her. I thanked her for going above and beyond to make a difficult situation so much more bearable.

She smiled and said, "Knowing it will bring Seth joy makes it all worthwhile." Wanda gave us a gift that day in more ways than one.

The next day we were cleared to go home with strict instructions: "Absolutely no weight to be put on that leg until the surgeon can repeat x-rays in six weeks." They gave Seth a walker to bear the weight. What a sight he was as he hobbled down the hallway. He caught the eye of a guy who looked curious.

"So, what did you do?" I suppose he hoped for an exciting, suspenseful story of action, accident, and injury. Seth looked at me too exhausted to explain.

"He developed, among other conditions, a disease that has killed healthy cells removing the shock absorption layer of subcutaneous fat, therefore, causing trauma and edema of the cortical bone marrow. As a result, his veins and nerves are superficial (at the surface) because they no longer have the fat to protect them." Four minutes more of my verbal diarrhea and this poor guy's face started to flush and drain at the same time as I continued my mystery medical synopsis.

Awkward silence.

I'm sure he was sorry he asked. Then, most unexpectedly, Seth broke the silence.

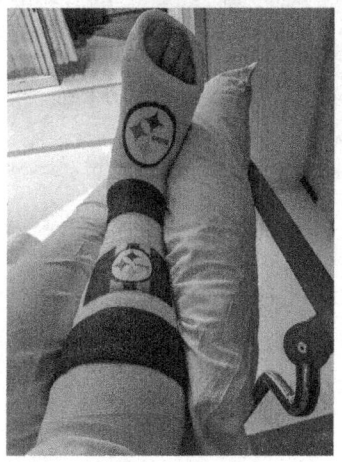

"Cool cast, huh? Steelers . . . Black and Yellow all the way, baby!"

The guy immediately discussed the football season, players, and their team's chances. A beautiful commonality of the human spirit overshadowed the complexity of Seth's conditions. Wanda's casting gift meant so much more than she could have imagined. Not only was it a creative distraction, it became another thread of connection Seth used to build bridges.

BRACE FOR IT

Jill, our wonderful Prosthetist/Orthotist, continued to care for Seth's every need pertaining to his leg braces. She was a joy, from helping Seth pick out the latest designs, to casting his legs every year, to maintenance. For years, we could count on her to take care of the continual adjustments and modifications for Seth's latest flare-ups. She helped Seth feel comfortable, stay active, and live his best life, one set of leg braces at a time.

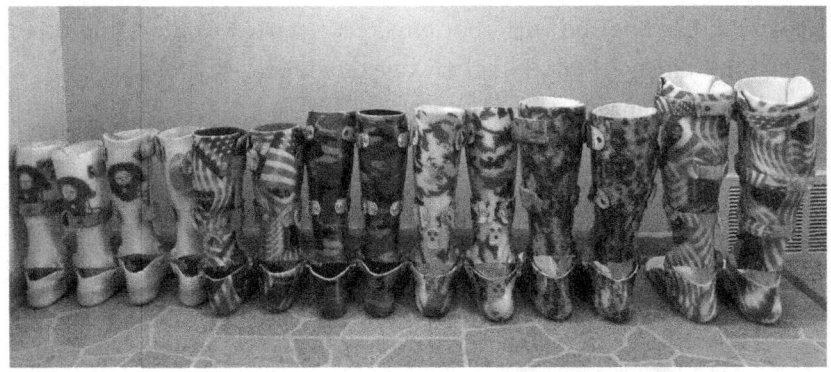

CHAPTER EIGHTEEN
IN THIS TOGETHER

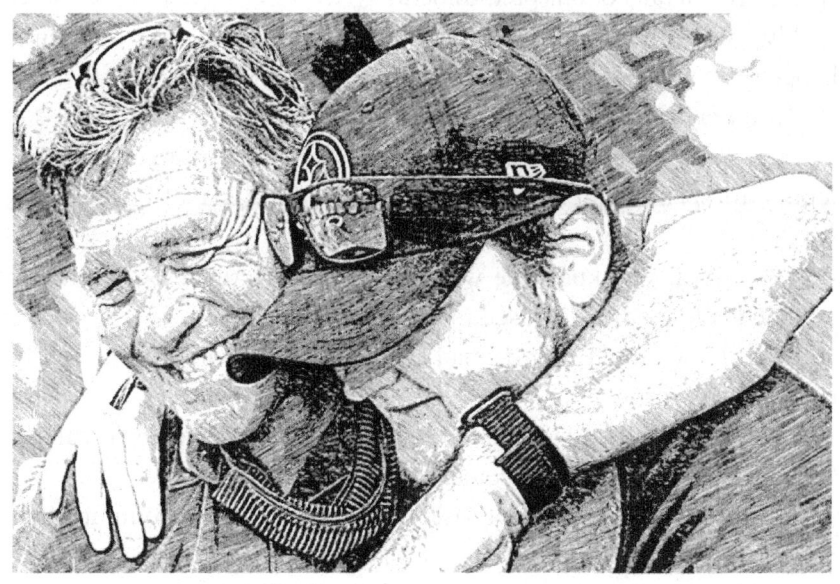

Live simply, love generously, care deeply,
speak kindly, leave the rest to God.
–Ronald Reagan

A WORK IN PROGRESS

A jolt of the steering wheel took me by surprise, followed by a thump, thump, thump. *What in the–?* I went from carefree humming to the radio to the panic of the unknown. I scanned my mirrors . . . nothing. Halfway between southeastern Wisconsin and central Minnesota seemed like the middle of nowhere. *Lord, help us.*

I veered toward an oncoming exit as our vehicle hobbled toward a small service station. The car began to shake. *What am I going to do? Will we be late for our appointment?* My exhaustion enhanced the anxiety and frustration for what was unfolding. The car barely limped to an air pump. The sign read AIR $1.50. Gah–I looked around for loose change in the console. More frustration. I got out to find the tire bulged and hissing. *How could this happen?* I dialed Donnie's number to vent. I spewed the details of our predicament.

My gentle husband gasped and said, "I prayed this wouldn't happen!"

"You prayed this wouldn't happen?"

"I'm sorry, Babe. I've been pricing tires, but we just didn't have the money to spend right now. I prayed they would make it one more trip."

"You mean you knew we were riding on bad tires? So, now I'm stranded! What am I supposed to do?"

Seth chimed in, "Don't be mad at Dad, Mom. It's not his fault. It'll be okay. It'll work out."

I ended the call and attempted to take matters into my own hands. "Stay here. I'm going to get something that might work."

I walked to the automotive aisle of the gas station, determined but clueless. *Twenty-two dollars for one can of Fix-a-Flat? Now I know where the term 'highway robbery' came from!* I headed toward the car to see a man and woman talking with Seth. Worried about strangers talking to my son, I hurried my stride. My mind was put to ease by their genuine concern and desire to help.

The man looked at the can in my hand, then into my eyes, "Go take that back inside and get your money back. That won't help. You need a new tire. Do you have a spare?"

My expression went blank.

"Do you mind if I look in the back of your car?"

I shoved our luggage, medical bags, and boxes of pop tabs to the side. I felt the need to explain where we were headed as I pushed items around, looking for any evidence of an emergency supply kit. I was ashamed to admit that I had never changed a tire. Lo and behold, a hidden trap door revealed a tool and crank to lower the spare tire. Woo-hoo!

The couple promptly went to work as I strode back inside to return my purchase. This stranger got on the ground, got dirty, and didn't stop until the spare was on. His effort to change out the tire was peppered with expletives, but we were so grateful he stopped. I thanked him repeatedly and offered to compensate them, but he refused. I begged him to at least take the refunded twenty-two dollars I held in my hand. He told me to "pay it forward" and modestly brushed off our encounter as being at the right place at the right time. Seth and I believed God sent this couple just for us.

Within the hour, we were back on the road. Since we couldn't drive over fifty miles per hour on the temporary tire, I had more time to think about what had happened. Seth was right. I felt bad about the way I spoke to Donnie. Even so, God didn't forsake us. His abundant grace (undeserved favor) far outweighed my sin.

Donnie had always provided for his family. He was the hardest-working man I knew. He understood the importance of having a dependable car and the challenges of transporting someone with significant medical issues. Donnie worked long hours to make the car payment and did all the maintenance he could. Why had I blasted him with the brunt of my wrath? I was ashamed of myself.

Then, I thought about Seth's response, both past and present. The way he handles adversity could only be from God. Despite fighting a losing battle every single day, he doesn't focus on the bad. He never tries to blame others for the afflictions he faced. He doesn't want anyone's pity, and he has never considered himself a victim. So why should I? *Lord, I am so sick of myself!*

So, I ate humble pie, and with God's help, I determined to try and be better. My rant and repentance humbled me as I turned my focus on the blessings and the lessons. Having a tire blowout while cruising at seventy miles per hour could have caused an accident–or worse. We could have been stranded in the middle of nowhere. Remarkably, I made it to a public place safely. Two people arrived willing to be inconvenienced and worked for no other reason than to be kind to strangers. And, remarkably, we did make it to Rochester on time.

As I recounted the events of the day, I saw the fingerprints of God. I don't claim to know much about guardian angels, but I have had my share of interactions that have been a godsend. I thanked the Lord for His goodness and patience with me as a work in progress.

Seth, Seventeen Years Old

Our dear friend Laura urged for the umpteenth time, "Julie, you and Seth have to meet Lucy! Seth and Lucy have both endured incredible suffering yet have a beautiful light to share with the world through their unwavering faith in Jesus."

Laura's passion for producing stories of faith and hope inspired her to recognize modern-day miracles. The sense of urgency in her voice had me super-intrigued. Laura had shared Seth's journey with Lucy, and Lucy was equally curious about Seth. After months of trying to coordinate our schedules, we finally met within God's perfect timing one beautiful spring day.

Seth and I planned to be in Rochester for the Ronald McDonald House groundbreaking ceremony. At the same time, Lucy drove in from North Dakota for appointments. Laura suggested we meet at the Canadian Honker Restaurant. We'd grown to appreciate this place for its delicious food, family tradition, and love for the community. The restaurant's giant rooftop sign, visible from the hospital windows, encouraged us more than once with its greeting, "Get Well Soon God Bless."

WE LOVE LUCY

As soon as we met Lucy, we knew this meeting was meant to be. Seth and I felt an instant connection with her. We understood one another, finished each other's sentences, and knew struggle and victory. Seth always felt awkward meeting in restaurants because he didn't eat solid food. With his feeding tube taped to his cheek, Lucy acknowledged that her cancer journey had also included a feeding tube. The beautiful way she dressed, complimented by a leopard-print silk scarf, portrayed the gracious way she now accepted life with a tracheostomy. Seth and Lucy talked about similar complex tests and procedures they'd undergone and how God brought them through. Lucy spoke openly about the difficulties in her life but also optimistically about the good she saw through it all.

Her tiny frame, her bronzed Filipino skin, and her youthful energy denied her grandmotherly age. Despite her cancer and extraordinary challenges, we learned later she celebrated her sixtieth birthday by posing as a warrior princess with a sword in hand against a background of the Badlands she had fearlessly climbed. We loved everything about Lucy, and I am only scratching the surface of her kindness, generosity, and the way she gave glory to God. Lucy, in my opinion, was the strongest, most remarkable woman I'd ever met.

It seemed to me that God intentionally crossed our paths for reasons I wouldn't discover until later. Seth saw in Lucy a beautiful example of someone walking a burdensome road while remaining faithful to God. She understood the stares, the ostracizing, and the depth of discouragement that could cloud the gift and purpose of life.

Lucy's enduring strength bolstered our faith. God painted a beautiful picture of friendship in a journey amid suffering. I wanted a word for that great feeling, that utter relief when feeling alone disappears because someone understands. We discovered that Seth, Lucy, and Albert all had multiple reconstructive surgeries on their heads performed by the *same* world-renowned doctor! What we shared went beyond mere friendship–it bound our hearts together. From Wisconsin to North Dakota to Minnesota, deep friendships and prayer partnerships formed that spring day below a giant rooftop sign.

As we left the restaurant, Lucy told Seth she had something for him. We walked with her to her car, and she pulled out a bag of pop tabs and handed it to Seth.

"This is a labor of love and support from my community."

"They know me?"

"Yes! And every week my prayer partners gather to pray for you!"

Seth was so moved. He asked, "Would you both like to come to the Ronald McDonald House groundbreaking ceremony with us? We're on our way there now."

Since both Laura and Lucy belonged to a beautiful part of our journey, it seemed most fitting. We'd just broken bread together, and now, it was time to break ground together.

"Friendship is born at that moment when one person says to another, 'What! You too? I thought I was the only one.'" C.S. Lewis

THE RONALD MCDONALD HOUSE EXPANSION GROUNDBREAKING, MAY 1, 2018

What an honor to be a part of this celebration, along with so many dear friends we made along the way. We knew everyone there: the managers, volunteers, executive officials, all the House staffers. We hugged a plethora of treasured friends developed over years of enjoying the benefits of the Ronald McDonald House. It was impossible to count how many worked tirelessly and gave generously to birth this day. It showcased a grand dream come true. When something is celebrated in Rochester, it's a town celebration. Everyone in the community gathers.

This was huge. Camera crews, tents for the public, and shovels decorated with children's hand prints in red, blue, and yellow lined a sandy area for the initial dig. Visitors received plastic hard hats with the House logo, and easels featured design ideas across the tent front.

All Seth wanted was for other families to be able to experience the warm hospitality that blessed our family. This incredible project exceeded Seth's dreams. The completion would mean a huge win for the patients and families of Mayo Clinic, Rochester, Minnesota.

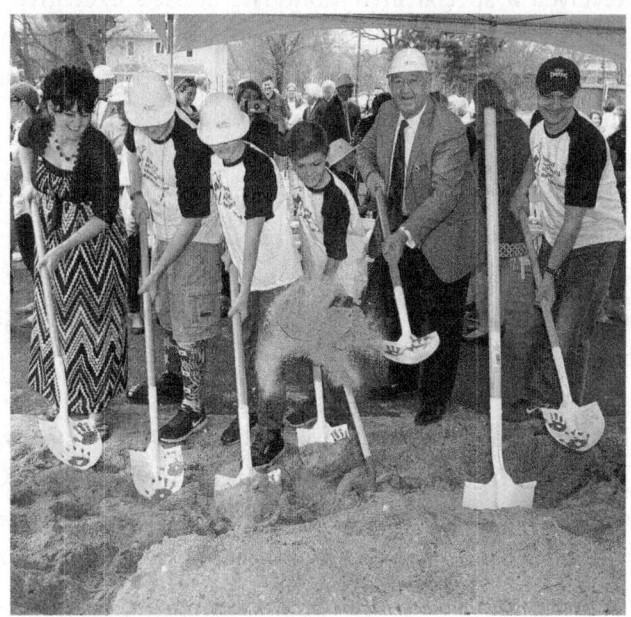

From Left to Right: Julie, Seth, Gabe, Luke, Mayor Brede, and Donnie "break ground"

LOVE TREMENDOUSLY, HOPE EXCEEDINGLY EXPANSION PROJECT

It was so exciting to watch the construction begin on the Ronald McDonald House. House warmer and best friend, Jeff, took us to the tallest accessible point for a bird's-eye view. Seth loved to watch the excavators, bulldozers, backhoes, and skid steers in action. It felt surreal that it was actually happening.

Along with other community members, Seth wrote his name and a special message on the first beam to be hoisted into place. Now, he looked forward with excitement to our trips to Rochester. With each visit, we could hardly believe the progress. So much heart was poured into this project, it motivated everyone in special ways. We would never be able to repay the kindness bestowed upon us through our years at the Ronald McDonald House.

One day, after the concrete was poured and the walls were going up, Seth received a special invitation. The house's executive director asked Seth if he would like a personal tour. Yes, Please! When we got to the site, Seth was shocked when the foreman of the construction company presented him with his own designated hard hat. It read, "Seth Bayles, The Pop Tab Kid, Ronald McDonald House."

I snapped photos throughout the construction and showed them to donors who couldn't write checks fast enough to help support his love for this fantastic place. The long-overdue expansion took the Ronald McDonald House from forty-two rooms to seventy. Twenty-eight additional rooms! The development and completion, from groundbreaking to the ribbon-cutting finish, happened in record time. Seth was thrilled and committed to continue to bless the house with tabs every time we made the trip for his routine medical care. Oh, and remember that Fortune 100 company whose employees supported the Ronald McDonald House in Rochester in honor of Seth? They gave 3.3 *million* dollars!

We look back in awe at how all of this came to fruition. What a heartwarming joint effort as so many came together nationwide. Once again, we experienced the power of community. God most certainly is able to do abundantly beyond what we can even imagine.

LIFE OF A TUBIE, FROM TEMPORARY TO PERMANENT

Although the purpose of the NG feeding tube previously placed was to give Seth's stomach complete rest, over time, his stomach did not regain function as hoped. Days and days were spent consulting with gastroenterologists, nutritionists, and feeding specialists. We tried new machines, feeding techniques, and specialty formulas. Imaging and function screenings, including swallow studies, were done. In the end, the team gave us grim news. We needed to pursue long-term feeding solutions. No one, no parent or doctor, jumps into a surgical solution. Every decision was carefully evaluated for risks versus benefits and included Seth's input. The entire scope of departments involved: specialists, dieticians, surgeons, etcetera, unanimously recommended the surgical placement of a gastrostomy (G-Tube).

I was blindsided by the advanced medical care thrust on me and Seth. This was a serious change of lifestyle to take on. I added gastro (stomach) and stomy (new opening through the abdominal wall) to my growing list of medical terms and hoped and prayed we could manage. I was a mother, not a registered nurse, but I was learning to manage the many hats of a mom.

Seth agreed a permanent feeding tube was his best option, and I was on board with him.

He joked, "If it means I can get this off my face, and I can shave easier, and, of course, everyone can see my handsome face better, let's do it!"

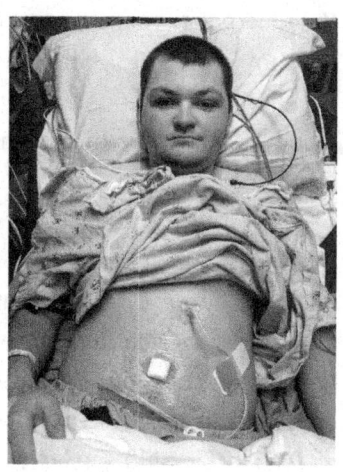

The surgeon visited Seth's room after he placed the G-tube and gave me his report. He found Seth's stomach to be abnormally small. It was up in his chest cavity. The surgeon had to "wrestle" it down to where it should have been, but it kept popping back up. Options for Seth were limited. The placement was not optimal but acceptable. The doctor was concerned about what the future held, so he wanted to keep Seth for several days of observation. How thankful I was that God directed this highly qualified individual as our son's surgeon.

Seth is one tough cookie. He pushed through the pain and embraced his new normal. He was eager to get home and get on with life. Even though he would still be relying on formula as his sole source of nutrition, his G-tube offered perks. It wouldn't clog like the nasal tube, and he really liked the newfound freedom of not having a tube in his nose and down his throat.

However, about three weeks post-surgery, I noticed Seth holding his side on several occasions. He shrugged it off, which is normal for him. One day, he mentioned the pain, but in true Seth style, it didn't seem to limit him. Then, it progressed to him asking me *not* to do his feedings. Since he receives 100 percent of his nutrition by tube, not hooking up his formula was not sustainable.

Each time I flushed his line, he would stiffen and wince in pain. Uh-oh. I called the nurse practitioner who worked with Seth's surgeon. She asked if the tube was functioning properly, and I told her it seemed to be. She made some non-invasive pain management suggestions, such as alternating an ice pack with a heating pad, but she didn't seem too concerned.

The pain intensity increased. And we were off to our local ER–again. Like before, they weren't comfortable with Seth's rare case, and the emergency room personnel weren't tube experts. They diagnosed a "tummy migraine." They discharged him with a couple of prescriptions for medications to coat the stomach and prevent acid. However, when I tried to flush his line, the pain came back with even greater intensity.

Over the next few weeks, I advocated: more calls, patient portal messages, ER visits, and new prescription trials to no avail. I talked with the surgical team but never the surgeon who knew Seth best. I alternated cool compresses with a heating pad. He took baths to try and relieve the pain. They prescribed lidocaine patches and more ulcer medications. All were no match for whatever was going on inside.

When I would push the issue, they always asked the same questions: Does he have a fever? chills? vomiting? No, no, and no. I was thankful for no signs of infection but frustrated that any further investigation was discouraged.

That evening, as I ever so slowly flushed his line, I noticed slight resistance. It wasn't flushing smoothly like a new tube should. I tried pulling back in an effort to free things up. Seth, at this point, put his hand over mine on the syringe.

"Mom, I can't take the pain anymore." When I looked down at the line, there appeared to be blood in it.

I broke the news to Seth that we needed to head to the hospital. He protested and predicted they wouldn't know what was going on, just like the previous trips. This time, I told him we would drive to Children's Hospital of Wisconsin. I was sure they had a bunch of kids with feeding tubes, and it was our best option.

A young woman in a white lab coat entered the small ER room and introduced herself.

"So, what brings you in this evening?"

I explained our dilemma again. This was the fourth emergency visit for this issue in the last couple of weeks. She was sympathetic but voiced what a complex case Seth presented. Transparent about her limitations, she admitted her lack of knowledge of Seth's overall care.

I tried my best to paint a picture of all of the symptoms, treatments, and prescriptions. Seth and I were hoping she could think outside the box and come up with something new. We needed a light-bulb moment. She said she would call around and consult with colleagues.

SAFE IN MY FATHER'S ARMS

When she came back into the room, I already knew by her expression–

"I am so sorry, the only thing I can do is write a couple of prescriptions for different, stronger ulcer medications."

In frustration, I asked, "Why would his pain be a seven or eight when I flush him? Wouldn't an ulcer hurt all the time?"

She nodded yet still lacked a satisfactory answer. I tried to put myself in her position, I really did. But few things are worse as a parent than watching helplessly and being unable to fix your child's relentless pain. My eyes turned away to disguise the tears that welled up while I gathered our belongings.

Seth had been prescribed *six* different ulcer and proton pump inhibitor (PPI) medications. Medicine, in itself, is hard on the gut. The last thing I wanted was more medicine. Seth had not had a full formula feed through his tube for two full nights now. I tried to make sure he was hydrated, but that only went so far. After we got home, I tried to push water into his tube to flush and for hydration. I had trouble even initiating a flush. It seemed stuck. When I tried pulling back the syringe, the tube became filled with a mixture of brownish (old blood) and bright red blood.

Poor Seth dropped in pain like I had never seen. He said his pain level was a 10 (on a scale of 1 to 10). He had never answered a 10 before. I tried not to show the depth of my concern.

I said to Donnie, "*Four* different hospitals and no one can figure this out!"

"I think you need to drive to Mayo. I'll work things out here with the kids."

I impulsively grabbed my phone and dialed Mayo Clinic. I glanced at the clock. It was after 10:00 p.m. I couldn't wait another day for a plan. The after-hours operator answered. I told her I needed to talk with Dr. Fornago in gastroenterology. She didn't ask if it was an emergency–she heard the urgency and said she would page her.

I had never done that before, but I just could not explain this *again* to anyone else. Within minutes, my phone rang. Her familiar voice at the other end of the line was comforting.

"Thank you for calling back. I'm sorry for having them page you so late. I-I just–" my voice quavered. "There is something very wrong with Seth's stomach. He's in a lot of pain every time I flush him. I know feeding tubes aren't your specialty, but his surgical team says it's a GI issue. GI says it's a surgical issue. He hasn't had formula in days. No one can figure it out. Will you please help us?"

"How long will it take you to get here?"

"Five hours."

"Are you able to get in your car and safely drive right now?"

"Yes!" I said without even thinking.

"I will see you first thing in the morning in the ER at Saint Marys."

My eyes locked with Seth's. "We're going to Mayo to get you help."

I expected he'd protest yet another trip, but Seth was beyond exhaustion. Standing near the door, Seth leaned on his cane that he'd wrapped in patriotic duct tape. Donnie put his son's jacket on like he did when Seth was little.

Seth leaned in to his dad's strength, and his body released the weight of the world. His dad held him and cried out to God as he prayed blessings over him.

The visual before me imprinted in my mind and on my heart. Too weak to stand, held by his father's loving arms, Seth found safety, comfort, and support. I saw a beautiful picture, not only of my son and his father but also of our Heavenly Father embracing a weary child. Learning to surrender my doubt, fear, unknowns, and exhaustion to my Heavenly Father seemed to be my daily lesson. I felt, again, God's unconditional love as it surrounded, comforted, and carried us.

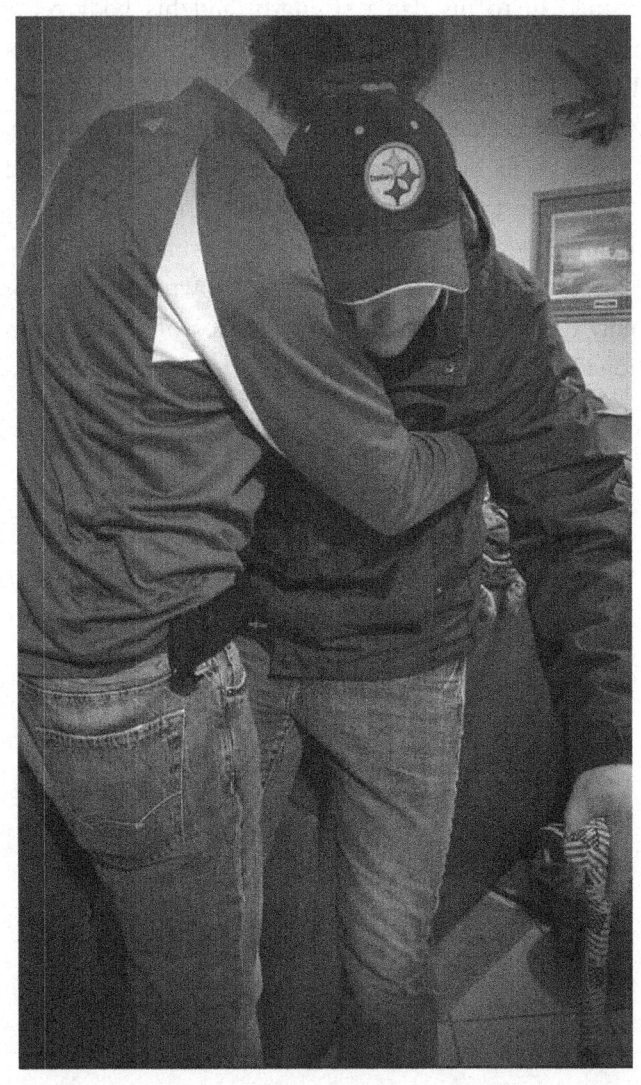

"A good father is one of the most unsung, unpraised, unnoticed, and yet one of the most valuable assets of our society."
–Billy Graham

CHAPTER NINETEEN
DIVINE PROVIDENCE

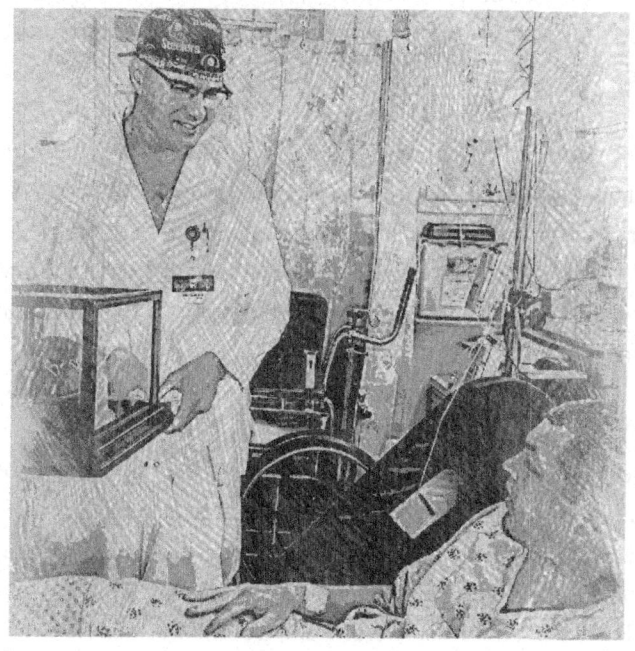

Kindness is a language which the deaf
can hear and the blind can see.
–Mark Twain

August 7, 2018

We arrived at Mayo's Emergency Department well before normal clinic hours. Knowing the attending resident physician didn't know us from Adam, I graciously answered his intake assessment questions. Even though Seth was exhausted mentally and physically, he was kind. By looking at Seth, one would never guess what he had endured in the last few weeks. The doctor attempted to flush Seth's tube as Seth tried to be brave. He gripped the bedrails of the gurney with every attempt.

Seth's pain threshold is higher than anyone I know. The doctor rocked the plunger of the sizable 60ml syringe back and forth. Dark red liquid filled his line.

"Look, that looks like blood!" I said.

The plunger finally freed as Seth clenched his teeth. The doctor considered it an accomplishment.

"Well, the tube is functioning, so you're good to go and continue with feeds as normal."

We were *not* good and nothing about this was normal.

"Seth, show him exactly where it hurts when we flush." He pointed to the spot.

"Every time I flush him, something is wrong." I explained what we had been through. "We have not been to multiple ERs and driven through the night in order to flush the tube and simply go home. Please, call Dr. Fornago."

He didn't want to bother a specialist and told me he had addressed and resolved things.

I kindly said, "You are *not* hearing me. Seth had the tube placed weeks ago, and there were complications. "Please page Dr. Rio. He did his surgery. He may have insight as to what could be happening."

"This doesn't appear to be a surgical or a mechanical issue at this point." He excused himself from the room. Seth looked at me and then closed his eyes. Tears rolled down his face from the weight of it all. Mama Bear stirred inside me. When the doctor returned, he began to set us up for discharge.

With unwavering conviction, I said, "I want an endoscopy done! I don't think we can get to the bottom of this until you are able to go in there with a camera and see what we are dealing with." Long awkward pause.

"I will have to check if, or when, that could be done."

After he left, I plopped down in exhaustion, mentally and physically spent. The second-guessing began to taunt me. *Maybe there isn't anything that can be fixed. Maybe it is just ulcers. Maybe I'm totally wrong. I'm just a mom. I'm just the mom. God, I'm just...so...tired, weary from the fight. Lord, please help!*

Waiting for word of a plan, we both dozed off. Metal clanging woke me. A technician raised the side rails and unlocked the brakes on Seth's bed. She said she was taking Seth to radiology. I was shocked and relieved. She said it would probably take about forty-five minutes. Seth awoke slightly and looked to me for reassurance. I smiled and nodded as I leaned over the rail and kissed his cheek.

I decided to grab a cup of coffee while I could, but within a few minutes, I received a call. They were looking for me–they found it! They found the problem! "Thank you, Lord," I said as I threw my cup in the nearest trash and dashed down the familiar hallway.

A nurse was waiting for me and led me back to the room. I saw Seth's gastroenterologist just as she promised. She apologized for all we'd been through. She explained the tube had pulled entirely out of the stomach and migrated. The bumper had buried itself inside Seth's abdominal wall so far that it was not visible. That's why Seth was in such pain with every flush. The force was burrowing the large, thick plastic retainer disk further into his abdominal wall.

Dr. Fornago looked at me with empathy and conviction. The seriousness of the circumstances couldn't be denied. "We have an emergency here. Seth needs surgery right away. Failure to recognize this has serious complications, including death. I am so sorry."

"But it's good that you found the problem, and you can help him, right?"

"I'm pulling together a team. If there's any good to come from this, we are learning so much from Seth's case. The thing I hope was learned by all today is–*Listen to the mom.*"

"Okay. Could you please page Dr. Rio? No one knows his anatomy better. I trust him explicitly."

"He's on the call list."

In the meantime, they admitted Seth to the Medical Intensive Care Unit. Regrettably, Dr. Rio was unavailable and unreachable. I assumed he was overseas on a mission trip where he often served.

Fear swept over me. *Oh, God, we need him! What are you doing?* My emotions swept in like waves. Then I remembered: *nothing* catches God off guard. He has a plan. Even though my head told me I needed to trust *His* plan, my mama heart was falling apart. We were forced to start from scratch with new doctors who did not know Seth at all.

A nurse entered to review Seth's extensive med list. At the same time, a team of doctors entered the room. With a clear understanding that Seth never did have ulcers, all ulcer medications were discontinued. The head surgeon introduced herself. She was confident, kind, and compassionate. She went over risks, scenarios, and backup plans if things didn't go well. Obviously, the team preferred the least invasive measures.

As I processed all of this, I chose not to be angry or bitter. God had been working on my pride and the way I reacted and responded to others. His Spirit was helping me let things go. Forgiveness and grace, so richly poured out on me, was what I wanted to give. Forgiveness could break down barriers and heal relationships.

The resident from the ER came in after the group left. He looked at Seth sleeping. Our eyes met in silence. I could tell he felt horrible about the way things unfolded downstairs. I broke the ice by talking about the hardship of rare disease. He seemed empathic. I knew he had a long road ahead in medicine. He was bound to see a lot of hard things. I shared our journey of faith and hope and trust in Jesus. He spoke openly about his relationship with God, and I was grateful we had that time. I thought of a C.S. Lewis quotation: "You can't go back and change the beginning, but you can start where you are and change the ending."

AUGUST 8, ROSIE AND DR. STULAK

The wee hours of the morning greeted us. After a rough night, Seth was only now falling asleep. It had been days of only briefly resting my eyes. I felt mentally and physically exhausted. On any given day, I sympathized with medical providers and parents of those with chronic illnesses over this common denominator. A fellow medical mom once joked, "When do I sleep? I close my eyes when I sneeze." I could relate.

I knew I needed to get up and get ready for the day. The surgical team would soon be making rounds, and I needed to be on my game– or at least look like I had my act together. Thankful for a change of clothes in the emergency bag, I dug around hoping to find some make-up or powder to try and conceal the puffy bags under my eyes. Then, I heard a soft knock.

A MAN CAVE MOMENT

The door cracked open and a male voice asked if it was okay to enter. A red-headed man in scrubs with a buzz cut and a five o'clock shadow emerged. He introduced himself in a quiet voice.

"I'm Seth's new nurse. My name is Patrick, but I'm known by everyone as Rosie (because of his red hair). Do you think Seth will mind a male nurse?"

I thought it was considerate of him to ask. I smiled and said, "Actually, I think he would appreciate it. He loves to talk about sports."

He smiled and I shared a bit about the complexity of Seth's case. He told me he would come back when Seth was awake. Morning light shone through the blinds. Soon, Rosie re-appeared and engaged his new patient in small talk as he did Seth's assessment.

"So, where are you guys from?"

I said, "North of Chicago." We found this to be the quickest way to describe our whereabouts on the map.

"Oh, are you a Cubs fan?"

Seth chimed in. "My Grandma Benson was a die-hard Cubs fan, but I'm a Pirates fan."

Rosie was taken aback, "Oh, why the Pirates?"

"Well, I'm actually a die-hard *Steelers* fan, but I also like the Pirates and Penguins, too."

I piped up to share a fun fact I'd just learned. "The only city in the nation where its professional sports teams share the same colors, black and gold."

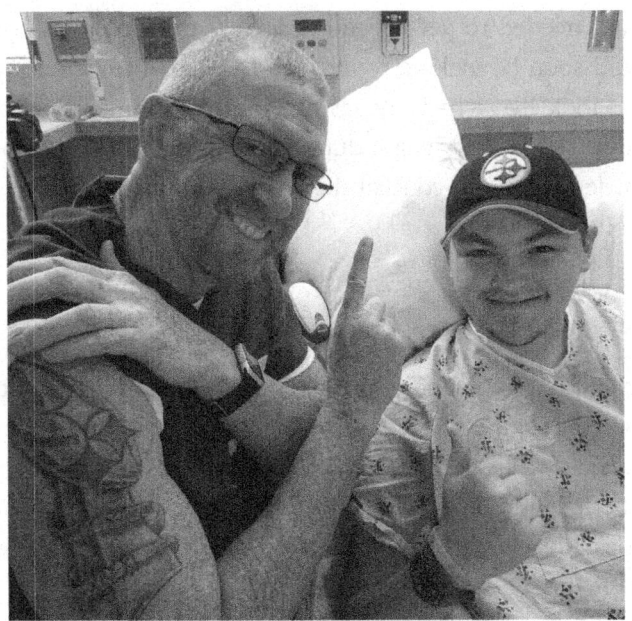

Seth and Nurse Rosie formed an instant bond.

Immediately, the tone in the room changed. Ha! A common bond sprung up. Rosie lifted his scrub sleeve to reveal a large tattoo of the Lombardi trophy with a huge, colorful Pittsburgh Steelers emblem across it. Seth could not believe his eyes. He immediately tried to sit up to get a better look. He shouted with excitement. Soon, these two guys were conversing like they were old friends. It warmed my heart to see this: Seth in a hospital bed filled with joy rather than despair.

Rosie said, "I need to call my best friend who is a doctor up in cardiac surgery. He's also a die-hard Steelers fan. I know he would love to come and meet you."

"That would be cool!"

Shortly thereafter, attendants came for Seth. As I always do, I kissed him on the cheek and assured him they were going to fix things. I reminded him how many people were praying at this very hour for him, having alerted our church's prayer team back home. He smiled and nodded.

In the stillness of the room, I prayed. It wasn't much of a prayer, but I knew God would meet me. All I had to offer was a weary, overwhelmed, but grateful heart. Soon, Rosie appeared. He asked about Seth, so I shared more about his journey. He seemed genuine in wanting to know Seth's story and how he could best serve him. After he left to take care of other patients, I slipped away to grab some coffee. I was never so grateful for a cup of hospital coffee in my life!

Rosie returned from his rounds to let me know he'd gotten ahold of his friend Doctor Stulak and told him all about Seth. Dr. Stulak wanted to meet him. Rosie told me that Dr. Stulak had something *super special* for him. He didn't tell me what, but with growing enthusiasm in the air, I knew something really great was about to happen.

Seth arrived back after a successful surgery. We were both relieved. Later on that evening, Rosie popped in to ask if Seth felt up to some company. Seth never refused a visitor. In walked a man in a lab coat, surgical booties, retro-styled glasses, a huge smile, and a Pittsburgh Steelers surgical hat. Seth quickly sat up and remarked how cool his hat was!

The interaction between the three die-hard Steelers fans was priceless. Seth's room suddenly became a man cave. They shared the immediate bond of "Steelers Nation Uniting." I had no idea of what was about to take place, but I pulled out my phone and hit record.

With a big smile, Dr. Stulak spoke words of encouragement.

"People like you are the true hero, so . . . accept something from me, please. Hold on a second." He left the room and returned holding a box covered with a hospital pillowcase. Ooh, we were intrigued.

"This has been in my office since . . . I started on staff." Dr. Stulak removed the cloth to reveal a football in a wooden and glass display case. Seth sat up in bed as Dr. Stulak placed it within his reach. "A signed football by Ben Roethlisberger. It doesn't need to sit in my office. It needs to be in your house."

Seth sat completely speechless until he could muster up the words, "Oh, thank you! Thank you so much!"

Later, we found out it was a wedding gift from Dr. Stulak's brother, which made it even more special. Who would give away such a personal gift to a complete stranger just to make their day? This guy couldn't get any better in our book, so we thought, but he did. We found out Dr. Stulak was a cardiac surgeon who did heart transplants among other things. The selflessness of his calling, devoting endless hours in life-saving surgeries, was apparent. But on top of that, he gave one of his most prized possessions to someone he had just met, my son.

We saw in the selfless hearts of these two servants, two of many examples, of what made Mayo Clinic so great. We became sensitive to the incredible people medical professionals are. We were privileged to get a peek behind the scenes of what they give in order to help thousands of patients year after year. We saw them sacrifice comfort, sleep, and family time for demands, stress, and high expectations. Taking care of such rare, complex patients is never an easy feat.

We wouldn't soon forget this day, a day when Seth had a very complex, urgently needed surgery performed, but also a day when we witnessed the very best of humanity. I loved seeing God orchestrate details and bring people together. I was convinced life held no coincidences, only divine appointments. Rosie was a floater that day. He wasn't supposed to be in that wing or in charge of Seth's care. He didn't usually take such assignments, but he agreed to go where he was needed. God had a plan for these three men to meet. But, the story didn't end there.

I asked the doctor's permission to share the sweet moment on our Facebook page. He hesitated to draw any attention to the gesture but agreed. His act of kindness resonated with the public. The post was viewed and shared thousands of times until it caught the attention of the Pittsburgh Steelers quarterback, Ben Roethlisberger's social media manager. She shared it with Ben, and they partnered to be a blessing and encouragement. She contacted me and not only mailed special gifts but also a video from Super Bowl champion Big Ben himself.

Ben videoed a warm greeting and message from the Steelers locker room to Seth and Dr. Stulak. The next time I brought Seth to the clinic, I surprised him, Rosie, Dr. Stulak and friends, by playing that video on the big screen in the doctors' conference room and unveiled Ben's gifts. Ben's message ended with, "Doc, thanks for all you do. You're a true hero. Seth, keep up the good fight, brother. Pulling for you. Praying for ya. And thanks for your support. Alright pal, talk to you later." Their reactions were priceless.

To some, it may seem like the football and Pittsburgh Steelers excitement is just too much hype. I get it–I used to think that, too. But sports have become such a blessing over the years. I've watched the camaraderie of the man cave excite, unite, and serve as a much-needed distraction from the daily grind of chronic illness.

I don't know much about football, but I found out a neat fact about the Steelers. Pittsburgh officially adopted the Pitt family motto: *"Benigno Numine."* It's a Latin phrase that means "Divine Providence." What better description could there be for all of this?

CHAPTER TWENTY
THE BIG 18

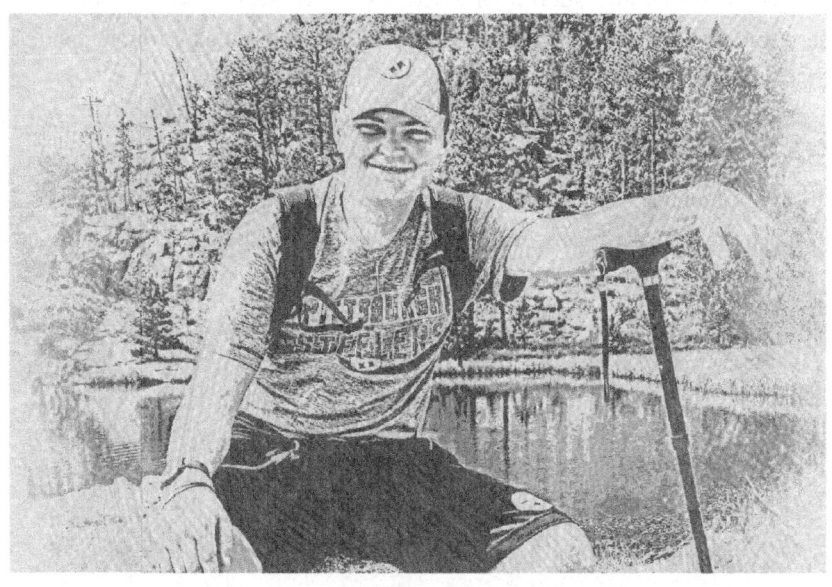

Every day we get to decide what we'll give to the world
and what we'll take from it. Love big; pack light.
–Bob Goff

With the realization that tube feeding wasn't going away any time soon, I wanted to use the opportunity to boost his immune system. I had no idea of the complexity that had developed inside Seth. Prior to this, I didn't even know there existed an entire department and specialists in Home Enteral Nutrition (HEN) dedicated to sustaining lives through a liquid diet. Despite all the cards stacked against him, I was determined to give Seth the best chance to not just survive but thrive. I researched the healthiest liquid nourishment on the market.

A relative of a friend was a knowledgeable doctor with expertise in this area. She didn't know Seth's particular situation, but she did know of an excellent product. A premium plant-based, organic, specialty pureed formula with no: GMO, artificial ingredients, gluten, sugar, dairy, soy, or corn. Oh, it would break the bank, but I was convinced it would provide the best nutritional support for Seth. I did the research and gave our nutritionist at Mayo the information. She wrote a prescription and letter to the insurance company, yet warned, "as long as he can tolerate it." I was filled with hope. I didn't know, however, as she did, that even though something was healthy, Seth's system wouldn't necessarily accept it.

Excited to receive the first shipment of foil pouches, I followed precise instructions for the proper administration of the formula. The cost of an ideal blender was beyond the reach of Donnie's blue-collar salary. Friends who understood our dilemma and dealt with food allergies for their own children, gifted us with the best blender money could buy. They gave glory to God that He could use them to meet our needs.

Disappointment, however, swiftly followed my first attempt. We learned the hard way through the horrible pain Seth endured that this was *not* sustainable. Seth's stomach couldn't process the fiber, and the formula sat in his stomach unable to be broken down. His distended belly looked like he was nine months pregnant. He rolled from side to side in agony as I phoned the doctor.

She said, "I knew he couldn't tolerate the fiber, but you were so hopeful. We tried."

"I just wanted the best for him." I now questioned what that was. I wrestled with regret, frustration, and despair.

"There are many families facing this dilemma. Please don't be discouraged. More wholesome alternative formulas without the fiber are in the trial stages that may work for Seth one day."

It was a tough blow. No chance of good, life-giving foods, at least for now. In the meantime, the team instructed us to go back to the original formula. They suggested we try changing Seth's continuous feeding schedule to all night rather than all day. We elevated his hospital bed at home to a forty-five-degree angle to assist with flow. Seth was pleased not to lug a backpack full of formula around all day.

This also did not go as planned. At the sound of gurgling, I lunged out of bed. Seth was vomiting, choking, and possibly aspirating (breathing in vomit). I yanked his CPAP mask off. We were both scared. This confirmed he could *not* formula feed at night (into his stomach). It was just too risky and another disappointing setback.

LESSONS FROM A HOSPITAL BED

We grew to dread our time at the hospital, which became a monotonous game of hurry up and wait. We read a little book by John Piper, *Lessons from a Hospital Bed*. I began to reflect on how we spent our time at the clinic and was convicted of how much time I'd wasted. Had we been paying attention to anyone around us, or did I slide into a sleep-deprived mode of simply wanting to go home? I didn't want to miss what God was doing at the clinic.

Because of the days added to this current hospital stay, I was out of clean clothes. Laura called and offered to pick up our clothes and launder them. It was humbling to be in such a position, but she wanted to help us and I needed clean clothes. I ate humble pie and accepted her offer. Instead of being irritated about having to stay longer, I thought about how grateful I was for her friendship. I wanted to focus on being more grateful rather than hosting a pity party over life's minor inconveniences. I began to see more opportunities to appreciate all the people God sent to help us along this challenging journey.

Laura returned with our laundered clothes neatly folded. She had hand-washed and air-dried my delicate bra so it wouldn't be ruined. She brought me coffee, just the way I like it, no cream or sugar, just light ice, for the right temperature. I felt so cared for. If that wasn't enough, she *thanked me* for allowing her to serve us.

I started to see all the blessings in the smallest of details. God surrounded us with people who came alongside us. Where actions speak louder than words, over the years, God sent an army of helpers who showed through their actions, "I got your back." How could I have missed the obvious? Seth and I started to talk about how grateful we were for the staff, who were likely also exhausted. I'm sure they wanted to go home to their families–everyone from the cleaning staff to CNAs who came in to clean bodily fluids and change sheets without complaint. From the healthcare workers who watched monitors all night to the kitchen staff who sent up ice cream and popsicles. Everyone was there to serve us.

I turned off the television, put away the phone, and looked for opportunities to express our gratitude. Seth started to engage with everyone who walked in. We had tucked small gifts into our bag. Giving them away made Seth feel he was repaying them in some way. One of the cleaning ladies said she was going to cry, she was so overwhelmed with gratitude by a small gift.

Encounters like this led us to pray and thank God for the people we met. Seth always kept a notebook and his favorite pens with him. On this visit, he wrote a thank you note to his surgeon. It took him hours to write and rewrite it in his best handwriting free from mistakes.

We were shocked to receive a reply from the surgeon thanking us for being positive despite a difficult journey. I never expected anyone in the busy medical field to take the time to encourage *us*. He wrote, "Thank you for being a positive light even while going through such hardships. Your light shines bright!"

What an encouragement his response was to us. I was blown away that the God of the universe chose to use the most unlikely vessels of His grace–a hot mess mama and a kid who just wanted to go home–to encourage such an extraordinary individual. Once again, God was up to something. He wasn't changing Seth's situation but was *transforming* us in the process. As Seth often said, "It's all God!"

We were grateful for the investment so many made in our lives. Despite busy schedules, many went out of their way to be there for us. Dr. Stulak and Nurse Rosie often surprised Seth by showing up after a long shift. On more than one occasion, they intercepted Seth as he headed into the operating room. Seth's face lit up like a Christmas tree as they talked about the Steelers and the projection for the season in the hallway. For a moment, they helped Seth forget about his latest medical dilemma.

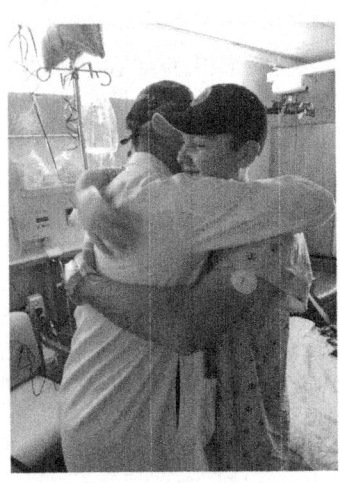

One day, Dr. Stulak came to Seth's room and asked about his latest project. Seth was selling T-shirts to sponsor children coming for the Children's Heart Project. Without skipping a beat, Dr. Stulak said, "I'll match every dollar you raise, Seth."

Seth lit up-hugs all around! My mama heart overflowed with emotion seeing these two bring out the best in each other. This beautiful partnership showed me another example of the power of community playing out in our lives. Now, a child with a heart defect, who may have died without intervention, was able to come to Mayo Clinic for life-saving heart surgery. Hallelujah!

God always worked out the details, connections, and timing. God took a trying situation and turned it into a thing of joy and purpose. God showed us we didn't need to leave the country on a mission trip to make a difference. We discovered plenty of opportunities to serve others and work together for good, right where God put us. We continued to meet Lucy whenever we could coordinate appointments in Rochester around the same time.

Lucy shared with us, "I used to go to my treatments, then back to my room or home. I didn't want anyone to see my scars. Then I met this young kid with a cane, leg braces, and feeding tube taped to his face. He wasn't trying to hide it. He was living life! I realized all he had endured in his young life. It stirred my heart and inspired me. I made a choice to no longer feel sorry for myself. I would go out and walk, even in the mall, I no longer walked with my face down, I held my head high. Meeting Seth changed my life! He's my little hero."

The feeling was mutual. Lucy was a warrior and hero of ours! Through her ongoing health challenges, she inspired and encouraged us. Our kindred Christian spirit grew a love between all of us; we were now family. We were so grateful we didn't have to walk this journey alone.

Kim and Frank continued to open their home to us, and our friendship grew. When Jeff was in town, he continued to show up for Seth's appointments, surgeries, and procedures. Donnie continued to work hard and hold down the fort at home. The children continued to pull together and help each other. It's hard to recount all of the people who walked beside us.

Looking back, I didn't verbalize my appreciation to the children as I wish I had. The two eldest spent lots of fun time with the babies. By the time Drew was twelve, he was cooking full meals for the family. Later, he learned how to cut the kids' hair and run errands while Donnie worked. Janae mothered her younger brothers with care and compassion. Gabe and Luke, my two little cabooses, made the best of the situation. Even with typical sibling rivalry, I appreciated how everyone stepped up. Bayles Bunch, your mom appreciates you!

Our treasured Rochester friends continued to put their boots on the ground hosting families who traveled there from all over the world. These dear friends allowed us to be a small part of what God was doing through Children's Heart Project. We prayed for God to allow us to spend our time at the clinic wisely, and he answered our prayers.

One day, I watched Seth confidently meet a new group from Bolivia. I found myself at the back of the group, watching Seth interact with a smile from ear to ear and an occasional nod and giggle. As the group followed Seth and Jeff through the halls of Mayo Clinic, they looked at ease walking and enjoying the time together. Even though the Bolivians didn't speak English, everyone shared the language of love.

We had come full circle. Seth, once a new, reluctant patient himself, and myself struggling with the long hours at the clinic, now welcomed others and calmed their fears with his contagious joy. I recalled a time when we'd forgotten our smiles. Now I felt God redeeming the time we lost.

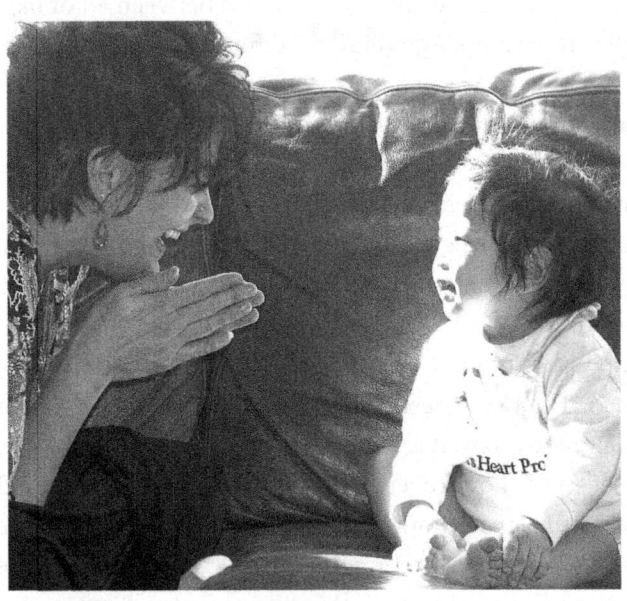

AUGUST 2018, MT. RUSHMORE OR BUST!

It had been a summer filled with trips, but not the fun kind. With approximately ten trips to emergency rooms, as well as long commutes to Mayo, it wasn't the kind of "summer break" a kid goes back to school and brags about. I suggested to Donnie an impromptu family road trip. Mt. Rushmore was a close second to the Grand Canyon for Seth's Make-A-Wish trip. The family liked the idea of heading west together and seeing sights we hadn't seen before. At this point, any sights would be better than the inner walls of the clinic. Seth and I found ourselves, again, in day-to-day care at the clinic with extra appointments.

Seth was exhausted, but what got him through were plans to camp in South Dakota the following week. He couldn't wait to see Mt. Rushmore. He pictured the scenes from one of his all-time favorite movies, *National Treasure: Book of Secrets*. We just needed to get through the week of medical monotony.

Finally, we were in the home stretch on Friday afternoon. Our last appointment was with our medical quarterback, Dr. Fischer, who regularly summarized the play-by-play from the team. Earlier, I had noticed a spot of *new* blood seeping through Seth's clothes. I didn't know what was going on, and Seth wouldn't let me get a good look at it. I think he knew it was bad and didn't want another hospital stay. Typical Seth. I asked his doctor to take a peek. As the doctor got up, Seth flashed me the death stare.

After a quick exam, the doctor rushed out of the room without explanation. When he returned, he told me Seth had a ruptured cyst that needed surgery. He'd left to call Dr. Rio, who agreed to put him on his surgical schedule first thing Monday morning. Seth admitted the pain was excruciating but had not shared that up until this point with anyone.

As Dr. Fischer discussed details and pre-op instructions, I respectively interjected, "But we won't be here Monday. We'll be at Mt. Rushmore."

"This really shouldn't be put off."

I paused to gather my thoughts. I had profound respect for this world-renowned doctor, and his opinion always held great weight. I knew he was always looking out for Seth's best interest. I shared my heart. I understood the risk, but I also strongly felt the importance of keeping my promise to Seth and the family about this trip. I learned to pick my battles, and this was one worth fighting for.

"Okay. Seth needs surgery, and I am in agreement with that plan. But we also *need* this time together as a family. We didn't even know this was here until today. I don't think it would be unreasonable to push the surgery ahead a few days."

Dr. Fischer stated the facts for the record, "Seth's risk for infection is high. This is an open wound that could easily abscess."

"Then I probably shouldn't tell you that we are camping." I might have cried if I didn't titter while stating my own facts for the record. We knew each other long enough to be open and honest, had mutual respect, and rarely agreed to disagree. "With all due respect, you know I am *not* refusing medical treatment. I promise I will call to schedule surgery the moment we're on our way back. It will be after Tuesday, which is Seth's eighteenth birthday. After all, you only turn eighteen once, right?" I flashed a cheesy grin hoping to lighten the mood.

At this point, Dr. Fischer knew he couldn't convince me otherwise. Another sigh—

"Alright. You need to keep this area clean. Use bottled water. You'll need to flush the area and wrap it in sterile gauze several times a day."

I listened intently to his words and nodded. "Yes, we will make it work. We'll be in touch."

Early the next morning, Seth and I eagerly took off from Minnesota headed for the Black Hills. At the same time, Donnie and our four children still living at home, began the thirteen-hour trek towing our pop-up camper. We were excited to eventually meet up in an area of the country we had never before experienced.

Seth and I arrived at Custer State Park, South Dakota, shortly before sunset. Greeting us at the entrance was an iconic buffalo resting right next to the welcome sign. We thought it was a statue until it moved! The scene in front of us seemed surreal as mule deer, elk, and wild turkeys crossed the road in front of us. Far from the burdens we carried at the hospital, time outdoors in God's country relaxed our minds and bodies. Like a balm to our souls, the change of scenery refreshed our spirits. I was so glad we came.

Mt. Rushmore was everything we envisioned and more. Colorful flags representing all fifty states lined the walkway to the mammoth monument of four prominent faces in American history. When we climbed up to the viewing area, it was breathtaking. Although difficult for Seth in the moment, surrounded by the view, he felt a sense of peace.

Our son Drew planned all the details, including a picturesque spot to celebrate Seth's birthday. He led us on a thirty-minute drive to Sylvan Lake. It was absolutely perfect. It reminded me of a Bob Ross painting, *Happy Little Trees*, with all the high-rise scenery reflected in the lake like a mirror. The majestic handiwork proclaimed, "This is God's doing." Seth loved the rock formations. The earthy rust, moss green, and terra cotta speckled boulders stood out against hundreds of shades of green in the trees that towered in the background. Seth struggled to find a flat spot to sit, even falling in the process, but it didn't deter him. He settled on a boulder and celebrated the accomplishment. He told me he would remember this day!

My mind reverted years back to the conversation we had with the doctor in Madison. He told us to go celebrate and make memories with our son because he didn't know where Seth may be for his ninth birthday. Here we were nine years later! Seth had reached the milestone of adulthood. I soaked in the moment filled with gratitude. It may have been difficult to fully appreciate the gift of life in the day-to-day trials, but this trip enabled me to see from a different vantage point. The time spent as a family in the quiet and beauty of God's creation rejuvenated all of us. With memories of this spontaneous trip lingering, it was time to return to the clinic and finish the race.

It took time to get Seth settled. Support pillows, blankets, a foam wedge formed and cut to accommodate his seatbelt, plus positioning the CPAP breathing machine, so he could sleep for the nine-hour journey back to Mayo Clinic took some creative arranging. Because of the cyst, the feeding tube, and his arthritis, his positioning was limited, so I did all I could to help him ride comfortably. The truth was Seth never complained once. He wanted to go on this trip so bad, he did whatever it took. The rest of the family packed up several days' worth of camping gear and headed home to Wisconsin.

On the way, I stopped to print a family photo to slip into a thank you note for Dr. Fischer. Back at the clinic, he asked about the trip. The smile on Seth's face said it all. I thanked Dr. Fischer for his grace and understanding and handed him the photo. He smiled and studied the family as he gathered his thoughts.

"Thank you. This means a lot. I'm glad you went. I'll keep this on my desk."

I looked at Seth, and his face was beaming. All was well, and that was especially important to all of us.

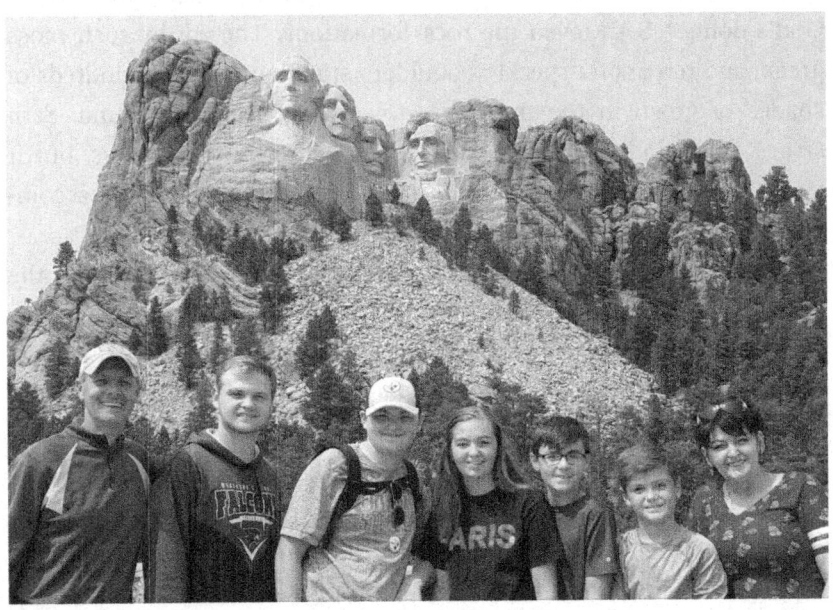

Next, we met with Dr. Rio. We thanked him for his willingness to shuffle his schedule. He was gracious and explained the entire process and what we could expect.

"I'll need to hollow out the area. You will need to pack that empty area several times daily with debriding gauze. My otherwise healthy patients have taken months for a cyst half this size to close."

As usual, nothing with Seth was simple or easy. Once Dr. Rio got in there for the excision, he realized it was essentially two cysts, larger and deeper than anyone had foreseen. Afterwards, he forewarned us of the long road ahead. Dr. Fischer shared in hindsight he was glad that I persisted in taking that major road trip *before* surgery. No way could Seth have endured the seventeen-hour drive to and from Mt. Rushmore after surgery. Now, the memories we made as a family would be especially important on the rough road to recovery.

The next year proved to be rough. Seth's room looked like a wound care supply closet. Like many times before, his body was working against him. Finally, after much prayer and hard work as a team for nearly *two* years, the hole caused by the cyst closed. Victory at last! We didn't realize how the pain and wound care had affected so much of all our lives, not to mention Seth's. To our dismay, another cyst appeared tearing open his flesh. We would have to start aggressive wound care all over again.

As Seth continued down the path of progressive degenerative disease, his back pain sometimes took his breath away. Corticosteroid injections offered localized, minimal, temporary relief. Soon, it seemed like every other joint, muscle, bone, and tendon had succumbed to this disease. His rheumatologist suggested we may need to consider adding a *biological drug* to Seth's treatment regimen. Now on top of the aggressive oral meds, I had to learn about biological therapy risks, plus the low-dose chemotherapy chemicals. It was so complicated it made my head spin.

I hated the predicament we were in. I hated what this disease had done and was doing to my boy. I also hated the number and strength of drugs Seth was on. Staggering and upsetting, quite frankly, it kept me up at night. I could barely recall the days of rarely giving Seth *any* over-the-counter medications. I felt I owed it to Seth to provide him with a non-pharmaceutical (alternative therapy) option at home. I set out to do something crazy. I petitioned our state to approve exactly what Seth needed at home–an inline heated, hydro-jet therapy tub. That way he could use aqua therapy safely. It was our only hope to avoid adding pain meds while working to improve his quality of life. Oh, how desperately I wanted to give my son the tools he needed to decompress and experience pain relief without side effects.

Those employed at the state level told me it would be a challenging, uphill battle. The grueling process of nearly a year of in-home assessments, bids, paperwork, proving medical necessity, and medical reviews at the state level made me question whether I should pursue this further. It drained so much of my time and energy needed to continue caring for Seth and the rest of the family.

As I drove back to Mayo Clinic for what felt like the millionth time, I had too much time to think. I started to succumb to a pity party. *Why does everything have to be so hard?* My mind recalled something Seth and I talked about earlier when we were prone to host such parties. We discussed all that Albert, Lucy, and others had been through. Some we'd met from around the world didn't even have water or electricity in their shacks! Our lives seem like a cakewalk in comparison. Right then and there, I surrendered the fight to God. Being still, remaining calm, and trusting God to fight our battles did not come easy for me. I'm a mom–I wanted to fix things. But I knew I needed to let go and let God . . .

"The Lord himself will fight for you. Just stay calm" (Exodus 14:14).

CHAPTER TWENTY-ONE
THE ADVENTURES OF FLAT SETH

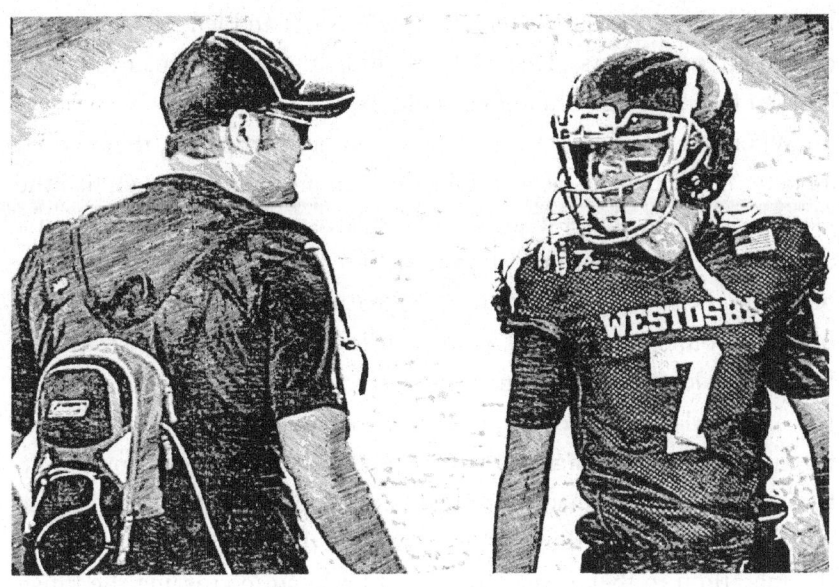

Do all the good you can, By all the means you can, In all the ways you can, In all the places you can, At all the times you can, To all the people you can, As long as ever you can.
–John Wesley

In November of 2018, Team Seth registered for the fast-approaching Madison Marathon. This was Seth's favorite marathon and favorite medal. He looked forward to the rush of competing and enjoying all twenty-six miles in his race chair with his team of "Angels." However, with each surgery, it became increasingly clear that Seth's marathon days were over, at least for the foreseeable future.

It was a struggle to let go of Team Seth, who prayed together, enjoyed each other's company, and spurred one another on. But we needed to be fair and let Seth's Angels know they should find another team captain. Such a heartbreaking reality.

We assumed the team would find a replacement captain or maybe even free themselves from the travel and physical commitment altogether and stay home. We still find it hard to believe what unfolded next. The series of selfless acts by Angels Karla and Jen will forever be etched in our hearts. They kept their commitment, ensuring Seth crossed that finish line in a spectacular way.

When Jen and Karla learned Seth could not participate, they crafted a poster board cut-out of Seth taken from a photograph, much like the *Flat Stanley* book series. Flat Seth, all twelve inches of him, sported a royal blue "Seth's Journey" t-shirt with a Steelers ball cap. He wore black shorts to his knees with his signature red, white, and blue leg braces. Around his neck, he wore a yellow, red, and green strap that held a previous marathon medal. Sporty sunglasses covered his eyes. Jen and Karla were a colorful duo themselves, and both wore black leggings with Seth's signature red and white striped socks pulled up to their knees. They made sure Flat Seth, safely strapped into his race chair, experienced all the feels and thrills of the race. From the start of the marathon to flying past the capitol building to crossing the finish line, Flat Seth was photo-ready for every selfie taken by his Angels. Flat Seth had a busy day: He directed traffic, went to church, and played in the leaves. He visited Camp Randall Stadium, survived being licked by a ginormous flat dog who stood along the sidelines, jumped in unison with a crowd of strangers, and, the greatest thrill of all–

crossed the finish line with Jen and Karla after twenty-six miles *together*!

All these memories were captured mile by mile in photographs filled with bright smiles, then compiled in a book his "cool aunts" gifted to Seth. And if that photo documentary wasn't enough, Jen and Karla insisted on giving Seth the prized medals they earned. On the back of the photo book, they inscribed this message:

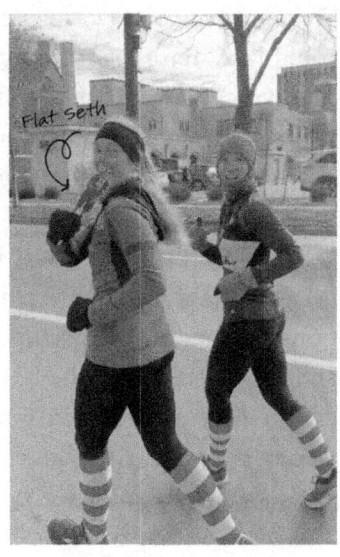

"Seth - You are an amazing young man! You have inspired us and so many others in many ways. We pray that one day we can make an impact on the world as big as the one you make. You make us and everyone you're around a better person! You have a tremendous heart that is never-ending. You have taught us to trust and have faith. You have taught us that no matter how much you have or what troubles you have, you always have something to give. . . .We love to run with you and, if you can't run, we will run for you. . . . We hope you know just how important you are to us Seth buddy. . . because it's, like, a lot!!! Love you! Jennifer and Karla"

As Seth's cognitive struggles increased, we became concerned. Things he knew in the past, he struggled to not only recall but make sense of. Although his younger siblings helped him, it was tough for him to accept.

One day Seth asked me, "Mom, will there be a day when I don't know you anymore?"

My heart shattered, but I didn't want to fall apart in front of him. "Seth, you don't need to worry about anything. God hasn't brought you this far to leave you now. He's got this!" He nodded. "Your whole family–all of us–will be by your side, no matter what."

Then, I went to my room and cried my eyes out. The fear of the unknown is the hardest.

A NEW TEAM AT BAT AND A GODLY MENTOR

We returned to Mayo for another neuropsychological evaluation that could take up to eight hours. Since Seth was now of age, this evaluation took place on the adult side of the clinic with an entirely new team. This would be his third full testing and assessment at Mayo. I silently hoped somehow things would miraculously change for the better.

That, unfortunately, was not the case. I knew it in my head, yet it was still disheartening to read the doctor's findings and recommendations. Seth needed assistance for the rest of his life. I cried and grieved and questioned what the future held for all of us. Then, I remembered a John Piper quote. "Occasionally, weep deeply over the life you hoped would be. Grieve the losses. Then wash your face. Trust God and embrace the life you have."

This quote spawned a turning point in my thinking. It gave me permission to grieve. Even if healing never came and the reality crushed us, my faith in God would not be destroyed. I wouldn't waste any more time crying for what I had hoped. This was my son, and I was blessed and proud to be his mother, *come what may*. Despite Seth's lack of self-sufficiency as a young man, with God's grace and abundance poured out over his life, it was enough. I still had a purpose. Seth still had a purpose. Our family still had a purpose. We had a lot of life left to be lived. Even if–

Seth watched Pastor John's sermons, pondered his daily devotions, and read all the books by Piper that he could get his hands on. Seth copied, underlined, and highlighted Scriptures, especially those about suffering. He kept the books and notes next to his bed. When he couldn't sleep due to pain, he'd put on his headlamp and drew comfort from reading. Despite his cognitive setbacks, God helped Seth glean strength from Piper's teachings. He was like a sponge soaking up the truths from Scripture. Piper's transparent and personal examples of physical suffering inspired Seth to not give up.

Unbeknown to us, dear friends of ours wrote to John Piper at Desiring God to share what they knew about Seth and how the ministry had impacted his life. Pastor John signed and forwarded a copy of his book, *Don't Waste Your Life* to be delivered to Seth. Seth was beside himself when he read the inscription: *"To Seth! Sorrowful yet always! Rejoicing! 2 Cor. 6:10"* If that wasn't exciting enough, I received an email from Scott Anderson, the CEO of Desiring God. He asked about Seth and wanted to know if I could bring Seth to the Desiring God international headquarters the next time we were in Minnesota. John Piper wanted to meet Seth!

I was so grateful for this opportunity for Seth. I knew what a huge encouragement it would be to him. I told Seth we had been invited to tour the Desiring God international headquarters but kept the meeting with Pastor John a surprise. At the finish of our next visit to Rochester, we headed up to Minneapolis. We arrived at the address, a modest building in the back of an industrial area. I was pleasantly surprised at the lack of pretentiousness. I saw a beautiful humility in that. Seth was eager to step inside and see where the resources he had devoured for years came from.

Scott greeted us warmly at the door and treated Seth to a special personal tour. Then, we came to the conference room.

As Seth approached the room, Scott said, "Occasionally, some pretty special things can happen in this room."

Just then, Seth saw John Piper waiting there for him.

"Hello, Seth!"

"Oh. my. goodness. This is amazing. Oh, it is such an honor to meet you. Oh, my goodness. I *love* watching your videos and reading your books."

Pastor John humbly replied, "God is good."

Seth immediately responded, "God is great!"

It was neat to watch Seth and John Piper interact with one another. They both were in total agreement with God's goodness.

We will never, ever forget the special prayer he prayed over both of us.

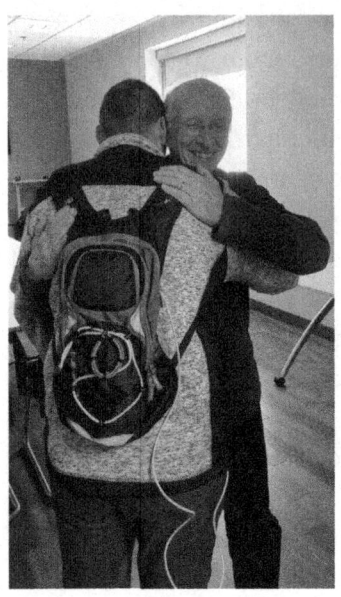

An emotional meeting with one of his faith mentors, John Piper.

As soon as Pastor John began praying, I was overwhelmed. His teaching through various media had so ministered to me over the years that when I heard his voice in prayer for Seth in person, my tears and sniffling didn't stop until he finished. I thank God for that meeting. Meeting someone whose teaching brought Seth so much hope and strength in dark evenings, gripping bed rails in pain, meant more to Seth than anyone imagined. In our eyes, it was not about putting a man up on a pedestal. It was about putting God in his proper place and giving *God* the praise and honor He so rightly deserved.

God used - and continues to use - Pastor John's calling, his gifts, and his sacrifice through this ministry to bless Seth. Seth grew closer to God because John Piper chose not to waste his life. This challenged Seth to not waste the gift of another day. He was beyond grateful to receive a special edition of Piper's collected works. Scott and John also told Seth to choose an array of Piper's books to give away. Seth loved to connect with people and give gifts, and those books were very special gifts for him to give.

AND THE BEAT GOES ON

Pastor John needed to catch a plane, and we needed to head back to Rochester for other exciting ministries we were honored to be a part of. A fund-raiser was scheduled for that evening benefiting Operation Christmas Child at Autumn Ridge Church. Samaritan's Purse had brothers and sisters from around the world in town. We had spent time off and on for weeks with a group from Uganda who were in Rochester through Children's Heart Project. We also looked forward to an Operation Christmas Child shoebox recipient, originally from Rwanda, who was going to give his testimony that evening.

Enya, a fellow volunteer with both Operation Christmas Child and Children's Heart Project, worked hard to put this event together. She lived in Rochester, and we stayed at her home on several occasions, and our families quickly became friends. Light 45 was scheduled to perform, but Seth didn't know of a more personal highlight brewing. A "drum-off" between Seth and his close drumming friend, Critter, would be showcased. For weeks there were posters displayed around Rochester promoting the event. It was quite a big deal, and Seth felt like a rock star! He was excited to be on the big stage and raise money for several causes close to his heart. We shared a time of fellowship with friends, new and old. Seth couldn't wait to give copies of his favorite Piper book, *Don't Waste Your Life*, to new friends from around the United States and the globe.

Critter later said this about Seth:

> From that day on Seth and I became drum brothers, playing the heartbeat of God together. When I was getting to know more about Seth, I found out what he was dealing with in his personal life. I was shocked how he always had a smile on his face, never complained, and always shared the love of God. Seth reminded me of a modern day Job–from the Bible . . . . Even through Job's hardest time, he never cursed God but stayed faithful to him. Seth is a true example of this, staying faithful with God, sharing the good news with people, and being a light to the world . . . . I am truly honored to have been able to share the stage with Seth (and) get to know him.

Seth continued to look forward to his tribe at his fundraising events. He was ecstatic that this year the Children's Heart Project fundraiser would be held at his old grade school. It was a summer weekend event of fun and Seth's Drumming for Dollars. It was incredible to watch Seth and his former music teacher, Mr. Murphy, play together for charity. It was extra special since Mr. Murphy was solely responsible for putting Seth on the drums in the first place, and they shared a special bond. Now the two of them were drumming to raise money to save the lives of children across the globe.

Countless individuals helped make this beautiful event a huge success. The event raised thousands of dollars in just two hours–enough to sponsor a child to receive life-saving heart surgery! These were the gifts that kept on giving.

LIFE COACHES

The sport of football was growing on me, not due to the game itself, but the team spirit. What the high school football coaches and team did for our family will never be forgotten. Coach Grube, also Seth's art teacher, asked Seth if he would like to become a manager for the football team. Oh, yeah! Anyone who knew Seth knew what a huge part football held in his life. He loved every single aspect of the game. Even though he couldn't physically play, now he had a place in the thick of everything the game offered.

Seth's PT assistant, Mr. Lorentz, was also one of the football coaches. Coach Lorentz pushed Seth toward the goals set by Seth's medical team. He encouraged Seth to press on while checking his oxygen levels and pulse. They would spend four years together, following this daily routine.

Seth continued his role as manager while adding the role of team videographer. The football season was undoubtedly a highlight for Seth. Although he was exhausted most days, he pushed himself to be on the sidelines and at the end zone to film every game unless he was in the hospital. Seth gave them his best, and they rallied around him like family.

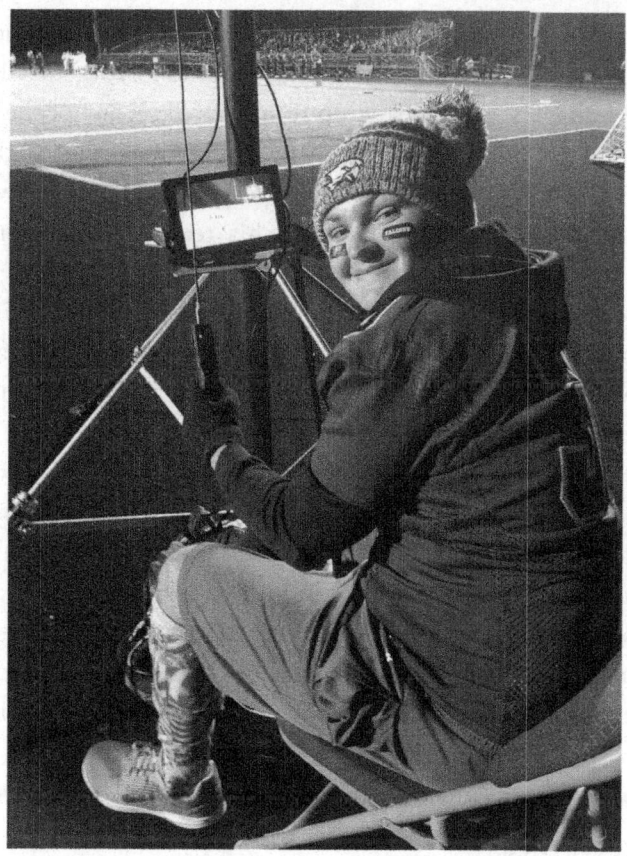

Head Coach Mr. Mengel, also his history teacher, developed a unique bond with Seth. Mengel's quick wit and sarcasm inspired Seth to enjoy history class. He'd come home and tell me some of the day's top laughs. Even though much of the class work was above his academic level, we made the decision to keep Seth in the class.

One day, I asked Coach how Seth was doing. I wondered if we made the right choice. He told me Seth was doing great! He was social and loved interacting, listening, and participating when he could. When others were studying material that Seth wasn't able to follow, he would quietly open his backpack, get out his Bible, and study on his own. I didn't know this. Based on what Seth was going through, nobody questioned it. Despite so much stacked against him, Seth was thriving and inspiring others in many ways.

Coach Mengel taught his team sportsmanship, inclusion, and respect. He taught them to celebrate and honor others who were enduring struggles. Seth looked up to him as did many of the players. I'm sure Coach was behind the many inspirational videos the team sent Seth, including the team singing *Happy Birthday* to Seth while he was in the hospital. Seth considered his team an extension of his siblings.

Out of the overflow of what had been poured into him, Seth joyfully gave back. Seth volunteered with the youth football league. He was able to model the positive leadership skills he learned from his coaches and countless other examples.

Seth spent many of his summer days up in the press box filming the youth games. He paid attention to detail by zooming in on the individual plays, so they could be viewed by the team later for teaching. When Seth wasn't behind the camera, he could be found on the sidelines encouraging the players, especially his two favorite players and younger brothers, Gabe and Luke. They learned so much about the game but, most of all, about good sportsmanship and working as a team.

POINT AND SHOOT

Mrs. Switalla, better known as Mrs. S, gave us the gift of photography. Mrs. S used her time, talent, and her trained eye to bless parents. She worked long hours at the school, then volunteered her time photographing students at various events. Come rain, shine, snow, or sweltering heat, she was there. After returning home from the events, Mrs. S spent countless hours downloading, editing, and posting on her social media page for others to enjoy. She never asked for anything in return. I was in awe of such dedication and sacrifice.

On the difficult days, when the unknowns of Seth's future weighed on me, her photos helped us focus on the good times. We cherished the memories she captured on and off the field, but, more importantly, we cherished her friendship. She and Seth spurred one another on. She wrote this note to Seth:

"Seth, You are a true inspiration to so many people, myself included. I admire your positivity and humor, even when you face much adversity. Your determination to do unto others makes me want to be a better person. Thank you for always being a positive role model. I know you have changed and touched so many lives through your efforts and helping them to live better. God bless you and your family for all you do. —Much love to you, Mrs. S."

BLANKETS OF LOVE

We love when we catch a glimpse of how God weaves our journey together with others. When Seth was about ten years old, a videographer from a local Rochester news station, came to do a story on Seth at the Ronald McDonald House. We hit it off right away and stayed in touch over the years. We had no idea he was dealing with his own health challenges and was now enduring dialysis several times a week at Mayo. Up until this point, we knew nothing about the world of dialysis.

We arrived at the clinic on a mission to cheer up our friend, but we weren't prepared for what we saw after we made our way to the lower level toward the unit. As far as the eye could see, a long corridor was lined with lounge chairs each holding an individual hooked up to a collection of machines, monitors, and cords. The huge machines reminded me of front-loading washing machines. The noise and the visual of spinning and cleaning (filtering the blood of the patients) was something I had never fathomed. These people's lives depended on and revolved around this process for several hours three times every week!

I fought to hold back tears. Our hearts were so heavy for this burden and the blessing this process offered to extend lives. Seth wanted to make a difference and bless those going through medical hardships. Out of great empathy, we asked him what we could do to make his life and those going through dialysis easier. He immediately mentioned blankets. He explained how cold and fatigued the dialysis process makes patients. Such a small thing to ask.

When we got to the car, we sat there for a moment to regain our thoughts. We couldn't forget what we had just seen. Confidently, Seth voiced that collecting blankets would be his new mission. It was the very least we could do. We posted the request on Seth's social media page "Seth's Journey." His goal? Collect one hundred new blankets for the Dialysis Unit in honor of our friend. Seth wanted to hand them out for Christmas, but it was only a few weeks away, so the clock was ticking.

As in the past, countless individuals came together in love and exceeded Seth's goal. Seth was busy! He picked up blankets at homes, at schools, and received boxes daily on our doorstep. Some gave money for us to purchase blankets while others made blankets. A dear woman in her eighties, who lived down the street from us, adored Seth and followed his journey. Whenever she read about one of Seth's latest endeavors to benefit others, I'd often receive a message, barely legible by her arthritic hands, asking me to call her. Often unable to leave her home to gather supplies, she offered, instead, to provide whatever resources we needed. She was another notable example of how everyone can do something.

Bristol School initiated a blanket drive in Seth's honor. Paris School joined the mission. Seth's younger siblings: Janae, Gabe, and Luke, worked with classmates to knot fleece blankets in different colors and patterns. We saw the power of community in our small Wisconsin towns create a ripple effect of love and care. We packed a U-Haul trailer with over five hundred blankets and towed it behind my SUV one week before Christmas.

The gracious nurses allowed Seth to pull a wagon he brought from home filled with blankets through the Dialysis Unit. He was blessed to go from patient to patient wishing them a Merry Christmas. We were met with much gratitude and some amazing stories. One older gentleman receiving treatment shared that this was his one, and probably the only, Christmas gift he would receive. Our hearts broke for him. He was as grateful to receive it as we were to give it. We were able to gift the nurses a small gesture of thanks for all they do and left them with about one hundred blankets for the patients that came on alternate days. We still had hundreds more to deliver.

We prayed God would show us where to distribute the remaining blankets. Best buddy, Jeff, hung with us the entire day as we drove around town stopping at various locations. A Mayo staff member we had gotten to know over the years along with her son helped us unload the bags of fluffy, vibrant squares of hugs.

We drove that trailer to several buildings dropping off blankets at the main Mayo Clinic campus, Methodist Hospital, Jacobson Building, and the Proton Beam Therapy Center. We couldn't end the day without visiting our favorite and most inspiring doctor, Dr. Fischer. We brought the remaining dozens of blankets up to the pediatric wing for the children. It seemed fitting that we shared this labor of love with Dr. Fischer's unit. Although he was too modest to share himself, we found out he spared someone he didn't even know the burden of dialysis by donating one of his own kidneys! His selfless example repeatedly inspired us to give, love, and serve others more.

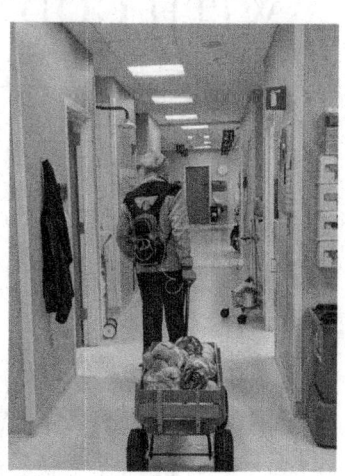

Seth delivering blankets of love!

By the end of the year 2018, we witnessed the fabric of our lives woven together in a colorful tapestry with many friends, new and old, all for God's glory.

CHAPTER TWENTY-TWO
WITH GOD ALL THINGS ARE POSSIBLE

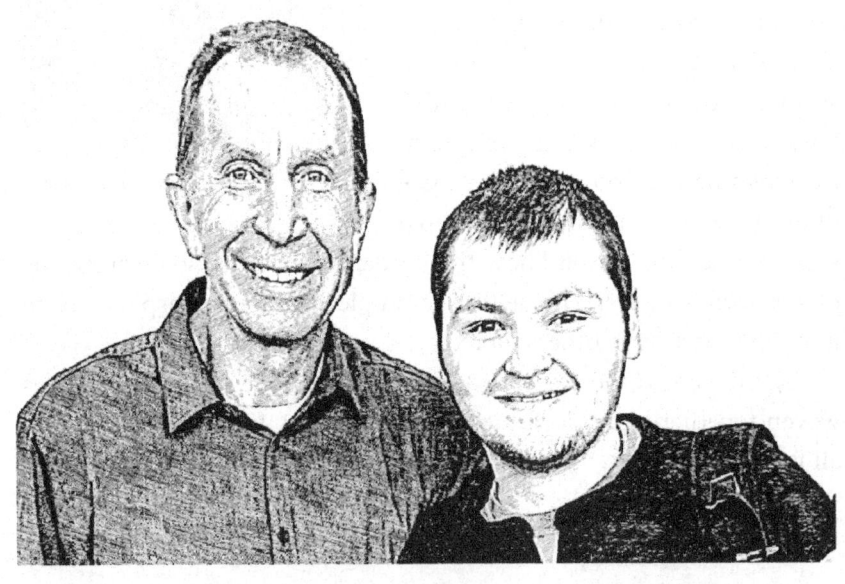

God doesn't expect you to be happy about what has been torn
from your hands—whether it's a marriage, your health, a job, or
someone you love—but if you are willing to trust him,
he can turn trash into triumph.
–Levi Lusko

Mayor Ardell Brede and Seth enjoyed several big moments together after the "Key to the City" presentation. They had many common bonds, including a deep faith and a heart to serve others in the community. We loved seeing each other at different charity events and kept in touch while apart.

TAKE ME OUT TO THE BALLGAME

Mayor Ardell, who had season tickets for the Rochester Honkers baseball games, arranged for Seth to throw out the first pitch for a special home game. He even ensured Seth had a cheering section at Mayo Field that day. In his usual seat behind home plate, the mayor invited Seth to sit beside him as his special guest. I sat beside them with sons Gabe and Luke, Seth's best bud Jeff, a French exchange student we were hosting in our home at the time, and seven other Rochester friends. On a sunny day in July, dressed in a teal Honkers jersey the mayor had previously given him, Seth was psyched. It didn't matter that we'd just spent the day plodding through five appointments at the clinic, sports recharged Seth's batteries. Cameras captured his signature smile as Seth posed with the mayor, a local radio personality, and Slider, the team mascot. As he walked out to the mound, the press box announcer introduced Seth to the crowd using a synopsis of some of Seth's trials and accomplishments. Many came out to witness and celebrate Seth throwing out the ceremonial first pitch.

Watching Seth front and center on that pitcher's mound, with the crowd cheering for him by name, was emotional. We embraced Rochester as our home away from home, and the citizens embraced us back. I saw a beautiful picture of the loving and supportive tribe Seth had been blessed with through the years along this journey. Those relationships, known and unknown (from his social media page in the US and worldwide), were priceless.

"NOTHING GETS WASTED IN GOD'S ECONOMY."

In all this, I've repeatedly seen God's favor in those who haven't had an easy life. How can I describe the selfless servants we've met in the families of those living with complex medical needs? It would be unfair to limit their description to a few words. Seth and I have been the recipients of the most loving, beautiful, compassionate, resilient, faith-filled, and generous souls. I have learned so much about faith, perseverance, bravery, endurance, overcoming, making do, being content, self-sufficiency, and humble dependence. Let me add: thinking outside the box because there's no box to check, advocating, and striving to be better rather than bitter. What has been most profound for me is watching other families who walked a similar extraordinary journey and yet work tirelessly to make life better for others.

The roots of our faith grew deeper trauma by trauma as we saw what I could only believe were miraculous details and the power of God's network. These could not, and will not, be brushed off as mere coincidences.

Seth had, and still has, notebooks and binders of words he carefully penned that have had a profound impact on him. None of the words were his own, but God used His word (the Bible) and the words of others to bolster Seth's courage day after day. It always seemed to be exactly what he needed.

Off and on throughout the night, I made my rounds into Seth's room to check on him and make sure he had his CPAP mask on. I often found him reading in the wee hours of a new day excited to share something that really resonated with him.

"Hey Mom, listen to this." Seth read from his worn copy of *Don't Waste Your Life* by John Piper, that he'd read countless times, "Desire that your life count for something great! Long for your life to have eternal significance. Want this! Don't coast through life without a passion."

Seth's infectious excitement seemed to light up the dim, still room.

His love for God, His word and plan for his life, even in the midst of painful, sleepless nights, was an encouragement to me.

Equally significant in our lives, we loved our pastor, Dr. Mike Bullmore. He has been our pastor, teacher, and an extended family member for nearly two decades. I can't help but think that Seth developed a love for God's word, the gospel, and people due to Pastor Bullmore's impact. Our family has benefitted from his character, integrity, and faithful teaching more than anyone else in our lives. He recently said this.

> I love the privilege God has given me to be a pastor, and I love with a special kind of joy the privilege that God has given me to be a pastor to Seth and his family. During my twenty-five years of pastoring, I've repeated many things to the people of CrossWay (church). One of those things is, 'Nothing gets wasted in God's economy.' Over the years, as I've watched Seth grow from a boy into a godly young man, I have witnessed God keeping his promise to turn all things for the good of those who love Him. If I could, I would heal Seth in a heartbeat. But God knows better, far better, than I do. Someday, Seth will enjoy complete freedom from any disease. But for now, God is using Seth's situation to accomplish his good purposes in many ways—some very apparent and, no doubt, many unseen—and Seth is calling attention to the greatness of his God by entrusting himself to God's hand. And in due time, God will raise him up.

SETH EXPLORES HOSPITAL CHAPLAINCY

Ever since Seth was little, he had hoped to become a pastor of some sort. One day, Seth felt pretty discouraged because he knew his brain could not retain things like before. As time passed, he accepted the unlikely possibility of continuing education, especially seminary. Having realized that, he knew God would provide, equip, and reveal where he was to serve.

As Seth shared this with his beloved doctor one day, Dr. Fischer told Seth not to get discouraged. He suggested hospital chaplaincy might be the place God was calling him for vocation. Seth thought this was a grand idea! Even though hospitals had been a source of pain and agony over the years, Seth wanted a place to serve others. He felt confident he could minister from his own experiences with empathy and compassion. It was as if Dr. Fischer spoke life into dry bones. His wise perspective refreshed Seth. We set an appointment for Seth to meet the hospital chaplain of our local hospital. The chaplain allowed Seth to shadow him as he made his rounds for several hours. Seth was quiet and soaked it all in until a woman in the cancer unit gave him an opportunity to open up.

She told him, "I'm getting a methotrexate infusion. It makes me sick, and it burns going in."

Seth nodded his head. He knew that burning, sick feeling all too well. "Yeah. I get the same chemotherapy drug injection weekly, but just in a low dose."

"How long have you been on it?"

"Over a decade now. But God has been with me every step of the way."

I was in awe as I stood in the back of the room watching this unfold. Silence fell as she teared up.

She looked Seth in the eye and in a quivering yet confident voice declared, "If you can be on this poison for so long and still have joy and purpose, I can and will get through this!"

I could see their shared circumstances combined with her new sense of hope and surrendering the hard things to God created a bond between them that neither could have anticipated. She shook Seth's hand, thanked him for coming, and wished him well.

Seth also had a second opportunity to shadow the chaplain at Saint Marys-Mayo Clinic. It proved to be another great learning experience for Seth. The work was intense, mentally and physically harder than Seth anticipated. He was exhausted at the end of the day. The amount of seminary and higher education, studies in ethics, legal end-of-life decision-making, and conflict resolution counseling would be extensive. The on-call schedule, the extensive walking, and the potential germs made Seth think this may not be where God meant to use him.

As Seth came to understand he might not be called to go through seminary, he accepted that none of his sufferings was wasted. He told me he believed God was using what he was going through to share hope with others.

In light of Seth's search for a meaningful career, he knew he needed something that did not require driving. To apply for jobs, he needed a legal ID. One weekday, we found ourselves at the Division of Motor Vehicles waiting for our turn to go up to the window. Excitement permeated the room as teens poured in to take their driver's tests. Seth wasn't there for a driver's license like most young adults. He stared off into space. We waited only to secure a state ID for identification purposes.

It's easy to focus on what you cannot do instead of all you *can*. The struggle is real. Driving at this time would pose a danger to himself and others due to epilepsy, dizzy spells, and blackouts, to name a few. Seth had been robbed of much, but the things that truly mattered remained.

He lives a life with no regrets.

He lives with bold faith in Jesus.

He lives with great joy and appreciation for the small things.

He lives life with great passion and purpose.

He loves and serves others fiercely.

He makes a positive difference.

SETH'S NEW SUPER POWER

Seth's stomach continued to struggle to function properly. We had switched formulas, but it became clear his body needed more help. His team highly recommended a peptide formula that would be easier to digest. His team said if anyone needed it, it was Seth. They were prepared to fight insurance all the way to get this life-sustaining formula for him.

As Seth's disease progressed, days dragged into weeks of appointments, consultations, and recommendations.

The team unanimously recommended the option of bypassing his stomach. The downside meant Seth would still feel hungry and wouldn't experience the sensation of feeling full. The team kept Seth involved in all of the discussions and the pros and cons. Ultimately, the choice was his.

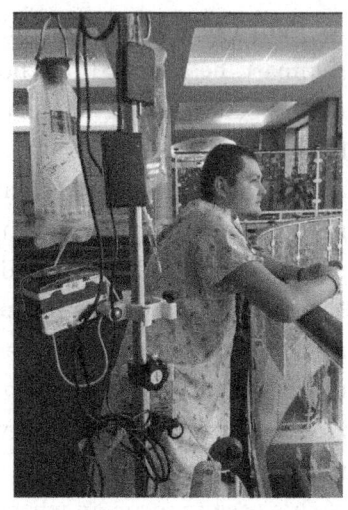

With all options presented, Seth chose to go from a gastrostomy tube to a gastrostomy-jejunostomy tube. A "G/J" tube administers nutrition straight to the part of the small intestine called the Jejunum. The "G" portion allows for the stomach to vent air and drainage and administer medications, while the "J" portion is primarily used for feeds.

The enteral specialist apologized that this wasn't offered sooner. Seth seemed to have fallen through the cracks when he transitioned from pediatric to adult care. He had suffered so long with pain, distention, nausea, and vomiting. Yet, he was young, and we had wanted to try every possible option with a glimmer of hope things would get better. Unfortunately, they didn't. A new option to bypass his paralyzed stomach would allow Seth to feed all night without the formula regurgitating or the danger of aspirating. He would no longer need continuous feeds during the day. For Seth, it was a no-brainer. No more backpack!

I eat while I sleep . . . what's your superpower?

SPRING 2019, UNEXPECTED NIGHT AT PROM

Seth had reservations about attending his Junior/Senior Prom as a junior that year. He explained it as a night of primarily eating and dancing. And since he couldn't do either, it kind of put a damper on attending. Prom, therefore, did not hold the excitement and anticipation that it did for most of his classmates.

One day shortly before prom, Seth's teacher called.

"You might want to encourage Seth to go to prom. There's something exciting brewing!" She was a bit vague but stirred my curiosity.

I didn't mention this conversation with Seth, but Donnie and I encouraged Seth to go. We told him we would attend and bring him home if he got too tired. We shared the excitement of picking out a tuxedo for the occasion, and soon Seth was eagerly anticipating the special event.

Donnie got choked up as he placed Seth's Pittsburgh Steelers cufflinks into his crisply starched double-cuff shirt. As his parents, we hadn't known if this night would ever be possible.

Seth asked his dad, "Are you crying?" They both laughed it off as Donnie pulled his son close for a hug.

Shiny, elegant gold and black decor lined the banquet hall. An overwhelming number of students and staff greeted Seth as he entered. I don't think I was truly aware of how many lives Seth had touched. Despite not feeling his best, he acknowledged each person with a big smile and a hug. Nearly five hundred students and adults filled the hall. The evening's emcee rose to the microphone to make an announcement. She seemed to glow with excitement.

"Aaand now, for the moment you've all been waiting for– The 2019 Prom King is . . . SETH BAYLES!"

The room exploded. Deafening shrieks thundered as Donnie and I watched hundreds of young people jump up and down, throw fists, high fives, clap, and shout in celebration. Seth was in total shock. He stood stunned in disbelief as the prior prom king placed a gold sash across his chest and a crown on his head. They also announced the Prom Queen, who was a good friend, but Seth was still processing his surreal moment. A moment that encompassed so. much. love. A celebration of unity and the impact of one life.

Although it was a great honor, I also saw a bigger picture. It was so much more than being voted Prom King. It was the student body accepting Seth for who he was. His faith, his positive spirit, and his kindness made everyone feel valued. Now this packed hall reflected all that back on him. God in him became a light to everyone whose path he crossed. What a great ending to Seth's junior year.

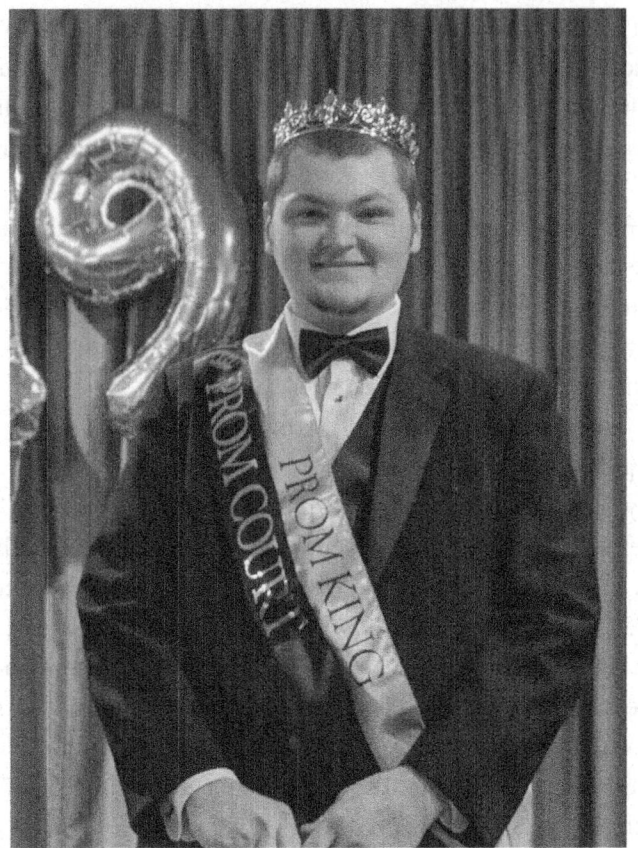

2019 Junior/Senior Prom King. With God, all things are possible!

CHAPTER TWENTY-THREE
LOOKS CAN BE DECEIVING

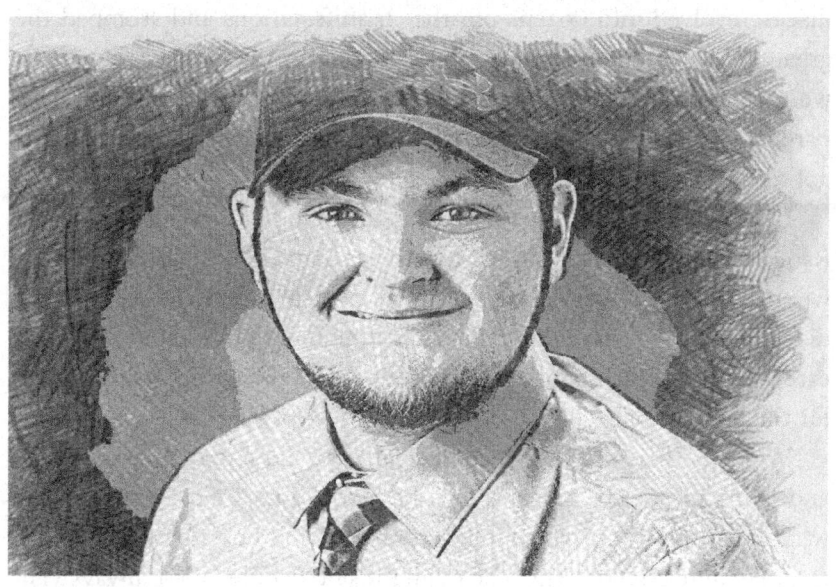

Everyone you meet is fighting a battle you
know nothing about. Be kind. Always.
–Robin Williams

Seth was now eighteen years old. By God's grace, Seth had now lived a full decade after doctors questioned whether he would survive this rare disease. We are forever grateful for the foresight and willingness of Dr. Ned and his team in Madison, Wisconsin, from 2008-2009. I will never forget their tireless battle to stop Seth's body from self-destructing. Even though there was insufficient documentation on what we could expect, doctors told us to expect the disease to be both progressive and degenerative. But, unfortunately, the disease had a mind of its own and changed course time and time again. No one could have anticipated that "progressive and degenerative" would mean head to toe.

The very beginning stage of the disease process that ravaged Seth's seven-year-old body was listed with the National Organization for Rare Disorders (NORD). If that wasn't bad enough, it didn't stop. The disease evolved into dozens of other manifestations and stumped the greatest world-renowned specialists. The more medical professionals we saw, the more admitted they'd never heard of a case like his. As a parent who at one time knew nothing about specialized medicine, I got a crash course.

If someone reading this doesn't understand "a day in the life" of Rare Disease, consider yourself fortunate. Some don't understand why we must go out of state for specialized medical care. Believe me, if we didn't have to, we wouldn't. There is a high cost to this level of vital care–and I don't mean just financially. It's a huge sacrifice, and not just for the patient.

When Seth isn't receiving medical care, he's pursuing normalcy and living life to the fullest. Since he "looks fine," most don't realize what he goes through to simply "show up," and he's totally okay with that. He understands. The war raging inside people is not always visible. Seth doesn't want anyone's pity. Sometimes, even we need a gentle reminder to give grace and understanding, be patient, and not judge. We never know what someone is going through or dealing with. We can never predict what type of day Seth will have or what unexpected issue may arise which means we have to cancel plans.

Each new day can bring new symptoms and new concerns. With new concerns comes a long list of new consultations with a variety of specialists at various locations. We are often shuffled around because we are stuck in an abyss of the great unknown, unspecified. I know medical providers can't be expected to know everything. But seeing one new provider after another who cannot help is disheartening.

Growing up, Dr. Ken was our go-to for the family's medical needs. Routine visits, broken bones, etcetera. As he tended to the medical situation, he'd talk about his experiences as a medic in the war. When he delivered me, my parents compensated him with fresh chickens and eggs from their farm. Every office visit, my mom brought a gunny sack of whatever was plentiful from the farm at the time: fresh sweet corn, currents, strawberries, potatoes, or peas. Dr. Ken never knew what was in that mystery bag, and he loved it.

I am grateful for how far the medical field has advanced. Without it, Seth wouldn't be alive. But sometimes, the current vast healthcare system seems unduly specialized, rushed, and impersonal. Having said that, however, we are also immensely grateful for the specialists who have devoted their lives to becoming experts in their field. Because Seth lives in a body with vast facets of dysfunction from head to toe, his medical team is extensive and growing.

To those who ask, "So, who does Seth see for the care of his diseases?"

Here's a list, in no particular order, to give an idea. These are off the top of my head, so I may be forgetting some. Like the scrolling list of credits at the end of a movie, here are the specialists/specialties who have been a part of Seth's medical journey.

Pediatrics
Complex Care Coordinator
Diagnostic Medicine
Adolescent Medicine
Adult/Family Medicine
Internal Medicine
Naturopathic/Chiropractic

Dermatology
Immunology
Epileptology
Allergy
Emergency Medicine
Endocrinology
Hematology/Oncology
Home Enteral Nutrition (HEN)
Nutritionist/Dietitian
Interventional Radiology
Nuclear Medicine
Gastroenterology/Hepatology
Dysmotility GI
Esophageal (upper) GI
Colorectal (Lower) GI
Otolaryngology/Ear, Nose, and Throat
Speech-Language Pathology
Genetics/Genomics
Rheumatology
Anesthesiology
Nephrology
Infectious Disease Specialist
Ophthalmology
General/Pediatric Surgeon
Cosmetic/Reconstructive Surgery
Physical Medicine/Rehabilitation and Physiatry
Physical/Recreational/Occupational Therapist
Pain Management
Neuropsychologist
Neuropsychiatry
Cardiology
Pulmonology
Wound Care Specialist
Child Adolescent Psychiatry
Urology

Orthopedics
Orthotist
Neurologists - nearly a dozen in various neuro subspecialties
Spine Center
Dental/Oral surgeon/Endodontist
Sleep Medicine/Sleep Apnea Specialty
Pathologists
Pharmacists
Social Workers/Case Managers
Disability specialists/consultants for various federal and state long-term care programs

Not only have we seen a plethora of providers in both pediatric and adult medicine, but I am also certain there are many more we don't know who worked behind the scenes on Seth's case. We are grateful for the tribe who collaboratively worked to enable him to be where he is today–alive!

We are indebted to all those who have prayed for wisdom, comfort, peace, and healing over the years. God is faithful! We are forever grateful for every doctor, nurse, assistant, intern, resident, tech, pharmacist, receptionist, insurance specialist, food service worker, hospitality team member, transporter, screener, scheduler, business office personnel, parking attendant, and volunteer that has served Seth at various medical facilities.

Seth's care reflects the very essence of a team approach. Although it has meant hundreds of thousands of miles in travel on our part, we acknowledge the options available to us as a blessing. We've met so many from around the world who don't have the access we have and who are far worse off suffering without prospects or hope. So, we are grateful. And that gets us through the tough times.

TENS OF THOUSANDS AND COUNTING

Over the years, many have asked Seth about his medical conditions. He struggles to communicate his unique and complex journey. We were elated to discover an organization called Beads of Courage. It's a non-profit organization dedicated to improving the quality of life for children and teens coping with serious illnesses. Mayo Clinic Rochester was one of over three hundred hospitals worldwide that participated in the Bead program.

For each injection, seizure, therapy session, testing, clinic visit, milestone, admission to ICU, hospital discharge, ambulance ride, or dozens of other treatments in between, the patient receives a specific bead. These are more than beautiful pieces of glass on a string. Each bead represents a tangible depiction of what Seth has endured over the years. Each patient creates necklaces of their unique journey. We added the "I can do all things through Christ who strengthens me Philippians 4:13" medallion front and center of Seth's collection.

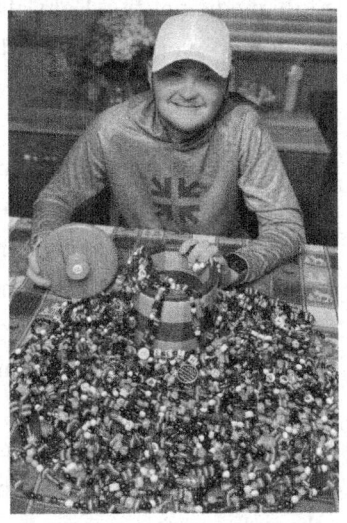

We don't know how to express the depth of gratitude we have for everyone who has served Seth since he was seven. He has accumulated several thousand beads from his medical journey–but it is mind-boggling to think it took *tens of thousands* of individuals to support the services those beads represent.

Talk about the power of community!

I have learned and grown so much through this journey. My son's invisible diseases have taught me about judging others unfairly. It's easy to make erroneous assumptions based on mere appearance alone. Seth may look perfectly healthy on the outside, but looks can be deceiving.

Looks Can Be Deceiving

Look fine
Not fine
Destruction on the inside

Organs failing
Life altering
No cure

Invisible disability
Put on a brave face
Put up a good fight

A censorious stranger yells from afar
Why are you parking in a handicapped spot?!
Too Lazy to walk? You should be ashamed!
Words sting
Looks of disgust cut deep

I long to tell you his story
But you turn away
Uninterested
Unaware of the suffering

If only You could feel my son's
Anguish
Exhaustion
Affliction
Discouragement
If only you could walk a day in his shoes–

But God...
Understands
Sees

Cares
Knows
Comforts
Protects
Loves

In Him
The broken are made whole
The weary are refreshed
The weak are made strong
Hope is restored
In Him we will
Extend grace
Smile
Help others
Exercise compassion
Exemplify joy
Show kindness
Love
Forgive

God has a plan

Invisible disease
Not Invisible to God

"Looks Can Be Deceiving" by Julie Bayles

CHAPTER TWENTY-FOUR

SENIOR YEAR... IT'S COMPLICATED

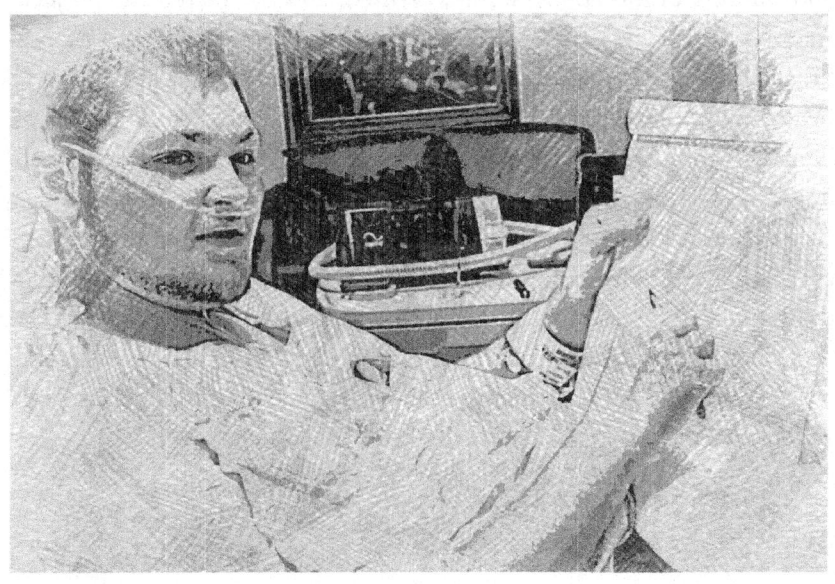

Is there any word more powerful than giving? Thanksgiving.
Forgiving. Care-giving. Life-giving. Everything that matters in
living comes down to giving.
–Ann Voskamp, *Be the Gift*

Fall 2019

Seth started his senior year and celebrated his nineteenth birthday in the same week. The school created a senior perk to purchase the right to "own" a premier parking spot. Seniors could paint it any way they wanted. The school called to tell us a parking place had been set aside for Seth, paid in full. Even though Seth didn't drive, he had the opportunity to express himself like the other seniors.

After Seth got over the initial shock, he began to plan. He wanted to display the superhero Seth's Journey shield and his favorite scripture. Along with his big ideas came limited energy. A crew rallied. From those who donated the cost of the spot to friends who helped with the design. Grandma Sue, an artist, helped transfer the design, and the rest of the family set up, painted, and completed the project. As we cleaned up, the sun began to set. I snapped a photo of our finished work to show Seth. Someone noticed the glow of a cross overhead between layers of blues, bright corals, pinks, and white clouds of light stretching across the sky. It was like God winked at our job well done.

I witnessed another example of how God can use whomever, wherever, whenever, and however he so chooses. Even myself, who can't draw a stick figure. Since I drove Seth to school, there would be no car to cover this work of art as students drove in and out. The verse and cross were a visible testimony, even on the asphalt of a public high school parking lot.

A CALL TO 9-1-1

Seth doesn't always listen to his body. Like other teenagers, he wants to keep up, but he doesn't always realize his limitations. One day after school, I found Seth sitting in his recliner, staring straight ahead. I sat down beside him and asked if he was okay. He attempted to talk, but his speech wasn't cohesive. Random syllables spilled out but were choppy and painstakingly slow. My stomach twisted in knots. I tried to get him to finish a thought, but he was fumbling and trying to get out of the recliner and go somewhere.

I barely managed to support his weight and transfer him from his recliner three or four steps away before he collapsed onto the bed. Was he having a series of seizures? He was coming in and out of whatever this was, conscious but unaware. I tried desperately to hold a conversation to arouse him to consciousness. He'd never seized this long before. He wasn't making sense. I could tell he was trying hard to speak—then would fall back in exhaustion and stop talking.

"What are you trying to tell me!" I was scared. Was he having a stroke? "You need to get up. We need to go to the hospital."

He didn't respond. He hates going to the emergency room. He always fought me. I was hoping he would snap out of it and object, but he didn't. I won't go into all the details that signaled red flags, but I knew we had an emergency on our hands.

"Seth, if you can't get up, I have to call for an ambulance!" I got a partial nod in agreement.

We had one designated outside door that led directly into his room, used only for emergencies. It gave ambulances and EMTs swift and easy access to help us. Since there are several houses on our property, I told Janae to go outside and lead the EMTs to our house and the entrance to Seth's room. Janae, who hoped to one day train as a firefighter or an EMT, remained calm and collected, her God-given gift. I was grateful for her. Within moments, EMTs entered with their bags and immediately surrounded Seth's hospital bed in the center of his room. Before I knew it, a sheriff's deputy appeared and stood just inside the door. All the commotion aroused Seth enough that when John, the captain of our fire department and friend, leaned over his bed and said, "Hey Seth," he acknowledged him. It was a comfort and blessing to have John there, and I told him so.

"I heard his name come over the radio, and I wanted to be the one to drive him."

His connection and desire to serve Seth personally meant the world to us. Captain John was one of many who came to visit Seth in the hospital over the next several days. We were usually out of state at a hospital, so it was a blessing to be close to home. Seth's dad and siblings visited daily to sit with him which gave me time to go home and shower. They watched a few football games on Seth's iPad. It was wonderful for us to be together, even if it was in the hospital.

Coach Mengel came to the hospital and brought along his playbook. He explained that he wanted Seth to draw up his own play for the homecoming game right there from the hospital bed. He would call it the "Seth Special." Seth perked up, and after grabbing a pencil, he started to draw a unique play of his own. He'd been watching and filming the guys for four years. He knew exactly what he wanted to propose. Coach and Seth's unique bond sealed the deal. Their love for the game, as well as the respect they had for one another, was as much fun to watch as the football game itself.

Seth seemed to have a different lens than I did about people. Maybe it was because he had such a real-time grasp of the frailty of this life. He had a magnetic personality and seemed to draw people in. Then, they fed off that and it worked both ways, so Seth made friends wherever he went. He had been known to hug strangers, he always has. He knew each day was a gift. It's not something I taught him. He just genuinely loved God, loved people, and lived life–even if it had to be from a hospital bed.

THE HIGH SCHOOL RALLIES

Even though Seth had to miss the October homecoming dance, parade, and activities because he was in the hospital, the school, teams, and classmates continued enthusiastically supporting him. A classmate sent us a video snippet of the homecoming pep rally. The coach can be heard addressing the packed bleachers on both sides of the cafetorium.

"As many of you know, Seth can't be here with us . . . I went to visit him last night in the hospital and asked him to draw up a play. We will be running that trick play, second quarter, for Seth, and hopefully, we can score in his honor."

We heard an explosion of cheers as the student body screamed their approval. Word spread fast throughout the school and social media posts. We received photos from Mrs. S of students sporting "Seth" on their wrists. Students took the initiative to go beyond wristbands. Seth was mesmerized by the photos that kept coming. The cross-country team wrote "#for Seth" on their calves. Someone sent us a picture of a banner crammed with well wishes. The eruption of support reminded Seth we were all in this together. He was so grateful he didn't know whether to smile or cry. The school told me they'd never seen an outpouring of this magnitude before. It was just as good for the school as it was for Seth. We were amazed over and over again by the power of community.

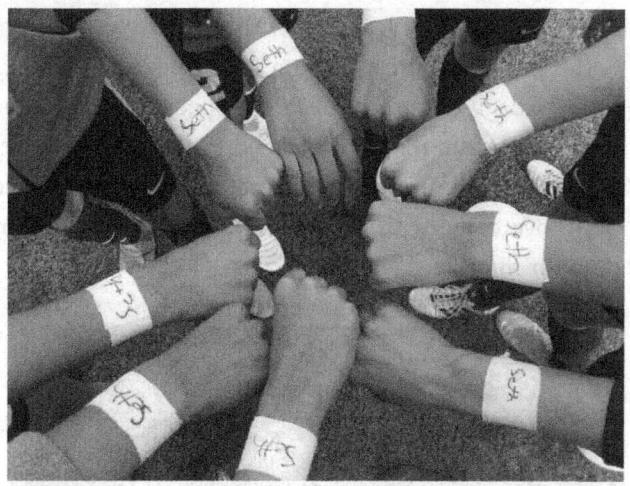

Many people in the community came to visit. Many others called and wanted to visit, but Seth had limited stamina to receive visitors. He was on oxygen and felt tired. Local medical professionals collaborated with Mayo working tirelessly to unpack this latest emergency. Seth's list of complications now included a (mini) stroke. We were thankful for the swift action and collaboration between the EMTs, the local hospital staff, and Mayo's input that helped Seth recover.

THE GAME PLAN

After nearly a week in the hospital, the doctor came in to discuss the game plan. Unlike when Seth first arrived by ambulance, he could now communicate his desires to the doctor with certainty. Seth told the doctor how important it was to him to make it to his high school football game.

The doctor hesitated for a moment, nodded his head, and with a big smile said, "Well then, we better get those discharge papers rolling and get you outta here."

Seth's goal was to make it to the last home game before he graduated high school. And God gave Seth the desires of his heart. We packed ourselves into the bleachers with the rest of the crowd and watched Seth soak it all in as he ran the endzone camera. In the second quarter, Coach called for the "Seth Special." When the Falcons made a twenty-yard gain, the crowd leaped to their feet and went wild. We saw Seth celebrating from the endzone as his play unfolded before his eyes. Seth, overcome with emotion and gratitude, stood by as the team lined up for high-fives and hugs.

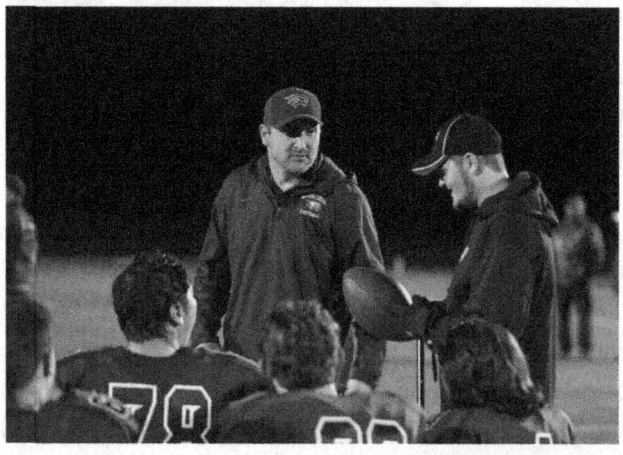

Coach Mengel and the team present Seth with the game ball.

At the end of the game, Coach Mengel huddled up the team. He waved Seth over, and the team gathered around with Seth in the center. Coach then presented the football to Seth. It was the first time Coach had ever given away a game ball to anyone.

What a night. The scoreboard didn't reflect a win, but spirits rose to a higher victory. The coach was so proud of how this team conducted themselves, came together as one, and supported each other. They also celebrated a young man who brought people together and inspired a community. Seth felt honored and overwhelmed by all the love and support. But no one truly understood what it meant for him–and for us–to simply have had the opportunity of reaching this milestone, a moment received as a true gift from God–to be alive!

NOVEMBER 2019, A NEW FIRE TO EXTINGUISH

As a mother of a child with complex, chronic issues, I could never let my guard down. One day could be as different as the next. Out of nowhere, Seth began having regular throat spasms. He felt like his throat was closing, making it difficult to breathe. I would find him pounding his chest with his fist in a panic. Seth had trouble finding words for the symptoms he was experiencing. His descriptions were, at times, difficult to interpret. He rarely complained about pain or problems with a mechanical breakdown of his bodily functions, so it was always a challenge to understand what he meant. Leading questions where he could give a one-word response were not helpful. I used simple questions hoping for a clear reply as I tried to figure out what he needed.

Seth had a long-standing relationship with his ear, nose, and throat doctors. The team had walked Seth through many difficult journeys. Like the handful of nodules he had developed in each lung, he had vocal nodules of unknown origin. The doctor regularly scoped Seth's throat with a camera to monitor any developing issues.

The ENT doctor we saw for these new symptoms referred Seth to consult with an esophageal gastroenterologist for the esophageal spasms since the ENT scope only went so far. We had a regular gastroenterologist who dealt with Seth's stomach issues. We had a motility gastro doctor who specialized in patients with gastroparesis (paralysis of the stomach). We had a lower gastro doctor we were referred to for bleeding that developed in the *lower* GI tract. Now we needed an *upper* gastroenterologist to deal with the esophagus. The scheduling staff told us there just weren't enough providers in that specialty. The waiting list was at least six months long. I systematically called to see if there'd been any cancellations, even though it could mean Seth and I would have to be on standby and willing to drive at a moment's notice. Months went by to no avail. While the spasms continued untreated, a bigger issue arose.

JANUARY 2020, A LIFE SENTENCE

We met with a new department for Seth's latest organ dysfunction. A month's worth of extensive testing did not reveal good news. Neurogenic bladder. Two words that would change and humble this young man for life. One more bodily function we had taken for granted was failing with no known cause and no known fix. The rare and mysterious features of Seth's conditions continued to develop with an unclear cause.

We were looking at a life sentence of catheter use. The nurse left us alone to process this latest development. The doctor came in several minutes later. She looked at Seth and was a bit taken aback. Then she looked at me.

"You would never know by looking at him . . ."

The doctor and I conversed, and then she turned back to Seth.

"So, Seth, how are you dealing with everything?"

Silence. I wondered what he would say. He thought for a moment. Then, he confidently responded, "God is great." It was as if Seth needed to say it out loud to himself. He needed to praise God through this storm.

The doctor nodded. "You have a very positive attitude about everything, and that is *so* important."

"It's all God. He has been with me since day one and gets me through each day."

The doctor and I were both moved by Seth's faith and positivity.

Seth left no room for pity - he wouldn't have it. I felt ashamed for complaining of far less significant things that had gone wrong in my life.

The physician's assistant came in holding a straight catheter and a tube of lubricant. "This is how you will need to relieve yourself about six times a day from now on. Mom, you will need to help at first. I will instruct you and walk you through—"

Seth politely but firmly interjected, "No, thank you, I'm good."

The nurse looked him in the eye and said, "But you're *not* good. You have to do this."

Seth looked at me in disbelief. I made a promise to Seth in the ER years ago: no more surprises. I would prepare him for what the next step was every step of the way. But this time I didn't and couldn't prepare him because I was just learning all of this myself. We had never seen a catheter before. Male catheters average fifteen to eighteen inches long (females average six inches).

His eyes were like, "You want to put WHAT in WHERE?"

The assistant explained, "The only alternative is a permanent Foley catheter. You could go with that and be done. It would be much easier than doing this six to eight times a day indefinitely." The choice was up to him. A permanent catheter meant he'd wear an external bag (likely hidden under his jeans) which he would need to regularly empty at school. Seth immediately refused. To choose intermittently catheterizing throughout the day wasn't any easier, but Seth has never taken the easy route.

"My mom will help me figure this out."

The assistant drained his bladder and trained us in the correct procedure. Because his brain signals did not communicate, Seth had no idea more than 600 ccs of fluid had been retained.

The PA spoke honestly about the challenges Seth could expect.

"It will be hard to get used to. You will bleed, clot, and it will hurt. Your body won't like it and will fight back with spasms. But it will get better, and it's far better than potentially causing kidney failure and eventually needing a kidney transplant."

Seth methodically nodded and acknowledged the medical details and instructions as he had for years. As we began to leave, he turned to her.

"Thank you. I really appreciate it."

"You're so welcome. I truly wish you well."

Seth asked to sit for a bit. I could tell he was grieving the loss. I cannot imagine how he felt as his body lost control of one system after another: his brain, various autonomic dysfunctions, his stomach, his bowels, and now, his bladder. This increased the complexity of managing his diseases individually and as a whole. Seth didn't complain. He didn't say anything. He just stared out the window. Sometimes silence and time is what's appropriate.

I gave him all the time he needed before we headed home. I anticipated the trip home would be drastically different from the trip there. At least now Seth had the tool he would need to relieve himself. We needed to put into practice the training we received and do so in public bathrooms. However, we immediately found ourselves in a challenging situation on the drive home.

Since Seth was an adult male who needed my assistance, we were at a loss for which public restroom we could use together. The hospital offered single special needs restrooms, but once we were on the road, imagine our dilemma. I told Seth we had no choice but for him to come into the women's restroom into a stall. He was not willing to surrender his "man card" to do it. I sure as heck wasn't going into the men's room at a truck stop past the urinals to go into the stall with him. I had no idea of the struggles that families regularly encounter when trying to provide support for an adult with complex needs. Now I could empathize. We tried several places but couldn't find a single private or family restroom on the road. Seth was miserable, so in desperation, I pulled over, so Seth could discreetly walk into a wooded area. This motivated Seth to practice at home repeatedly until he could manage on his own.

I also didn't realize catheters are by prescription only, so it's not like we could pick one up at our local store. The request needed to go through insurance and then a urology supply company. This was in addition to the medical equipment, oxygen, feeding supplies, and wound care companies I already dealt with monthly to supply all his needs.

Insurance fought us for weeks due to the cost and quantity even with doctor's orders, prescriptions, notes of extenuating circumstances, and medical necessity. What an injustice for anyone to be denied the ability to be able to perform the most basic bodily function. And depending on insurance, we couldn't even purchase out-of-pocket until this got resolved! We had to *wade and wait* through the process. I worked day and night and talked to everyone who would listen at the local and state level before finding a company that worked with us. We finally got our first monthly shipment (240 catheters), but believe it or not, the fight would start over again when the approval expired in one year.

Every single day patients, parents, caregivers, and guardians have to battle for coverage/denial, shortage/backorder issues, and recalls for a litany of needs: healthcare, dental, medications, durable medical equipment, incontinence and wound care supplies, tube feeding, oxygen, therapies, in-home services, and more. It's a full-time job. By God's grace and an obsessive amount of coffee, I pressed on. I would not stop until my son got what he needed to live.

MARCH 2020, THE COVID CATASTROPHE

A growing concern over a little-known virus referred to as coronavirus or COVID-19 suddenly took the world by storm and turned life as we knew it upside down. Everything we had come to know about the healthcare system changed overnight. For those with chronic medical conditions, it made a tough situation impossible. Let the nightmare begin. Facilities across the country were told to cancel all procedures. Due to the prospect of a bed and ventilator shortage, they reasoned that even routine procedures and treatments held the risk of exhausting resources. In addition, authorities didn't want to risk overloading the healthcare system as they waited for the influx of coronavirus patients that reports projected.

I tried not to be anxious, but the fear of not knowing when my son's treatment would resume was paralyzing. We prayed for those who were sick, for the families, for the exhausted workers, for our nation, for wisdom, for fear to cease, and for the return to normalcy.

We knew of heart-wrenching stories of those battling cancer who couldn't get their regular treatment and those who died alone. I had a newfound appreciation for the staff and world-renowned medical care that we had come to take for granted over the years. My heart sank every time the phone rang. Although I didn't want to face it, I knew the inevitable. Specialty department after department delivered the hard news. They called to cancel Seth's appointments. I knew it was selfish to plead with them, but I couldn't help it. This was my son. I'm sure it was just as hard for them. I tried to see it from their perspective.

I felt like we were in the Twilight Zone. Individuals introduced themselves as calling from Mayo Clinic, yet I could hear dogs barking and babies crying in the background. I realized they must be working from home. To add to the confusion, they admitted that, quite honestly, they didn't know much about what was going on.

I asked, "Are appointments going to be rescheduled? How long will it be? When should I call back? Who's making the decisions? Who can I talk to that would know?"

Every answer to all my questions was "I don't know." They told me restrictions and mandates were "fluid" depending on the latest infections and facility capacity numbers. Even those were misleading and inconsistent. They received morning briefs on a daily basis concerning what they were to do for each day.

I knew they were doing their best and their hands were tied, but we both agreed things could have been done better. Everyone was scrambling as this unprecedented pandemic revealed weaknesses and inefficiencies no one could have anticipated. The lack of solid information and unforeseeable plans made everything more complicated and difficult for everyone.

Details, statistics, and recommendations evolved rapidly. So quickly, local government officials couldn't even unpack them, let alone the caregivers. Procedures, mandates, and restrictions changed daily. Growing confusion, fear, and frustration permeated the nation. People were glued to their televisions. Restrictions were not in writing because they depended on many variables. Everything seemed to be up in the air, and Seth didn't do well without things explained to him in advance. We just had to wait it out. I remembered reading a quote from Ben Patterson once that said, "At least as important as the things we wait for . . . is the work God wants to do in us as we wait."

While we waited for the initial appointment for Seth's esophagus, his health was declining, and the throat restrictions happened more frequently. It was as painful for me to watch as it was for him to experience. His eyes watered as he struggled to breathe. The fact that he already had reduced lung function made the situation terrifying. We had more questions than answers.

And then the world shut down.

CHAPTER TWENTY-FIVE
LESSONS FROM QUARANTINE

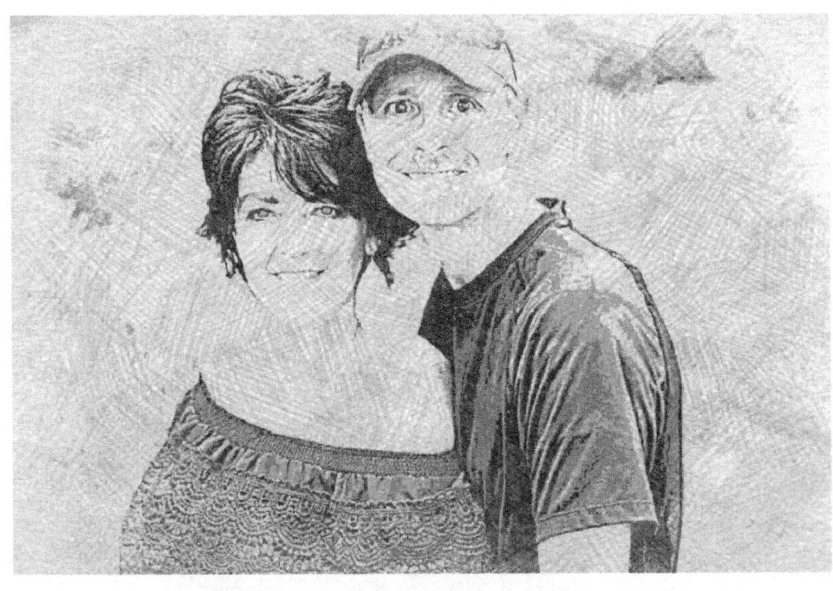

When asked if my cup is half-full or half empty, my only response is that I am thankful I have a cup.
–Sam Lefkowitz

A MANDATE ISSUED

We received the dreaded email. On March 17, 2020, our governor mandated schools to close indefinitely. With that communication, Seth's senior year of high school crashed. In an instant, the Class of 2020 was robbed of significant closure–no good-byes, no locker clean out, no long-awaited senior activities.

Several weeks had passed since the lockdown forced the closing of schools, businesses, and "non-essential" services. We were living out history in an unprecedented global event. Political voices created confusion, distrust, and division adding to the national stress level of uncharted medical information. The special needs community fell under particular stress. They needed routines for psychological calm, so the massive changes dished out an impossible hurdle for families in the special needs community to overcome. Rules and procedures–and common sense–flew out the window.

Our primary concern in all the upheaval focused on keeping Seth safe as best we could from germs, ensuring he had all of his medications, administering treatments, and helping him keep up with his studies toward graduation. Every week, Seth's teachers dropped off his schoolwork on our front doorstep. Donnie and I knew it was equally vital to calm fears and fight for normalcy for the rest of the family. All of a sudden, they didn't see their dad due to long hours. They couldn't meet with friends, go to school, or go anywhere unless it was absolutely necessary. The interstate was deserted, and the two highways at the corner of our farm were silent.

We entered the world of virtual doctor visits. I appreciated the germ-free option, and it saved us the commute to Minnesota. The drawback, however, meant Seth didn't have access to his regular therapies. Seth's deconditioned state from being homebound had become increasingly apparent. Inactivity made his joints stiff resulting in limited mobility. The domino effect meant his pain was constant. He wanted to do his schoolwork in bed due to overwhelming fatigue.

I couldn't bear to watch Seth decline, so I contacted his physical therapy coordinator, and we came up with an in-home program. Seth was not happy. He assumed quarantine meant taking time off, but I knew he needed to keep pressing on. I picked up exercise equipment and started Seth's home therapy with him several days a week. I woke Seth like any other school day which was difficult for him to understand.

"Why do I have to get up? Why can't I just sleep in?"

"I would love nothing more than to spend my days in bed. We all want comfort and ease, not the hard things. But easy isn't always what's best for us."

I pushed Seth in his wheelchair up to the table and instructed him to use the hand bike, a tabletop exercise. He needed it to increase cardio and upper body strength. Seth begrudgingly rotated the pedals with his arms and hands for a few minutes until he was exhausted. I knew he was fatigued, but I also knew we had to trust God to supply all of Seth's needs and strength. Isaiah 40:29-31 came to mind. "He gives power to the weak and strength to the powerless. Even youths will become weak and tired, and young men will fall in exhaustion. But those who trust in the LORD will find new strength. They will soar high on wings like eagles. They will run and not grow weary. They will walk and not faint."

A few weeks later, in addition to the untreated throat spasms, Seth developed a cough and other complications. I was concerned, but the last thing I wanted to do was take him to the ER during this crazy time. I phoned the after-hours doctor for a professional opinion.

"You need to head to the Emergency Department right now. You will both need a mask."

"Seth has a mask, but I don't have one."

"It can be anything. They just want your mouth and nose covered. Also, they might not let you in. Be prepared for that battle. Bring your legal paperwork. It may or may not help, but it's the best chance you have."

Donnie helped Seth get ready while I checked online for "the quickest way to make a mask." I grabbed a pair of my zebra-patterned leggings and cut off one leg. I placed two rubber bands over it, one on each end for ear loops. Then, I tucked the extra material on each end toward the middle, and voila! In thirty seconds I had a designer mask.

SETH SPEAKS UP

I called our local hospital and learned there was a five-hour wait, so I decided to drive thirty miles to a larger hospital. As we made our way around to the emergency room, it was like we were transported to some sort of sci-fi movie set. Large white tents stood in front of the doors manned by people in white hazmat suits. We saw security everywhere and several checkpoints with signs giving warnings and instructions. I stopped the car as someone approached and tapped on Seth's window. It scared him half to death. I rolled down Seth's window as the Michelin Man leaned down to peer into the car.

The person (whether male or female, we couldn't tell) communicated as best they could from behind their hood, neck gaiter, mask, goggles, and face shield.

A muffled voice asked, "Who's the patient?" When I motioned to Seth, they put up their hand and told him, "Stay seated." They scanned Seth's forehead with a thermometer. "Step out of the car. You can pick him up when we call to say that he is done."

"NO! I'm NOT going! Mom, don't let them take me!"

I leaned over to explain. "I have Power of Attorney for Healthcare for my son, and there are extenuating circumstances for why he needs me with him."

"Do you have the legal paperwork with you?"

"Yes, right here."

"Pull up and park ahead. I have to get special clearance."

Special clearance to stay with my son? I felt like we had entered into a world I no longer recognized.

As they left, Seth started to panic. It looked like he was hyperventilating under his mask. With Seth's sinus tachycardia (high heart rate at rest), high levels of stress could push his numbers off the chart. He wore a daily patch that lowered his blood pressure, but this was far from an ideal situation. Seth did not handle new or unexpected circumstances well.

"Seth, what do you want me to do?"

"Let's get the Hello Kitty outta here!"

While we waited for clearance, I threw out a compromise. "Let's see what they say. If they don't accept us *both*, then we'll leave." That swift reassurance seemed to calm him, and he agreed. It felt like everyone was on edge and very tense. Everything was methodical, with no personal interaction, almost robotic.

Seth was a very social person. He was used to talking with people and acknowledging others. We could barely see the eyes of the human behind the protective equipment. I wondered how they felt. Scared? Overheated? Overworked? I smiled instinctively as I often did to show kindness and gratitude, but I think my mask concealed my attempt.

We did receive special clearance which I was not expecting. I was so grateful they led us past the waiting crowd and into a private room. We felt our concerns were heard and validated. The doctor came up with a game plan, and Seth was released to the comfort of home.

DONNIE

Throughout the quarantine, Donnie continued to work out of state as a manager for a grocery chain, sometimes pulling *ninety* hours a week without overtime pay. At one time, everyone in his meat department was out with the virus, and he was running the entire department by himself. Donnie returned home one night just before 10:00 p.m. As he started to undress to take a shower, I piped up.

"You can't do this anymore. You left the house this morning at 3:00 a.m.! I'm worried about you. Can't they get help? Can't they find someone else?"

"No. People are dropping like flies. I'll be fine. Plus, I have to put food on the table."

"Are you scared?"

"Not for me." He put his sweatshirt down and looked at me with tears in his eyes. "I can't help but think–it's my greatest fear–that I bring home this virus to my family. Especially Seth. It's on my mind all the time."

We held each other without words. Then prayed for God's protection and strength.

It was our thirtieth wedding anniversary. Only God could have known when I married Donnie what would fill the three decades leading up to this day. For years, I dreamed of going to Hawaii and celebrating on the beach–maybe renewing our vows. After Seth got sick and we couldn't leave him, I thought about making it a family trip. For many reasons, it wasn't meant to be, and I embraced the life we had.

Like many little girls, I dreamed of being swept off my feet by Prince Charming. We'd have a gazillion kids, a white picket fence, and a fun and happy life. When Donnie and I started dating, it was easy to picture a life together forever. Ah, young love! When I spoke my marriage vows to Donnie five months before my eighteenth birthday, I was a blank canvas. The words "For better, for worse, in sickness and in health" nonchalantly rolled off my tongue. Little did I know that meant commitment through suffering, sickness, shattered dreams, separation, and survival mode. Over the years, we endured many challenges and heartbreaking losses, multiple miscarriages, financial turmoil, and pain. We found out love wasn't so easy.

Now, here we were three decades later celebrating the day we got married, sitting in a house full of kids and chaos, in quarantine and a mandated lockdown, during a global pandemic. We dug up old photos from the basement and reminisced. The kids giggled, hardly recognizing their parents–Donnie with a head full of hair and me, "Julz," with my big bleached blond hair. As they picked through the photos, Donnie and I slipped away from the house and took a walk on our farm.

Donnie was a good, hard-working man. He loved God and his family. When our son got sick, Donnie worked even harder to keep the family afloat. He never complained about wanting an easier life, at least not out loud to us. He sacrificed to make sure our family had all they needed. Through the trials and suffering, Donnie showed me true love.

Young love romance after the traditional "I do" matured into a commitment of life after the honeymoon. After fighting tooth and nail to protect our marriage, we walked together as two weak vessels depending on God. I never imagined this kind of trauma along with the work and love and fun of a houseful of kids. Truly, we were blessed beyond measure. It wasn't the life I envisioned, but we had a good life.

We hadn't spent a penny on our anniversary this year. Visions of a ceremony in Hawaii had long faded, but we renewed our vows day after day as we tackled life's jagged journey together. As the sun set over the prairie grass, Donnie and I lingered in the moment. He wrapped his arms around me and drew me close with a kiss. I felt a deep sense of contentment.

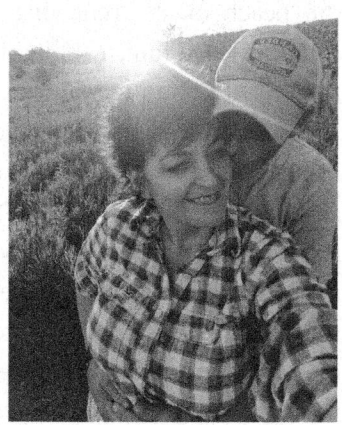

May 2020

School was still virtual, but school authorities allowed certain limited outdoor activities if the risk of germ transmission was low. The administration decided to schedule the traditional senior drive-through. This final Falcon experience gave graduating students the opportunity to drive in parade fashion through the high school parking lot while staff lined up to send them off.

Unfortunately, Seth lay in the hospital for this event and could not participate in the drive-through. Football Coach Franz was not about to let him miss out. He asked someone to shoot a video from Seth's perspective in a car, slowly approaching staffers who held signs and banners. As the car drove past, one by one the staff shouted their well wishes, "Congrats, Seth! Way to go! Good work, man! Whoo-hoo Seth!" The camera eventually panned to a contribution pail at the end labeled, "Seth's Journey," for the Ronald McDonald House. No way could I watch this without getting emotional. Seth watched from the hospital bed in awe that they went to all that trouble to include him. What a sweet memory to finalize the close of his high school years.

Finally, Mayo Clinic called to reset schedules. We were beyond grateful. The long-awaited consultation with the esophageal gastroenterologist gave us hope we'd get answers and some relief for Seth.

Through connections in the medical community and social media discussion groups, I understood the growing tension at facilities between the exhaustion, miscommunication, mandatory furlough, and added pressure of choosing who would make that first round to be rescheduled.

On our way to Mayo, I received a call. The doctor on the other end identified himself in a tone that took me aback. I knew that tension was at an all-time high for healthcare workers, but this call I could cut with a knife. This was a doctor we had previously met with who'd informed us that he was not the best candidate due to the extent of Seth's case. He had already made it clear in the office that he didn't know anything about motility disorders (digestive movement problems). I understood and appreciated him for being upfront with me. It's not ideal for any parties involved to accept a patient and move forward with care if the doctor doesn't think they can add value to the team. I respect any doctor who will admit that.

I pulled off the road to give him my undivided attention. He informed me that he was *canceling* our consultation with the upper gastroenterologist. This was especially disappointing for Seth's sake because we had already waited so long.

He said, "You have too many cooks in the kitchen - less is best."

Yes, I could agree with the sentiment. It may seem obvious to eliminate some doctors, but a more thorough look in Seth's file would reveal that it's complicated. Not every doctor listed, however, was an active part of his care plan.

Some doctors had walked into the exam room and simply said, "This case is too rare. I'm sorry you were put on my schedule. You will not be charged for this visit," and walked out.

I also understood studying Seth's extensive file takes an exorbitant amount of time. To further complicate things, when Seth transferred from the pediatric side of the clinic to the adult side, we had to start over. Patients were expected to coordinate care on their own with new doctors and new referrals. Details, specialists, testing, and care for the complex easily fell through the cracks, and communication was challenging even for someone without cognitive limitations. No one wanted fewer doctors, less testing, trips, and treatment than Seth and I. If only . . .

I listened and extended gratitude for his desire to simplify things. At the same time, my son was suffering without a voice due to his limitations. "All we want is to get to a specialist as quickly as possible. We need to get to the root cause in order to prevent further damage as well as get Seth relief."

I respectfully tried to communicate several reasons why I thought we should stick with the referral orders. I poured out my heart regarding all of the problems and concerns Seth had suffered as he waited. Our referring ENT was confident that Seth needed an upper GI evaluation.

As if the doctor on the other end of the phone had heard enough, he interrupted—

"I'm canceling this appointment, and I will be in charge of what happens next. I am putting in orders for a swallow study and medical device to be placed."

My mind was reeling. I asked about the role of this device, how it would be placed, and what difference in treatment that type of information would provide. I didn't like the fact that the device would need to be surgically placed to obtain data, and I told him so. Strangely, unlike Seth's doctors who have always cautioned *all* surgeries come with risk, this doctor downplayed any risk. He communicated it was inconsequential and in approximately five days it would naturally travel out of his system. I was still uncomfortable about having anything implanted that needed to "move through his system" when the movement through his digestive tract was slow or ineffective due to muscles nearly paralyzed.

I found myself in the middle of an awkward power struggle between me, the referring doctor's orders, this doctor, and–most importantly–my son.

"Please," I pleaded. "We have waited for this appointment for so long. Please keep the referral for the upper GI on the schedule. Both the referring doctor and I want their opinion and I think that's reasonable."

The doctor on the phone insinuated that I was "just a mom."

I politely but assertively replied. "I may be just a mom, but I know my son."

I felt the crushing weight of not being heard. My voice started to quiver. Still parked on the side of the road, I pleaded with a doctor who didn't know my son to listen to my concerns. The more I shared my thoughts on the matter, the more there seemed to be no room for negotiation. Out of frustration, I voiced that I didn't feel the benefit would outweigh the risks. His callous response was more painful than the situation at hand.

"Nothing will go further until this is done!"

There was a long, awkward pause. Seth's only hope was to get through the procedure to appease this doctor, so we could get the esophageal gastroenterologist back on the schedule.

I felt backed into a corner . . . defeated.

CHAPTER TWENTY-SIX
STUCK!

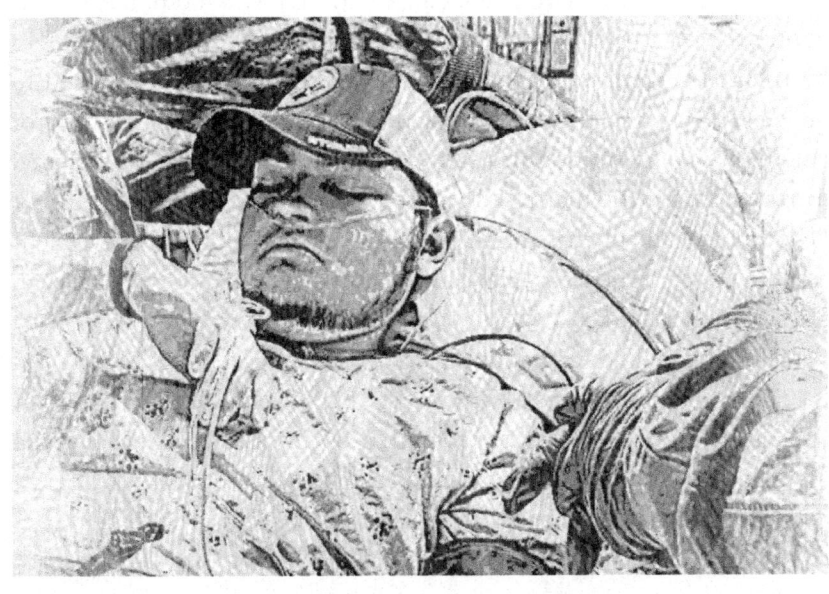

God continues to get me through the toughest times. It's all God!
–Seth Bayles

Ironically, I did not receive a follow-up call from the doctor who ordered the May 19 surgery. In fact, I have yet to hear from him. Instead, that doctor appointed a new GI doctor. So much for "less cooks in the kitchen." Instead of a phone call, the new doctor messaged me through the patient portal. In her message, she apologized that the device, unfortunately, malfunctioned. Instead of recording for ninety-six hours, it stopped after only one hour. Therefore, they had no valid results.

Wait, what? So . . . Seth endured this surgical procedure, the implanting of the device, and all the pain (not to mention wearing a monitor for days and the time spent documenting) for absolutely nothing? Talk about pouring salt on an open wound!

The doctor's message stated they contacted the company about the problem, and we would not be charged. This was of no consolation. She encouraged me to reach out to her if Seth felt up to repeating the procedure. I already knew the response before it came out of his mouth: "Absolutely not!" Although Seth's sentiments were mine, I tried to be gracious. After all, it wasn't her fault and couldn't be undone. It was what it was. She hadn't even ordered it - she was just the messenger. I reiterated if there was a small percentage that something could go wrong, chances were, it tended to happen with Seth.

Sadly, that was the element of rare we had grown accustomed to. I didn't share how marginalized the prescribing doctor made Seth and me feel. As for Seth repeating this, we didn't want it done in the first place. We needed to heal and move on. I had hoped this was the end of this fiasco. Little did I know–it was just the beginning.

June 7, 2020

Virtual events can have perks. We were able to watch the live broadcast of Seth's Senior Award Ceremony, from his hospital room in Milwaukee. The Central High School 2020 Senior Superlatives of "Best Personality" and "Biggest Heart" went to Seth! Previously in his sophomore year, he was awarded "Best Smile," and in his junior year, "Most Positive Attitude." Although he also received an academic medal, the academic achievements paled in comparison to the character traits Seth maintained while enduring his medical challenges. Donnie and I considered these traits more important.

Over the next few weeks, I rushed Seth to multiple emergency room visits. We used several local emergency rooms depending on wait time, equipment available, and other factors. He experienced new stomach pain, and his feeding tube kept malfunctioning. No one could figure out why. Each emergency visit got harder on Seth. They tried everything to free the obstruction. When they finally decided to change the tube out surgically, doctors had quite a time deflating the retaining balloon. Even after the deflation, they still struggled to remove the tube and then wrestled to insert a new one. This went on several times while Seth gripped the sides of the gurney and tried to breathe through the pain.

One doctor gave up. They called in a specialist to assist. As usual, everything about Seth's situation proved challenging. I asked to be in the procedure room since we had been through this before. They felt bad for all Seth endured. Four people were working on him at one time. I couldn't understand why this was happening. I watched as they bent the guidewire and then changed to a thicker gauge wire, which bent as well. Finally, he called in yet another specialist. I was worried the force might perforate the intestine, and then we'd really have a critical situation on our hands. As Seth lay on the fluoroscopy table, he was able to catch a much-needed break while we waited for another specialist to arrive.

As the doctor stared at the screen, I heard him say, "I just don't understand what could be holding things up. It doesn't make sense."

Suddenly, it dawned on me, "He had a device placed several weeks back. As long as we are here, would you check his abdomen to see if it's still in there?"

Sure enough, we saw it! I could only wonder what role the device played in all of this. I was trying to piece it all together. Was this device the cause of the repeated obstruction? If the formula was left to coagulate and harden, could it obstruct the end of the tube? The ER doctor considered it a definite possibility. I asked him to save the image for Seth's doctor at Mayo. All of this happened on a Sunday.

First thing Monday morning, I called his GI and explained the situation. I told her to look over the local hospital records for the imaging. She wasn't convinced that the trouble was caused by the device because she didn't see how it was possible for the device to still be in him. It defied logic. It should have long been expelled. Because it had been several weeks, I understood her skepticism. But, as I had told her, if a small percentage of something could go wrong, it would with my son. I reminded her that the device in question wasn't supposed to malfunction, yet it did.

After she reviewed the image, she messaged me through the patient portal. In her response, she concluded she saw "a button from Seth's trousers."

Really? I know what I saw. It was *not* a button. I politely disagreed since I knew there would be no good end to arguing.

It reminded me of other times when medical professionals didn't listen to or believe me. Since Seth's journey began at seven years old, things happened and caused pain that couldn't be seen. He could be the poster child for the mystery of invisible diseases. Even though my gut told me something was wrong, and Seth's body showed evidence, it was disregarded. I was so tired of being dismissed as "just a mom." I was so grateful for all of the good medical professionals who helped us along the way, but here, once again, I did not feel heard.

And my son was paying the price.

Over time, Seth's pain became more diverse. He'd been dealing with relentless headaches and back pain for months and was scheduled for a lumbar and thoracic magnetic resonance imaging (MRI) of his spine. Since the device should have been expelled within a week, he was cleared for the imaging. A thirty-day waiting period was protocol for any temporarily implanted device and assured a broad safety net for the patient.

Because of the situation, his pain, and the need for confirmation of the placement and function of his tube, they did an x-ray. This turned out to be a blessing in disguise because the device (that no one but me believed was still in him) was metal and showed up. The whole month since the implant was a train wreck. I would not schedule an MRI because with a metal device in him the magnetic pull of the MRI could cause serious damage.

The MRI was on hold, his back pain was on hold, he had a foreign object stuck inside him somewhere, and now his feeding tube is obstructed. Since the tube was his only source of nutrition, this became our new emergency. He couldn't seem to get a break.

At the local ER, we had to, again, abide by COVID protocol. Seth begged the staff to let me stay with him. From what we encountered, the new restrictions caused more harm than good. Separating families caused high levels of anxiety when family members needed each other most. What they called "fluid" policies seemed to defy common sense and reasoning. But we were gracious and kind to the workers caught in the middle.

Whenever I asked to stay with Seth through procedures, they asked if I had guardianship since Seth was over eighteen. Apparently, medical power of attorney no longer proved sufficient per their protocol due to restrictions.

Seth had to endure laying still on his back in the fluoroscopy room while a team tugged and pulled on his stomach, abdomen, and groin. No IV, no pain medicine. *Why does everything have to be so difficult?* I told them about the stuck device, so that they could be aware of that issue. After several hours, the team finally managed to insert a new tube. We were discharged the same night.

Within the next week, the same scenario. Same local ER. This time, the healthcare workers remembered me. They remembered I was gracious and thanked them for their help. This time they asked me to come back with him. Once in the procedure room, the attendants and I decided to schedule imaging right away to try and shed light on the root cause of the tube obstruction. They knew I would be able to identify the device.

It was now *five weeks* after the surgical placement of the device. It should have exited his body in *five days*. Poor Seth. This wasn't fair. The tech went into the back room to look at the x-ray. I explained to her what we were looking for.

She yelled from behind the wall, "I don't see it . . . . I don't see it."

Dare we trust a glimmer of hope that maybe he did finally pass that menace of a device? I suggested they pan up for one final look.

"I see it!"

The technician was gracious enough to let me go back there to confirm and take a picture of it. It looked like it had moved in the *wrong* direction, up toward the rib cage instead of down through his digestive system. Seth wore nothing but a hospital gown, so *no buttons* could possibly be identified. The device was as clear as day. The doctor could no longer refute this. I sent her a message with the picture. I circled the device and drew an arrow pointing to it. I also called the doctor and told her we needed to get this out of him!

All of this was so bizarre. I thanked God for walking beside us. I credited God for helping me advocate, giving me a voice on Seth's behalf, giving me the intuition to stall the MRI, and for staff allowing me to stay, despite restrictions. As we drove home, Seth lay in the car exhausted and weary.

"Mom, I want this thing out!"

"Seth, I hear you, and I am going to fight for you."

Now that they had evidence, they were transparent about not knowing what to do. However, they still weren't clear exactly where it was. The images were limited in dimension, and the human digestive tract is long, with much of it inaccessible.

The plan, as I understood it, was to work from the least invasive procedure of flushing it out to the worst-case scenario of cutting his abdomen open. A team was trying to come up with options in between. They planned to create a multi-step plan. If an attempt failed, they would initiate the backup plans.

June 24, 2020

Seth was feeling a lot of emotions. The news of his pending procedures loomed ahead, and the unknowns were difficult to process. On top of that, the challenge of the pandemic's "social distancing" and trying to read what others were comfortable with was very confusing. Seth was a hugger. Touch was his love language, but overnight that was not allowed, not even handshakes. The lack of physical touch and genuine interaction was especially difficult for him. Some doctors' offices had caution tape partitioning off part of the patient bench closest to the doctor's desk. In order to keep a distance in the elevators, tape on the floor boxed off the corners for individuals to stand.

Relationships became strained. People were easily triggered and offended. We wanted to respect whatever others needed to feel safe, but everyone had varied and strong opinions, which caused division, even within families. We were often in the wrong over simply needing clarification about what was acceptable. It was different everywhere we went. Smiles were hidden behind masks. Fear and doubt overshadowed people's eyes.

We heard the buzz about a special outdoor "Farewell Rochester" concert the Singing Surgeons planned. I told Seth about it, and he perked right up. Although we were exhausted after a full day of appointments, I knew we needed a diversion. So, the evening before the scheduled hospital admittance, Seth and I drove less than a mile from the clinic to the venue.

The weather was perfect. We basked in the glow of the warm, evening sun. A wooden fence draped with hanging greenery and colorful potted plants surrounded and hung throughout the garden patio cafe. Patio lights hung overhead as people gathered around tables or on the lawn. Seth took a seat as I plunked down on a blanket next to him. The intimate gathering with a small-town feel began to fill our emotional cup. Community friends we'd made in Rochester stopped to say hello. The personal connections combined with fresh air, sunshine, music, and smiles refreshed us.

The singing orthopedic surgical residents, who warmed the world's hearts with their piano and singing renditions of hope, covered the crowd in love through their concert. Our hearts were sad their residency ended, and they had to move on. As one of the doctors played the keyboard and the other sang their farewell tribute, Seth leaned in toward me.

"Mom," he whispered, "do you think it would be okay if I went up afterward and shook their hand?"

Seth hesitated because of the clinic protocol, and this was a doctor. However, he really wanted to express his appreciation. Since first hearing "Everything's Gonna Be Alright," their inspiring music blessed us over the months when we needed it most. This was our connection and I wanted to tell them.

I nodded my approval and smiled. At the end of the concert, Seth approached the singing doctor and stuck out his hand. Ignoring Seth's outstretched hand, he opened both arms for a big bro hug. There are those moments as a mom I could not possibly plan for, the ones that put a lump in my throat while fighting back tears. This was one of them, and tonight was a gift. God showered our weary hearts with His grace. He knew exactly what we needed to lift our spirits, fill Seth's emotional tank, and strengthen us for tomorrow.

The following morning, to attempt the least invasive method first, Seth was sent to a special wing of the hospital to receive a colon flush-out. We entered a small, stark room with a bed, a toilet and sink, and a wall of supply cabinets. The orders called for 1,000 ccs of plain warm water. The specialty nurse and I were in the room with him. Seth was determined to do whatever it took to get the demon device out.

The first attempt did not flush the device out. The nurse explained to us we needed to try again. Not how Seth wanted to spend his morning, but he readily complied because his mind was set on results. After the second flush attempt, the device had not yet been expelled. Attempt number three–no results to celebrate. Ugh. Let's try one more time. Each flush-out drained Seth, and he grew weaker as the attempts progressed. With only three steps from the bed to the toilet, I struggled to bear his now nearly dead weight. I grew more and more concerned. Finally, after the fourth fail, the older nurse turned to me.

"In all of my years of training and experience, (I know) the body is not meant to endure this much. But I'm not the doctor." The nurse locked eyes with me. "I have no choice but to call the doctor. I have never done more than four consecutively."

With the phone in hand, she said, "The doctor wants to move forward. Can you do that, Seth?"

Seth managed the words, "I don't quit that easy," as if he was trying to convince himself to press on.

After he bravely completed rounds five and six, the nurse went back to the phone. But again, the doctor insisted the nurse ask Seth if he could endure one more.

I went over to comfort Seth as he looked like he was going to be sick and rolled into the fetal position.

The nurse said, "Seth, they want you to try one more, but Seth, you can say no."

She read my mind. I encouraged Seth as he looked at me.

"You have been brave, and it's okay to stop. You're in control."

He slumped down on the gurney. "I can't take any more." He covered his eyes, trying to hide the tears. He spoke without moving, "It's not out yet, is it."

The nurse exhaled. "No, Seth, I'm so sorry."

Weak and frustrated, Seth's body began to tremble as he sobbed.

I insisted we meet with the doctor face-to-face. There was no denying the predicament we found ourselves in. Hours later, the doctor worked us into her schedule at the end of the day. With her hand on her chest, she said, "I am so sorry. I didn't realize this couldn't be reached this way."

"How could you not know? Where is this stuck?"

"It's hard to say," was her only reply.

Seth was discouraged that what he had endured was the *least* invasive. In his mind, at this point, being cut open seemed like the quick and easy way. The team was discussing a rather new procedure discovered in Japan just after Seth was born. Known as a double-balloon enteroscopy, doctors used it when both endoscopies and colonoscopies were not far-reaching enough to retrieve something or to stop bleeding. They needed to compile a team who was comfortable using this technology and willing and available to perform it asap. If they were unable to retrieve the device using this procedure, they'd be faced with the final, and most risky, step–surgery. Everyone on the team wanted to avoid that at all costs. It was the worst-case scenario for Seth due to all of his risk factors as well as the possibility of causing more harm.

We finally had a comprehensive plan, but the team insisted they needed more time to get all their ducks in a row. After that, Seth fell asleep in the office out of pure exhaustion. It was now Friday evening. They told me it would be best to take Seth home and let his body get some much-needed rest for what was to follow the next week.

Seth was thrilled at the thought of going home, even if we had to turn around and drive back in less than forty-eight hours. It gave me time to attend church with my family, which was my therapy. I needed that perspective and spiritual renewal for the week ahead.

Upon our return on Monday, Seth had to endure yet another deep nasal swab. I was so stinkin' frustrated that we had to then wait up to forty-eight hours for the results. Once we got a negative result, we could proceed. Poor Seth! Poked and prodded in so many orifices while dealing with this device trapped in his body for a month and a half. We couldn't wait to put this nightmare behind us.

CHAPTER TWENTY-SEVEN

SHE'S NOT A VISITOR, SHE'S MY MOM!

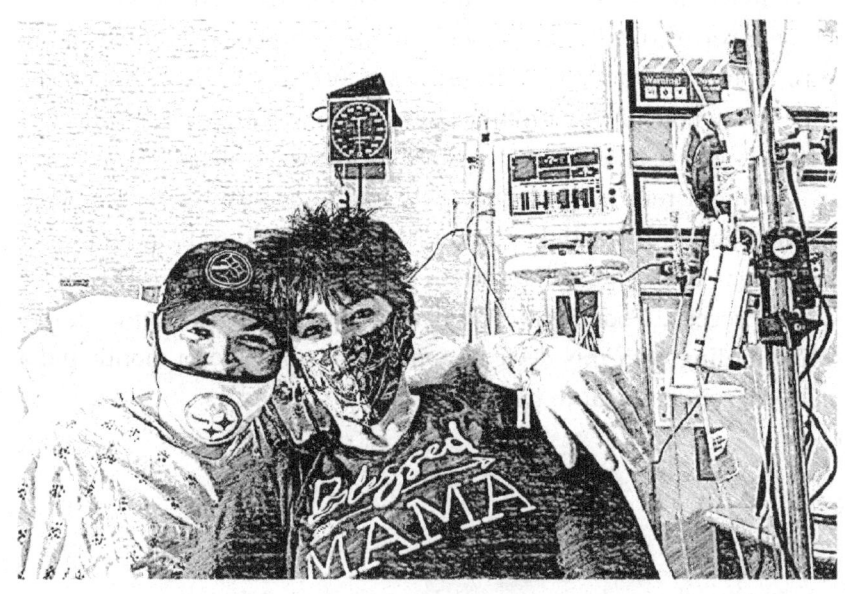

God does his deepest work in our darkest hours.
–A.W Tozer

End of June 2020

We settled into Seth's hospital room. He donned a standard blue hospital gown as he had countless times before. We met his nurse for the day. Her kindness shone through her big smile as she got to know us. She asked Seth several questions that he couldn't answer. Seth's difficulty communicating his complex medical history and extensive medication list made him uncomfortable. The nurse picked up on it.

"Seth, I can't even pronounce most of your medications."

Seth chuckled. "Me neither."

The nurse then turned to me. "Okay, Mom, let's do this."

We spent the next twenty minutes reviewing medications by name, dosage, and the last time he'd taken them. Seth giggled as he watched an old black-and-white sitcom on his iPad. He loved slapstick comedies, and a good belly laugh helped take his mind off things. When dear friends had given him that iPad years ago, they would have had no idea how invaluable it would be.

I brought all of Seth's tube feeding supplies since clinics and our local emergency rooms don't always carry exactly what we use. This efficiently avoided having to order them and wait. They also didn't carry Seth's specific catheters. Seth was not your typical patient, so I learned to come prepared.

I read of the risk factors, which included seizures, associated with the prep Seth required. A normal individual can experience seizures due to dehydration and electrolyte imbalance. With Seth already depleted from his procedures just days ago, I stayed extra vigilant about the possibility of an epileptic episode.

I assisted Seth to and from the bathroom several times. No longer my little seven-year-old, Seth, now towered over me at nearly six feet tall. This man-child of mine had become so weak, he leaned on me with little strength of his own. Understandably self-conscious about receiving help from nurses in the restroom, the nurses and CNAs were genuine and kind and often thanked me for my help.

After placing an IV, the nurse was given the go-ahead to start the surgical prep. They gave him the preparation to drink. Seth looked at me with wide eyes. He remembered quite well the events of the last surgical prep. His stomach couldn't handle the volume of liquid, and he ended up in the ER in excruciating pain. The events of that trauma came flooding back. He ended up projectile vomiting out of his mouth and nostrils simultaneously. He had bowel obstruction, trapped air and liquids causing severely dilated intestines, and had to have his stomach pumped. To make matters worse, the prep couldn't work because most of it didn't go where it was supposed to. It just sat in his stomach due to gastroparesis, i.e., delayed gastric emptying.

Thankfully, this time, instead of drinking the bowel prep, Seth had the benefit of a G/J feeding tube. I asked if the liquid could be administered directly to his "J" jejunal port to bypass his stomach altogether. They were unfamiliar with that but went to check. The doctor on call felt that was a reasonable alternative. It needed to be administered more slowly through a part of his small intestine, but it was doable.

In the past, I voiced my objection to the amount of radiation exposure on Seth. Now, because of this malfunctioned and stuck device, Seth endured at least five x-rays, several fluoroscopies, and a CAT scan. I thought by now his entire body might glow in the dark! Not only was it all so unfair, the injustices continued.

Around 3:00 p.m., our nurse dropped a bomb. "Due to coronavirus precautions, the facility adopted a strict no-visitor policy. Therefore, you will have to leave by 6:00 p.m."

Seth looked up from his iPad in shock.

"And, unfortunately, you cannot return until 10:00 a.m. tomorrow when visiting hours resume."

Seth started to panic. "But she's not a visitor–she's my mom!"

The nurse spoke compassionately, "I know, Seth. It doesn't seem right."

I could tell she felt bad. She said to me, "I am so sorry. I really want you to be able to stay. You've been a great help, and I believe you know your son best. It's just the new policy."

She was simply caught in the middle, so I asked if I could talk to a nursing supervisor with whom I could explain our extenuating circumstances. She was happy to do so. My mind was still reeling after she left. I still couldn't believe it. There had to be a mistake. The pandemic made everyone's jobs more difficult. I recognized many heroes in this new world we had to navigate. Everyone was struggling to handle the pandemic physically, mentally, and emotionally. I certainly did not want to add stress on top of anyone's load.

Soon, a supervisor entered and introduced herself. She reiterated this was, indeed, the new policy. When I started to explain our predicament—

"There are no exemptions, and from what I've been told, everyone needs to get used to it. This is the new normal."

So, I pivoted. I got on the phone with the doctor's office at the clinic that admitted Seth. I wanted to ensure they knew what was happening before they left at five o'clock. I was racing against time. Clinic personnel were shocked and unaware of the policy at the hospital. They worked up the chain of command, voicing their approval for me to stay and their disapproval of this policy. They told me not to worry. They would likely be able to pull some strings to keep me there. They knew how much Seth needed me and understood the complexity of his care. They vouched for me as the best advocate for him.

I was confident I had every reason for a qualified legal exemption. I just needed to get to the right person who had the power to approve it. I looked on the website to see if they had a form I could fill out. Information on the clinic website mentioned extenuating circumstances that were exempt from the No Visitors Policy but didn't list specifics.

I explained as discreetly as I could to the staff about the predicament. I always tried to maintain Seth's dignity by not having to repeat the particulars of his intellectual disability. Seth doesn't openly admit this to everyone. He does joke from time to time about "chemo brain," but that's the extent of it.

I spent the next several hours trying to petition for an exemption, an exemption the clinic side of the hospital claimed they knew nothing about. Since there was an obvious gap, I spent time educating those I talked to about their own "policy." I couldn't understand how something so highly enforced in the hospital could be so unknown in the clinic. How could these two entities that were more connected than any medical facility we had ever known, be so oblivious to what was going on? Everything seemed to be getting more and more difficult.

I tried to make things as easy as possible. I even called the pediatric wing of the hospital to see if it would be easier to admit Seth through their department. *Certainly, a mom is able to stay with her child on that floor.* After all, Seth was not cognitively nineteen years old. He was still seen in pediatrics and had a pediatrician as the head coordinator of his complex care. I'm sure that doctor would sign the orders. I didn't realize the extent of the situation until I was told, "It wouldn't matter."

"The rules are the same—parents are visitors, and visitors are not allowed from 6:00 p.m. until 10:00 a.m. due to increased virus risk. No exceptions!"

I was in shock. I understood the need for rules. In fact, I appreciated the rules, especially those that were there to protect vulnerable patients like my son. But I honestly didn't understand how making me leave now would be safer. After all, I was screened and had already been there all day. I had stayed in his room. I didn't leave to get coffee or food to limit exposure. Instead, the hospital was mandating me to leave, which would only expose me to outside germs. How was that better protection than allowing me to stay in his room? Why was I any more of a health risk to my son at 6:05 p.m. than I was at 5:59 p.m.? In my humble opinion, this lacked common sense.

I gave them countless reasons and examples - which were well-documented and could easily be verified in my son's file - for my need to remain with Seth as his supportive care advocate. I explained that he was deemed unable to make decisions independently. I didn't go into detail in an effort to preserve his dignity. Although I had Durable Medical Power of Attorney, I was told that the restrictions via executive order superseded prior accommodations.

I couldn't believe what I was hearing from the administrator, so I opened my laptop to search for executive orders. I read through the Mayo Clinic website to find and understand the legality of emergency powers given to the governor. A *"one size fits all" blanket ruling? A refusal to listen on a case-by-case basis to issues concerning a patient's needs and extenuating circumstances? Access to a patient's supportive care advocate is now banned? Is this compliant with the Americans with Disabilities Act, or was this a violation? What policy was I violating?*

Over the next nearly three hours, no matter what I pointed to on their website, I was told there was nothing in writing that they could show me. First, it was not a policy for the public, only internally. Then, I was told it wasn't their policy at all. Their hands were tied. Then, I was told it was a fluid policy that could change tomorrow based on cases and hospital capacity. I was then told it was an Executive Order from the Governor.

I believe we agreed that it was unfair and unjust to place those with intellectual disabilities at a disadvantage and to endure treatment without their supportive care advocate. I pointed to regulations on the Americans with Disabilities website, which stated emergency orders should not deny a patient with intellectual disabilities the right to have their supportive care advocate present to help them make informed decisions.

"Aren't you able to exercise discretion on a case-by-case basis with more than enough evidence provided and verified?"

I was told repeatedly, "NO. Our hands are tied."

Approaching the 6:00 p.m. deadline, and after three hours, when I realized we were spinning our wheels, I asked for another supervisor. Certainly, there had to be someone with the authority to make an exception. In walked the nurse administrator. I started from the beginning, stating our case and answering all of his questions. Very matter-of-factly, he ended the conversation.

"You must leave. This is an Executive Order. If you have a problem with it, take it up with the Governor."

All of a sudden, Seth spoke up. "If my mom leaves, so do I." This level of authoritative confidence was out of character for him.

Everyone I had previously spoken to had gathered in the room.

Someone said, "A voluntary hospital discharge is risky since Seth could have a reaction to the prep process," which I now had to administer myself.

The intimidation to stay and Seth's authoritative statement led me to clarify our position.

"This is *not* our first choice. This is Seth's choice. I am well aware of the risk factors for seizures, but so is high stress and sleep deprivation, which also lowers the seizure threshold. I just want you to know no one is "refusing" medical care or treatments. My son is simply choosing to do the prep for surgery elsewhere with his supportive care advocate. I will remain close and transport him right to the ER if there are any problems. We will be back first thing in the morning."

The staff left the room. As I started to gather our belongings that we had just set in the room, emotions came flooding in. I only wanted what was best for Seth. I was shaking. *Dear God, why? Why does everything have to be such a struggle?* I was nervous. I knew it would be a financial stretch to use the hotel connected to the hospital, but I called Donnie while scrambling to pack our things and asked him to book us a room. Donnie did not hesitate to agree. Seth was immediately relieved. He grabbed the phone and thanked his dad. I didn't know until we got to the room how upset Seth was with the way the conversation with the doctors played out.

As I hung up with Donnie, the surgeon walked in. He greeted and introduced himself to Seth in a warm and friendly manner. For a moment, I felt a glint of hope that the staff had agreed to a visitor restriction exemption. But he knew nothing of the events that had occurred. He was there for standard pre-op protocol.

"Seth, do you know what surgery you are having tomorrow?"

"To get this thing that's stuck out of me."

The doctor nodded. "I need to ask you something. I have to ask this of everyone. If while in surgery the need should arise, do you give permission to administer paddles and chest compressions?" The doctor spoke so quickly, I could tell Seth was trying to process what he'd said.

Seth hesitated—I was sure he didn't understand. Knowing the doctor was waiting for a response, he said, "I don't think so."

I watched as the doctor started to write on his chart. Mama Bear rose up.

"WAIT!"

This guy wasn't asking what flavor of gelatin Seth wanted after surgery. This was a major question, with a major decision to be made, with major implications!

"Seth, do you understand what the doctor is asking you?"

Seth looked at me, then at the doctor, then at the floor. He shook his head and spoke a quiet "No."

I said, "It's okay. You don't need to be embarrassed. What didn't you understand?"

He leaned in and said, "I don't know what that word compression means."

I explained in layman's terms what the doctor was asking him. "If during surgery, something went wrong, and your heart stopped beating, would you want them to use paddles and do CPR to try and start your heart up again?"

"Well, YES! Of course, (like DUH) I don't want to just DIE!" Seth couldn't believe this was what the doctor asked.

This confirmed my purpose in asking to stay with him. Didn't they understand the risk *they* were taking by separating a designated caregiver from the vulnerable patient? Seth had not understood what was being asked and was not able to make an informed decision regarding his care and wishes without me. At that moment, nothing was more important.

I shudder to think what could have happened had I not been there to intercede on my son's behalf. A "Do Not Resuscitate" order would have been placed in my son's medical record. I was firmly informed I could not return until 10:00 a.m. the next morning which would have been after they took him to surgery. Anything could have happened. The thought that I would be contacted by phone and told he didn't make it—and worse, they didn't even try to resuscitate him—sucks the breath right out of me. This experience stirred in me a deeper boldness to be a voice for those without one. From what I just witnessed, my son's life depended on it.

BFFS (BEST FRIENDS FOREVER)

To our surprise, the hospital called us at six o'clock–far before visitor hours began–for a six-thirty CAT scan. We were more than ready to get this nightmare over with. Our hotel was mere steps from Mayo Clinic, so I pushed Seth in a wheelchair over the walkway into the clinic and to the radiology department.

We finished up business at the clinic, and I drove Seth back to the hospital to be admitted. Seth settled into his room but seemed restless. Every time he heard a noise outside the door, he'd perk up to see who it was. He was hoping to see his best bud's head pop in with his legendary greeting, "Seth...E...Beeeeee!" To which Seth would respond, "Jeff...EEEEEEE!" This regularly anticipated reunion kept Seth grounded, reduced his anxiety, and gave him something to look forward to.

Although they were forty years apart in age, Seth and Jeff grew to be the best of friends. They really are a huge blessing and encouragement to one another. Over the years they prayed together, laughed until they cried, celebrated victories with great joy, and wept together when things were just plain hard. Jeff's friendship reminded me of Proverbs 17:17, "A friend is always loyal, and a brother is born to help in time of need."

Seth was holding out hope that somehow Jeff would be able to visit. Inevitably, I had to break the news to him after Jeff texted me to say they wouldn't let him in.

"Jeff can't come this time. He really wanted to be here."

Seth drifted off in a blank stare and fought back tears as the words sank in. When Jeff and his wife weren't away on medical missions, Seth had grown used to having Jeff by his side for his Mayo visits. Donnie always prayed with his son over the phone, but there is something to be said about an in-person presence. This would be the first time his best friend, spiritual mentor, and hilarious sidekick wouldn't be allowed to be with him. Then, my phone alerted me to a new text.

> Jeff: Where are you guys?

> Me: Alfred Building 5th floor Why? Did you get in?

Several minutes pass.

> Jeff: Tell Seth to look out the window.

There are no adequate words to describe what those moments before Seth went into surgery meant. But I will try.

This . . .
This is what it looks like to show up.
This strengthens our faith.
This is a reminder that even though we are far from home, we are not in this alone.
This is faith in action.
This is love from a fellow brother.
This is what the hands and feet of Jesus look like.
This is what "I know I can't be with you, but I see you, I feel you, I am here for you, and you matter" looks like.
This is what compassion for a young man with incurable medical conditions, complications, and unknown prognosis looks like.
This is what gets us through the tough stuff.
This has us thanking God for the helpers, those whom he has brought into our lives.
This changes our perspective.
This changes our tears of suffering to tears of gratitude.
This is what *anyone* can do.
This costs *nothing*, but time.
This. is. Priceless.

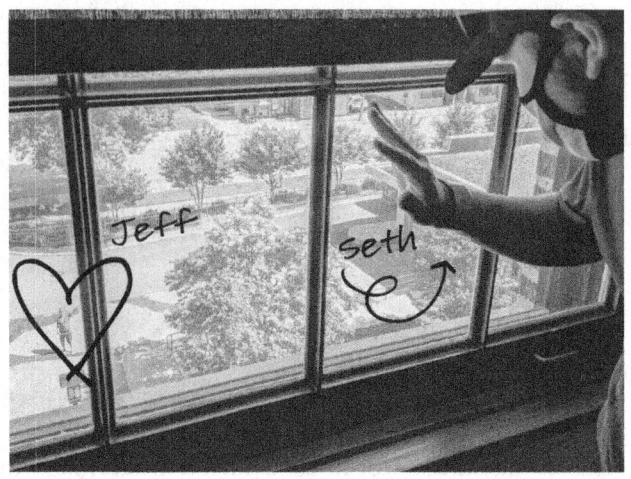

To those who loved us well, set the bar high, strengthened our faith, and inspired us to press on . . . thank you! I hope I can be that kind of strength and inspiration to others.

> Seth: Thank you so much Jeff it meant a lot. Love ya!

> Jeff: Love you too Ace!

Hundreds of people were praying behind the scenes. My phone was blowing up with pings and messages. While that brought great comfort, I was overwhelmed with everyone I had to respond to, plus the hospital morning was awakening to a beehive of activity. I was tying up loose ends with the clinic from leaving the hospital the previous evening. I had my phone on one ear updating the staff at the clinic and used Seth's phone on the other ear to talk with radiology at the hospital. As I struggled to juggle two conversations, a notification alerted me to a message from Dr. Fischer: "I hear you are having quite a time."

I stopped what I was doing and messaged him back. "You don't know half of it!" In all of the craziness, in all the fires I had to put out, I can't believe I forgot to notify him. I don't know how he found out, but I was grateful to hear from him. I didn't think he could have done much to change things, but what a comfort to know he was there and concerned. I knew he would keep close tabs on the situation.

My mind was racing with the whirlwind of the last few weeks and the worry of the procedure. Seth must have picked up on it.

"Mom, look at your shirt!" I had pulled on a black t-shirt without thought that morning. It read, "Blessed MAMA." Seth looked me in the eyes and confidently said, "You are blessed. God will get us through this. He always does!"

He was so right. Timely reminder: I *am* blessed, our family is so blessed! I needed the reminder that my circumstances did *not* determine whether I was blessed. My child was ministering to me in the trenches.

Because I am a visual person, I snapped a picture of us to remind me of this. What a powerful, timely reminder and gift my son gave me.

After they wheeled Seth to surgery, I sunk into the chair. I crashed and tried not to burn. I was trying to keep it together after all my son had been put through. I sat in the quiet of his room and let my body and mind be still.

Within two hours, they called me to the recovery room. Seth was in a post-op fog, so all I said was, "Seth, they got it!" With his eyes still closed, I saw him smile. I typed one brief post to hundreds of waiting prayer warriors and supporters:

"July 1, 2020, 11:34 a.m. They got it!! It's finally out! HALLELUJAH!"

CHAPTER TWENTY-EIGHT
FROM HOSPITAL GOWN TO CAP AND GOWN

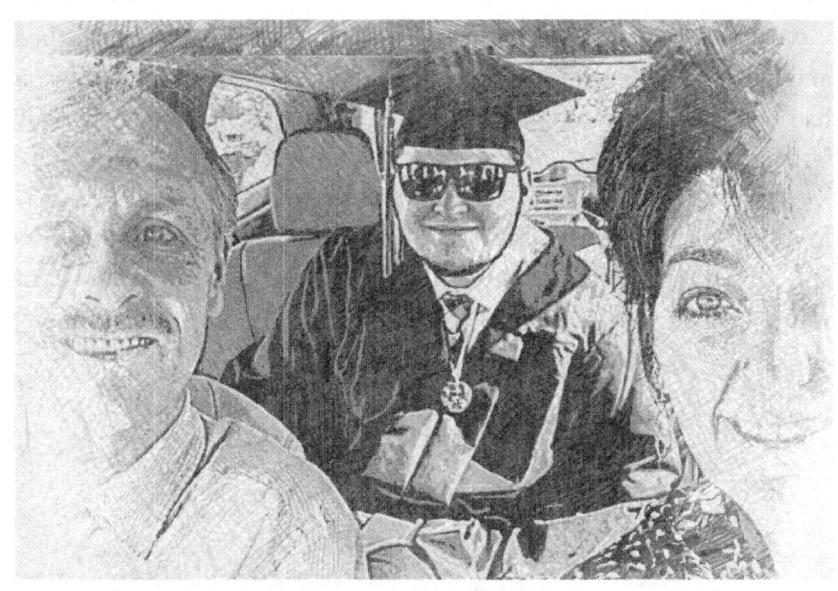

Never be afraid to trust an unknown future to a known God.
–Corrie Ten Boom

We were beyond grateful to be on the other side of this device debacle. As if the whole month-and-a-half process wasn't stressful enough for Seth, to consider a repeat was an absurdity. Privately, Seth adamantly told me he would not go back there again. This would take time from which to heal both physically and emotionally.

We were dealing with relentless feeding tube obstruction, muscle spasms, bleeding, excruciating pain, and formula backup because his muscles weren't contracting to move things along. His disorders were like a growing, rolling snowball. Depending on the doctor, I heard several educated guesses as to what was going on overall. More than one doctor believed there to be neurological (brain communication) disorders. This made sense because his stomach muscles didn't contract properly. He had already been diagnosed with a neurogenic bladder which I learned meant his brain and bladder were not communicating. Now, doctors thought the same might be happening with his bowel. That didn't even take into consideration the latest issues involving his esophagus.

Was there a common denominator? Doctors discussed possible causes: the malfunction of the vagus nerve (the longest cranial nerve in the body running from the brain through the digestive tract)? medications? the progression of his rare disease? It was anyone's guess.

Seth was seriously burned out after the last procedure and had no desire to return to Rochester. At the same time, his back pain limited daily activities and kept him from things he loved to do. After some time passed, he was ready to get answers. With the device finally removed, we could *safely* schedule an MRI of his back.

Seth moved from side to side as he tried to find a comfortable position in the back seat of our SUV. At six feet tall, and with all of his physical limitations, lying down comfortably for a long drive was a challenge. Another vehicle would be more comfortable, but since I put over forty thousand miles on our car a year commuting to medical appointments, fuel efficiency and reliability took priority. Seth was grateful when we finally arrived. He winced as he got out of the vehicle taking a deep breath while slowly straightening his stiff legs. As we waited for the elevator to take us from the parking structure to Mayo Clinic, Seth asked me a question.

"Mom, I feel like I'm eighty years old! What do you think I'll feel like when I'm older?"

In contrast, our beloved Uncle Bill was already in his 80s and still worked at his business seven days a week, gardened, and entertained in his home weekly. So, the sad part was, Seth may have been feeling even *older* than eighty.

I didn't know how to respond to Seth's question. Sometimes there aren't words. I could tell it was more than a haphazard remark, weighing heavily on his heart. He deserved a response, but all I could think of was to reassure him that he was not alone. I told Seth we'd be there for him. We talked about the unknowns. He smiled and nodded, and I saw the wrinkles on his forehead relax.

We made our way to radiology, a place we knew all too well. We were greeted by familiar faces as if it were a family reunion. Ever since Seth was eight years old, he'd experienced numerous MRIs. They weren't a big deal to him. He's not claustrophobic, and the monotonous hum of the machine relaxed him to sleep. The attendants tried to keep him awake and focused on their prompts.

The results of this lumbar and thoracic MRI, even without the clarity of contrast, revealed multiple unexpected issues, especially for Seth's age (not yet twenty years old). I read a new list of abnormalities in his file that covered more than a page. To make a long story short, after discussions with the spine center and various neurologists, they knew of no viable options to tackle the new complexities.

With no plan and no relief in sight, I decided to focus my efforts, now more than ever, on getting home hydro jet water therapy approved. I used the passion that came from watching my son suffer in agony to make sure his voice was heard. Two of Seth's top doctors wrote letters supporting my efforts. Month after month, I relentlessly pursued every step of the process for approval.

In the meantime, Seth's rheumatologist suggested we move

forward with the next level of treatment–biologics. He had spoken to us about this previously. Although we tried to avoid it as long as possible, he suggested it was time. I was prepared that the biologics would be brought on board only after there had been an inadequate response to conventional medications. It's difficult to define the complexity of biological drugs. I didn't fully understand it all, but as I understood it, unlike traditional pharmaceuticals, biological drugs could zero in on specific parts of the immune system. I was told they were used to treat a wide range of conditions — from autoimmune disorders to cancer. Although they are powerful and carry risks, we banked on their benefits to help stall further damage within Seth's body.

This new biological therapy was an injection I could administer at home twice a month. I was already used to administering Seth's weekly (low dose) chemo injection. Despite my lifelong aversion to needles, I learned to push past the discomfort to care for my son.

HELP IS ON THE WAY

Driving home from Mayo, I received a call from someone who was helping me with Seth's petition at the state level.

"Are you sitting down?" My heart fluttered as I pulled over to the side of the road. "It's been approved! The lowest estimate for a home hydro jet therapy tub, with inline heater, bathroom remodel, and installation will be paid in full."

I couldn't believe my ears, and I couldn't wait to tell Seth. I glanced in the rearview mirror to see him sprawled out across the back seat asleep.

"Thank you, God!" I cried with tear-filled eyes. "Thank you for fighting this battle for my son!"

A simultaneous influx of hope filled me with a sense of sweet release of toxic stress. I didn't realize the full weight of this burden until it lifted.

Our Seth would finally get some pain relief.

GRADUATION TIME

From all Seth had been through, Donnie and I stood in awe that he had come this far and would soon don his cap and gown. With so much suffering in the past, we focused on the blessing of finishing high school and what the future might hold. It was time for Seth to graduate!

The pandemic restrictions forced schools to rethink graduation logistics. Some chose to go virtual or live-stream. Others resembled a fast food drive-through where a school official handed students their diplomas through the car window. Some schools opted to simply mail diplomas. Our Westosha Central High staff decided to hold graduation outside in the fresh air with precautions.

Some in the community questioned the wisdom of allowing Seth to attend. We talked to Seth's rheumatologist about the risks involved in his participation. He had treated Seth for over a decade and knew his risk factors better than anyone. Together we weighed the benefits versus the risks and concluded Seth should be afforded the opportunity to participate in this once-in-a-lifetime occasion. Only by a series of miracles over the course of his life was this momentous celebration even possible.

Although graduation usually occurred in early June, by the time the staff sent surveys and organized logistics, the ceremony was scheduled for the end of July. We thought this day would never come because of the pandemic and Seth's health.

At home, Seth dressed in black dress pants, a white shirt, black and white tie, cap and gown, complete with an academic medal around his neck. Dressed and sporting a freshly sculpted beard and sideburns, he climbed into the back seat of the car. Of course, we had to take a selfie to mark the occasion.

Although we were extremely grateful to attend Seth's graduation, pandemic restrictions limited tickets to only two per graduate. Attendees wore masks and sat on marked Xs on the stadium bleachers six feet apart. Donnie and I were disappointed that Seth's siblings and other family members couldn't share this milestone, but we would celebrate with the family at home afterward.

Graduating students were instructed to wear masks for the processional and recessional but could remove them once seated on the field. Seth didn't mind bringing his beloved Pittsburgh Steelers to his graduation as he completed his attire with a black and white mask emblazoned with the team's emblem.

As parents and visitors entered the athletic stadium, the rich ruby-red gowns popped against the green artificial turf like eye candy. Rows of chairs spaced six feet apart on the field due to safety concerns would forever be imprinted in photos of the unprecedented times. It was obvious this was a well-thought-out event, and we were beyond grateful.

Seth sat down, pulled off his mask, and kept his sunglasses on. Thankful he was placed front and center, he sat next to Mr. Ellerbrock who was a long-time supporter of his journey, an encourager, and a friend. I watched as Mr. Ellerbrock turned to him and smiled. The crowd stood for the national anthem as the American flag hung still at the end of the field with no wind. At the opposite end, the scoreboard displayed 20:20 for the time and 20 for the home team, and 20 for the guests. My heart warmed as I thought about what creative staffer tuned in to such details for this Class of 2020.

We felt the heat of our midwestern summer day. The metal bleachers could scorch bare skin. The sun beat down on the black track around the field, and we felt heat waves rising off of it. The outdoor arena offered not one area of shade. Students began to fan themselves. I had spent so much time focused on the germ risk, I had forgotten about Seth's sensitivity to the sun. Being on methotrexate makes a person more susceptible to solar complications. On top of that, Seth had also developed heat intolerance. I quickly realized how it affected him when I noticed Seth started to sway. The smile plastered to his face turned limp. His face looked as red as his gown.

I leaned over to Donnie and said, "Seth doesn't look so good. He looks like he's gonna pass out!"

I was uncomfortable. I stood up, but what could I do? At just that moment, Mr. Ellerbrock turned and saw Seth's condition. He immediately grabbed his water bottle and handed it to Seth. Like Popeye slurping down his spinach, Seth revived as soon as he chugged the entire bottle of water. I thanked God for nudging Mr. Ellerbrock at the right time and giving him the wisdom to act.

Mr. Ellerbrock stood to give the address and present diplomas. It felt surreal to watch Seth walk across the outdoor stage and receive that diploma.

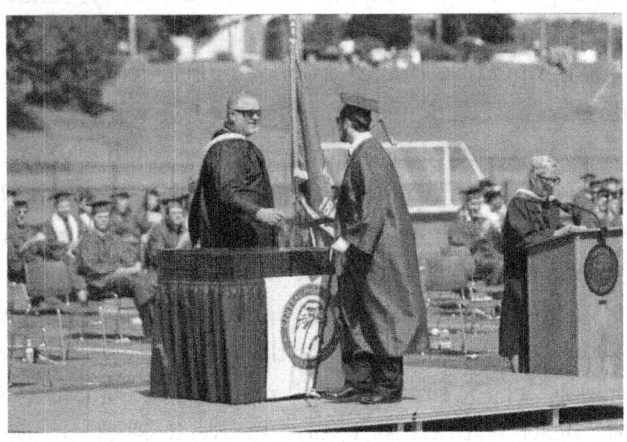

The school's beloved Mrs. Switalla stood ready to snap Seth's photo as he removed his sunglasses. When the graduates heard the final announcement, the majority of them took off their caps and flung them into the air. Congratulations, Class of 2020! In hindsight, 2020 was, indeed, a unique year to graduate.

The high school also put together a virtual commencement for those unable to attend. Our family watched it afterward at home. A lot of hard work went into pre-recording elements of the ceremony that could not be done in public. A multitude of speakers talked to the camera, to the graduates, and loved ones. A split screen showed members of the high school choir singing in unison and harmony from the safety of their homes. The school band did the same. Then, they announced each graduate with a slideshow photo and bio. Each graduate wrote thoughts and details unique to them. Here are Seth's.

Future Plans: I plan to spend my days part-time at Matthias Academy. . . . I would like to continue to help families in need going through various medical issues.

Favorite High School Memory: The Homecoming football game. Coach Mengel visited me in the hospital and asked me to draw up a play. He called it the "A Right Seth Special." I was able to get out of the hospital in time to make the game . . . . It was all a huge honor.

To My Classmates: Life doesn't always go as you planned. Trust God, stay positive & focus on the good things instead of the bad.

I will miss: High-fiving everyone.

The first half of the year was a whirlwind. Amidst a World Health Organization-declared global pandemic, we had three kids set to graduate: one from college, one from high school, and another from eighth grade. Because of a difference of opinion within our family circle, we did not celebrate with large family and friend gatherings typical of graduation celebrations. All of our children pressed on through their fears, uncertainties, and disappointments. It was a unique time in history, one our children may one day recall with their own children.

Our friends Kim and Frank in Rochester absolutely insisted on a party at their house during our next medical visit. They put together a backyard picnic at their home. Critter surprised Seth by driving in from Nashville, Tennessee, and gifted him with a set of his signature cymbals.

We had a blast hanging out with our second family at our home away from home. Nearly seventy-five of our closest friends came and went throughout the day eating popsicles (one of Seth's staples), sharing laughs, and celebrating life.

What I chose to remember most were those who strove for unity in a confusing and controversial time. With gathering restrictions in place, we were particularly moved by those who found creative ways to show care and support, and who stayed connected. They boldly reinforced the power of community.

GRADUATION DAY, JULY 26, 2020

In the hardest days
He perseveres...
Pressing on by God's grace
We prayed for this day
Longing for normalcy
For a few hours, he wasn't medically fragile
Bold
Courageous
Fearless
God with him
Joshua 1:9
This is God's strength on full display in weakness
Philippians 4:13
This is refusing to succumb to ongoing medical battles
At times life is difficult, painful
But it's a good life
Full of abundant blessings
We celebrate
There is purpose
We trust God's plan
For the best is yet to come
Today, he is a high school graduate.

CHAPTER TWENTY-NINE
"JUST THE MOM" CHANGING THE PARADIGM

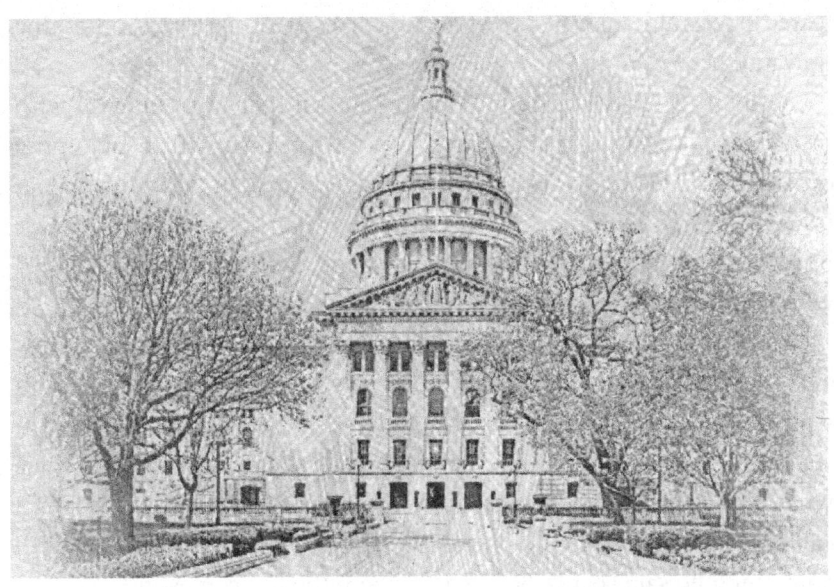

Alone we can do so little; together we can do so much.
–Helen Keller

Change. A word that bristles. I have mixed emotions and an ambivalent relationship with this word. I have found change isn't necessarily good or bad. I've seen disastrous results of some changes, but on the other hand, sometimes change offers valuable, constructive, and positive results. We've been on the receiving end of decisions made in haste and regulations that failed to consider all the people affected. For those with special needs who require extra assistance, adapting to change without warning or explanation often upsets established routines. It puts them at an unfair disadvantage with detrimental consequences.

The recent hospital experiences left Seth with new anxiety. At least he was now older and able to communicate his fears. The fear of confrontation and separation led him to insist I didn't leave his side. Seth worried about the ever-changing and unknown restrictions. He feared he would answer a question incorrectly or agree to something unwanted.

Seth struggled for years to comprehend all that was going on with him medically. His coping strategy was to converse with people on a different level. The majority of people wouldn't catch on to the deeper issues. Often, no one was the wiser. Rather than admit something was unfamiliar, or that he'd forgotten something, Seth used humor, agreed with what was said, or changed the subject to sports.

I encouraged Seth to be honest, but it was easier for him to simply agree. In one instance, Seth came out of the local procedure room with a different-sized apparatus surgically placed. When I inquired about it, the doctor said he asked Seth, and Seth said, "Sure." Seth had no idea what he had agreed to, and then it was too late to reverse it. When I called him out on the implications, he chuckled and replied with something he said regularly, "That's where the fun comes in!"

We had a real dilemma on our hands. Cognitive impairment wasn't always immediately apparent. We'd been told repeatedly by professionals, "He looks so normal." I think I understood what they meant. He looked healthy on the outside. Others often noticed his eyes sparkled, his complexion was clear and nearly glowed, and his bright smile disguised the invisible diseases within.

I worked to communicate, educate, and put into place measures for Seth to have the tools he needed in order to make informed, safe decisions. I believed we could keep people safe - even during a pandemic - without sacrificing the rights and responsibilities we had to individuals with disabilities.

I needed to ensure we had a plan in place *before* the next medical crisis arose. Based on our prior experiences with Seth, I knew that a medical dilemma could arise at any time. Avoiding another miscommunication was key knowing there may not be time to hash this out in the event of an emergency. I truly believed there was a common ground for all of us, who were essential to Seth's care, to continue to work together. We had grown to appreciate the facilities that served our son so well. We chose to assume their best intentions and tried to see things from their perspective.

Staff at Mayo Clinic wanted to better understand and address the needs and unique challenges of those with invisible disabilities. Therefore, I contacted the Office of Patient Experience as well as the legal team who worked with disability inclusion regulations and compliance issues. We wanted to help them help us and other patients in the future.

It was especially challenging for me to rely on the latest information because I had to monitor the regularly changing mandates in three states. We lived in Wisconsin. Donnie worked in Illinois, and Seth received medical care in both Wisconsin and Minnesota. State to state, facility to facility, there were always variances and various interpretations. We never knew what to expect. Federal mandates or recommendations were also part of the mix. It definitely kept me on my toes. I carried a copy of legal paperwork with me and had a copy on file with the various hospitals, but it wasn't a guarantee of avoiding pushback.

NAVIGATING MUDDY WATERS

I spent the next month using countless hours a day on the phone. I needed clarification on the ever-changing visitation rulings for Minnesota, so we could be better prepared. Where are these rules coming from? What should I expect when I take my son for medical care in Minnesota?

I talked with the governor's office directly who informed me he was using the recommendations of the Department of Health Services. His office suggested I call the Minnesota Department of Health. After calling to get clarification on what they recommended to the governor, I was transferred several times. Each time I was told I didn't have the correct department, and they didn't know the answers to what I was asking. *Am I the only one questioning all of this?* I then emailed both the governor and the lieutenant governor of Minnesota and filled out the appropriate form to request a meeting. I thought it would be a good opportunity to explain my perspective on how this executive order impacted mothers and children with special needs and those slipping through the cracks without a voice.

Why was something that affected millions of lives not readily available in writing? I wondered. My son's medical care now revolved around this, yet there seemed to be much resistance to transparency. I could get no one to verbally interpret or confirm the guidelines. So, I requested a copy of this "Executive Order" regarding the no-visitor policy. Those I talked to either communicated their lack of knowledge or sounded appalled that anyone was asking for specifics. Apparently, they had nothing in writing because things were "fluid." I was told to go back and ask the hospital about their visitor policy even though the hospital told me very clearly to "take it up with the governor" and the governor's office told me to call the Health Department. It was like a three-ring circus.

Hospital personnel told me their policy wasn't available to the public, only internally. Yet, the public was to whom the restrictions applied. Furthermore, if indeed such restrictions existed across the board, one would think there would have to be exemptions for certain individuals. I wanted to know how and where to file for such an exemption and was willing to endure that process.

One person at the Department of Health told me, "It is what it is–" then click and a dial tone.

I contacted the office of the mayor of Rochester, Minnesota. How I wished Mayor Ardell Brede was still in office. I learned the current mayor was on vacation and unavailable. I explained my situation to her office, and they gave me several phone numbers. I left messages but received no return calls.

I contacted members of Congress and senators even though I wasn't technically their constituent since I didn't live in Minnesota. A government official's office told me I was only one person, and there was strength in numbers. So I encouraged those who cared about Seth, especially in Minnesota, to call and write their elected officials and voice their concerns.

I found out every state has a Disability Law Center that was contracted with the state for issues that arose. What an amazing turn of events. What a blessing to speak with someone who listened and could not only empathize with our predicament but was willing to help us work to find an agreeable resolution. The Law Center agreed there was definitely a need for education and awareness for *all* people to be protected. They offered to take Seth's case at no cost. They emailed me the paperwork for Seth to retain an attorney for services.

THE LEGAL ARENA, AUGUST 2020

At first, I was uncomfortable with the thought of "retaining an attorney." This was *not* a lawsuit. That was never our intention. Having said that, however, and because of the unreturned phone calls, hangups, and unresolved issues, I quickly realized this was the only way things would move forward. I felt compelled that our most vulnerable deserved nothing less. Because Seth was now over eighteen, he signed for an attorney to represent his side of the injustices he had experienced. Together we would dive into laws, mandates, recommendations, emergency executive orders, and the potential excessive use of emergency powers.

Seth's attorney heard us loud and clear. Our intention was to be a voice for those without one and help make a positive difference. With each obstacle, I hoped and prayed our hardships were paving the way for the next person to help them avoid the traumatic battle. I believed nothing was wasted and even the darkest of our situations could be used for good. My passion and commitment was to be part of the change rather than merely complain from the sidelines. Although I tried to initiate change, in this particular matter, I was not making much of an impact as a solo voice.

I wanted to help draft clear and comprehensive paperwork that employees of facilities could refer to, so everyone was on the same page. Seth and I also desired to make it easier for employees to be allowed to do their jobs and not be caught in a legal crossfire of unknowns. I also wanted to make sure that those with special needs had the opportunity for facilities to be able to honor exemptions on a *case-by-case* basis. It wasn't just about my son anymore. Maybe, I wondered, I had been placed in this situation for this purpose.

Seth's attorney spoke on his behalf. The legal department came to the conclusion that the staff was wrong to deny Seth access to his support person. Although that was a great first step, that wasn't the end goal. I told Seth's attorney we don't need an apology, we need to come up with an agreeable resolution and solution for the future. The clinic committed to train and educate their staff on such issues.

I didn't want to make extra work. I just needed everyone to be on the same page when at one time I felt we weren't even in the same book. I spent a lot of time keeping a good, working relationship with the legal department. We worked together to protect rights and dignity while respecting clinical protocol. I began to see an effort to shift the paradigm.

I suggested a way to mark a patient's chart discreetly, so staff would know when someone had been screened and approved to be accompanied by their support person. They thought it was a great idea, but many factors must come into play to implement any new procedure. The legal department at the medical facility again suggested I obtain guardianship. The recommendation to obtain it by Seth's neuropsychologist years ago flooded my mind. I heard his voice in my head. "You will need this for when he becomes an adult."

I remembered the exact spot I was sitting when the doctor's office gave me the difficult news that my son would forever need assistance and not gain independence as he grew into adulthood. The reality of it was devastating. I had never cried in front of a doctor I had just met before, but I couldn't stop the tears. It hurt so deeply. The doctor assured me Seth would be fine because he had a good support system at home.

Even though the doctor had recommended I obtain guardianship before Seth's eighteenth birthday, I held out hope that maybe, just maybe, things would improve. We did another neuropsychological evaluation and then another. Oh, how I wanted to see improvement! But it only confirmed what I didn't want to accept. My heart sank. Seth would require assistance for life. It was so daunting to consider the length and depth of what that meant going forward.

Parents envision their children leaving and spreading their wings, but I was left trying to wrap my brain around what this would look like for Donnie and me in the long haul. As those around us became "empty nesters," we celebrated that right of passage with them, but Seth's future looked far different. This wonderful doctor even went to the trouble to help me fill out the guardianship paperwork. I couldn't do it. It hurt too much. I was overwhelmed by it all. He was so kind and compassionate. I thanked God for him.

Seth had many medical events that year. We were constantly putting out fires. On top of that, I had to compile all of his paperwork for him to reapply as an adult for Social Security benefits. In hindsight, I should have followed through with the guardianship petition. Instead, I shoved it in a drawer hoping out of sight meant out of mind. My heart was in the right place, being hesitant and hopeful, but in the end, it just caused more hardships.

Seth's Department of Health Services consulting nurse said, "Usually, we don't make these recommendations, but in this case, I strongly believe he needs you appointed as his guardian. You really need to go through this process."

She knew him best, so her words held extra weight. She was the deciding factor that pushed me to pursue guardianship. With the first phone call, I found out everything was more difficult because he was already considered an adult. *If I had only filed the documents with the court while he was under eighteen!* Hindsight, as always, is 20/20. As time went on, trying to help my son with his medical needs became more and more challenging. And then, COVID restrictions made things impossible.

I made an appointment for a third time, for the neuro-psych eval which consisted of one to two hours of an interview and questionnaire, plus six to seven hours of testing between Seth and the professional. Again. He walked Seth back alone as I sat in the waiting room. In the end, this new doctor came to the same conclusion as the previous neuropsychologist. The repetition of the report helped me to accept the reality of Seth's needs. Weeks later, I learned that the court might reject all three evaluations because they weren't done in the state in which we lived. So, we had to start over.

This time, I contacted the Aging and Disability Resource Center (ADRC) for the county in which we lived. Although I didn't know exactly what resources they had available, it was a great place to start. They got right to work. Standard protocol meant Adult Protective Services got involved, a guardian ad litem was assigned to Seth, and a new neuropsychiatrist was assigned by the state who did their own assessment. Seth had a legal team working on his behalf. And, yes, in case someone's counting, that was *four* neuropsychological evaluations all confirming the same results before the paperwork was filed to go before a judge.

Seth was just as relieved to get the ball rolling. As he told many individuals prior, "I just want my mom to be able to help me."

It was unfair for anyone to be forced to manage their healthcare when ill-equipped to do so, on top of enduring so much suffering.

"JUST THE MOM" CHANGING THE PARADIGM

A WORK IN PROGRESS

Our daily routine at Mayo was the same.
Every screening station
All three Mayo campuses
For months now
This, on top of them calling the day before our appointment, with the same questions. . .
He pretty much had it memorized.
After taking his temperature:
1) Why are you here?
2) Have you or anyone you have been exposed to tested positive for COVID? (No.)
2b) Have you been tested for COVID? (Yes, more than once.)
2c) What was your result? (Negative each time.)
3) In the last forty-eight hours, have you experienced any of the following symptoms:
Fever
Cough
Shortness of breath
Sore throat
Diarrhea
Respiratory distress
Chills
Shaking with chills
Muscle ache
Headache
Nausea
Vomiting
Loss of smell
Change of loss in taste sensation

At a routine checkup at Mayo, Seth went through screening for his last procedure of the day. He patiently waited and respectfully answered.

Then, he felt he had to break the somber mood with his Seth humor. He asked the screener with a serious face, "Is bleeding from the nipples on the list?"

The gentleman hesitated–suddenly, all the other screeners stopped and stared. You could hear a pin drop. Thankfully, the guy was a good sport.

He said, "Well, that's not on the list, so you're clear to go."

Oh my goodness, I could barely contain my composure! As we got further down the hallway, we laughed ourselves to tears. I could feel the stress melt away like Proverbs 17:22 says, "A cheerful heart is good medicine, but a crushed spirit dries up the bones" (NIV).

CARE FOR THE CAREGIVER

From an early age, I was a caregiver. I looked after my little sister while my mom worked and attended school. After I got married, my sister lived with Donnie and me while she attended high school. Sometimes, I drove my dad to and from the hospital for his cancer treatments. Donnie and I had our first child when I was nineteen. I was my grandmother's live-in, full-time caregiver until she passed. I care for my stepmom's medical needs while helping elderly neighbors. As a mother of seven, caregiving is in my blood. However, caring for someone with complex medical needs around the clock is by far my most challenging role.

Until recently, as many family caregivers do, I put others' needs first not realizing that my own health and well-being were just as important. I was on the brink of burnout, burning the candle at both ends. The job of a caretaker can be stressful and isolating. I learned some grim caregiver statistics. Unfortunately, 30 - 40 percent of caregivers die before the person they are caring for. One study found that caregivers have a 63 percent higher mortality rate than non-caregivers. The intensity of responsibilities chips away at the caregivers' health physically, emotionally, and spiritually. Also, conditions that don't lead to death, such as depression, are rampant. We caregivers often don't find time to go to our own appointments. We put them off because we're too busy, can't get respite care, can't afford it, or are just plain sick of scheduling appointments, fighting insurance, and sitting in clinics. As a result, ailments like breast cancer, which could be caught at an early stage, aren't found until the illness is much worse or life-threatening.

A medical journal headline read "Long-Term Caregiving May Shorten Life Up To Eight Years." Readers concluded that mothers who cared for chronically ill children often developed changes in their chromosomes that amounted to several years of additional aging. I recognized that caregivers, trying to put others first, were literally killing themselves. I wanted to find a way to help myself and use that to, in turn, help others. Caring for caregivers and helping them stay healthy became a special interest of mine. It was personal. First, I thought about starting a caregiver support group in my spare time–which was non-existent. That would be overwhelming to take on myself. I had to respect my limitations.

I networked with a fellow mom of a medically complex kiddo and joined an online group she started. Many moms from across the country signed up for mutual support and encouragement. Along with my page, I could add value and engage as I shared my experiences, encouraged others, and built relationships as time permitted. There was a local group that met twice a month through our county aging and disability services. I found many opportunities to connect with others for mutual encouragement.

One day, I attended the funeral of someone close to me. I'll call him Caleb. I hadn't seen Caleb since I was a child, but I wanted to pay my respects. As early as I could remember, Caleb had a severe mental disorder. After his parents died, he moved to a group home. With the help of many who supported him with his daily needs, he lived a productive life.

One day, a doctor covering for his regular doctor switched his medications. Things went horribly wrong. From what we were told, he became combative with people at his group home, and the police were called. Caleb ended up being transported to a 24-hour psychiatric facility. Before anyone could visit, the family received a call that he had died! Information on his death was mysteriously absent. After the funeral service, Caleb's long-time caretaker approached me to offer her sympathies.

She said with her eyes wide, "This should *never* have happened!"

Those words sent shock waves through me. What happened? We may never know. Either way, it seemed like a severe injustice.

I know that a burning question and paralyzing fear lives in the hearts of us parents of kids with special needs. What will happen to our children if they outlive us? Who will devote their lives to caring for the extensive needs day in and out? Who will go to the doctor with them and manage their medications? Who knows my child like I do? Who can sense when something is wrong? Who will continue to be his voice? Tears flow as I write this.

The journey of navigating my son's disabilities, as well as caring for elderly family members, has revealed injustices that changed me. I found a substantial gap between those needing assistance and services and a system that makes obtaining and receiving those services far too difficult. This has ignited in me a passion to help others. I felt compelled to be a part of the change I wanted to see. But how could I make a difference and still focus on my primary responsibilities with my family? Understanding my heart's desire, God opened a door.

Unexpectedly, I received a communication from our county executive's office asking if I would be willing to lend my experience and time to serve as a member of the County Commission on Aging and Disability Services. I was humbled and honored that she believed I could provide a valuable service to our community. After discussing this opportunity with my family, I accepted. The county board of supervisors confirmed my appointment, and I started my new role. I also joined the quality committee as well as the caregiver coalition.

I never set out to be an advocate. I didn't want to be qualified. This was not a club I wanted to join. My involvement was born out of necessity, and I stayed because of love. That doesn't mean the long term realities aren't daunting. When I am feeling overwhelmed, I search the Scriptures. They have never failed me. Proverbs 31:8 confirmed I was on the right path. "Speak up for those who cannot speak for themselves; ensure justice for those being crushed."

May God give me–and all who care for the needs of others–the strength, wisdom, and resources to do all He calls us to do.

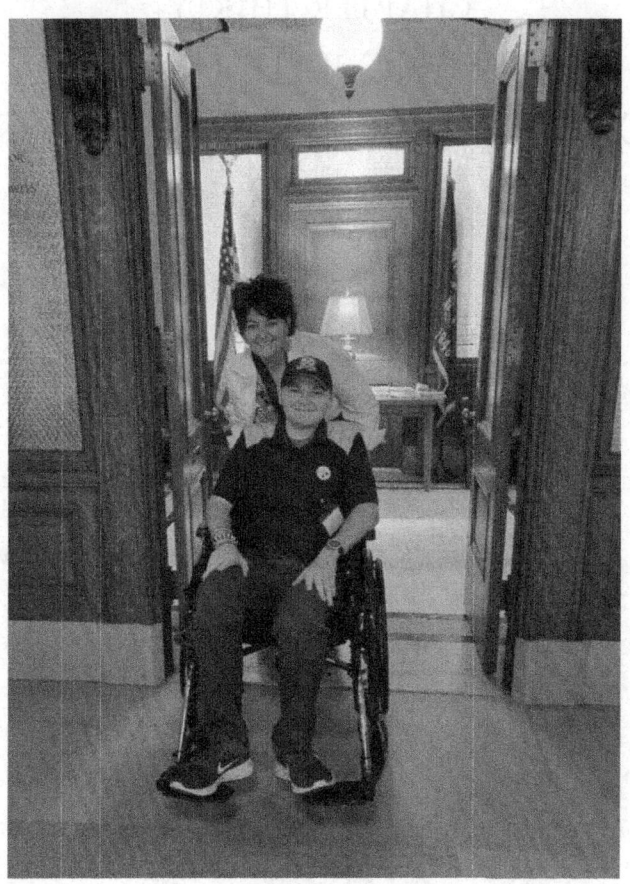

Seth and I after speaking with our legislators.

CHAPTER THIRTY
GRIEVING THE LOSSES, EMBRACING THE CALLING

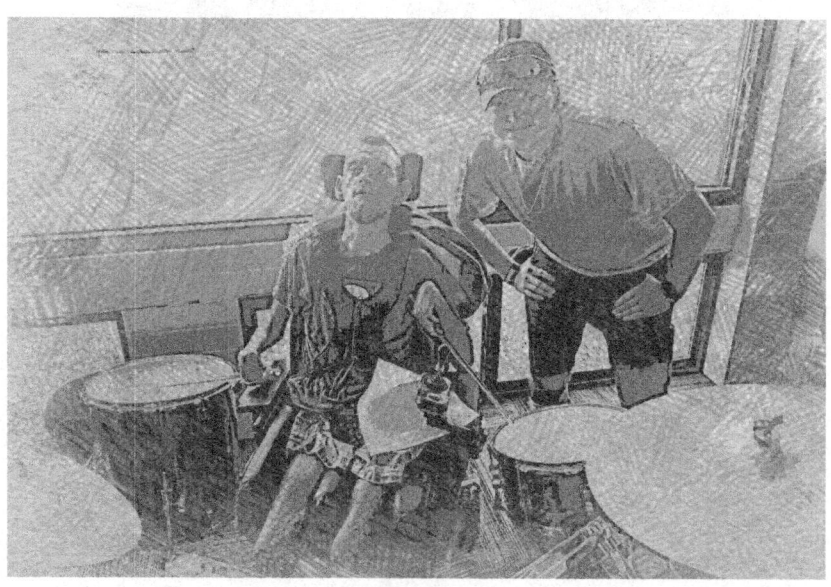

How far you go in life depends on your being tender with the
young, compassionate with the aged, sympathetic with the
striving and tolerant of the weak and strong. Because someday
in your life you will have been all of these.
–George Washington Carver

Seth's pain management doctor is a unique fellow for whom we have developed great respect. He helped Seth stay as active as possible and found ways to manage chronic, sometimes debilitating, pain without narcotics. Although I don't like the fact that Seth has needed this type of doctor throughout his life, there are benefits to a long-standing partnership.

The visits usually began with the same question.

"So, how are things going (pain-wise)?"

Seth and I always tried to share something good. This also helped Seth keep his mind on the victories rather than defeats. When things turned more conversational, our doctor, who always wore a bow tie, listened to Seth explain what was going on in his life and what brought him joy.

The doctor told us that Seth was one of the most positive patients he had ever seen. He said half-jokingly that he would like to take Seth on rounds with him. Seth chuckled. He said he would like him to meet his other patients as an example of remaining positive despite facing so many difficult challenges. That sentiment touched us.

"So, have you thought about what your plans for the future are?"

Seth confidently replied, "I want to help others who are struggling. I just want to encourage them and share the hope I have. God continues to get me through the toughest times."

What could have been seen as a vague and childlike outlook on life's endless possibilities was received by our doctor with much compassion. This dedicated anesthesiologist, who probably had a million other things to do, stopped what he was doing.

THE RIPPLE EFFECT

The doctor locked eyes with Seth. "I want to share a story and piece of advice with you. There was a man born sixty-two years ago with cystic fibrosis. His parents were told that his chances were bleak at best. He defied the odds." The doctor continued as Seth listened intently. "With each milestone he reached, people would say about him, 'I don't know why he's bothering; he's just going to die anyway!'" Tears welled up in my eyes as he continued. "They would say things like, 'College, what a waste!' That man became an anesthesiologist here, at the world-renowned Mayo Clinic. He was well-liked and respected. He went on to make a *huge* impact on countless lives. He made a difference, not only in his patients' lives but with the staff here who were better because of him. He recently passed away, but the ripple effect of his life lives on."

I could tell that man had a profound impact on our good doctor. And now, he was sharing that legacy and speaking hope into Seth. It was impossible not to think about the ripple effect.

"Seth, don't let *anyone* in this world tell you you're 'too sick' to make a difference! That doctor was also told he was 'too sick.'"

I wiped my tears as Seth nodded and received those words. The ripple effect of one had changed generations to come. We left that appointment challenged to embrace God's will and calling for our lives. We asked ourselves: *Are we making an impact? What legacy do we want to leave?*

I found this definition of ripple effect: "A situation in which an event or action has an effect on something, which then has an effect on something else." I thought of the classic Christmas movie, "It's a Wonderful Life." The main character, George Bailey, had no idea the profound impact his life had on the lives of others and his entire community. Sometimes God gives us a glimpse of the effect our lives have on each other, and it spurs us on.

GODSPEED, DR. FISCHER

We learned Dr. Fischer planned to follow a call to serve overseas. Like the changing seasons here in the Midwest, when one ends, it can be both bitter and sweet. Some are more difficult than others. We were heavy-hearted to watch this season of our lives come to a close.

Seth and I met Dr. Fischer on the sixteenth floor of Mayo Clinic to say our goodbyes. I worked hard to keep my emotions in check and professional while acknowledging the tremendous impact he so obviously had had on our lives for over a decade. We will never forget how it all began and how God answered my prayers. No doubt, God handpicked Dr. Fischer to be Seth's primary pediatrician and care coordinator at a time when we needed him most. Our paths were meant to cross, and we were better for it.

After some not-so-positive experiences, Dr. Fischer helped change our trajectory and restored our trust in the medical community. His care for us can only be described as immeasurable. Looking back, I wasted years focusing on why this was happening to our little, once-perfectly-healthy, boy. Dr. Fischer helped me see there is purpose in pain and nothing is wasted. Through God's mercy and providence, before Seth was born, God was orchestrating the details. He would place in Dr. Fischer a desire to specialize in rare diseases. I am confident we don't meet people by accident. God is in control and He has a plan.

As we parted ways, we trusted God was moving Dr. Fischer to exactly where He had called him. It softened the sting to think he would be the answer to someone else's prayers. Now, the ripple effect of his life of service and expertise as a doctor would continue across the ocean. We bid godspeed to our treasured friend, Dr. Fischer. We grieved this loss, then continued our journey.

In the spring of 2021, an article in one of the local newspapers named Seth Bayles as "Today's Teen." Nominated by his high school, Seth was honored to be chosen and highlighted among many schools. To the question, "What are your plans after high school?" Seth communicated what he felt his calling was.

"I want my life to reflect Jesus Christ in everything I say and do. I want to help others. I think it's important to not waste the life God has given me. I will continue to raise awareness for rare diseases and continue to give to charities that bless sick children and their families."

And that's just what he did.

THE VISION AND FIRST CLASS OF MATTHIAS ACADEMY

Seth attended the visionary fundraising event for Matthias Academy in Wisconsin. He immediately felt comfortable because he and the founder, Liz, had known each other for years. She was one of his "Angels" who ran alongside him in the marathons. She was also instrumental in fund-raising for Seth's own race chair. Liz once said of him, "Seth is . . . far different than any other young man I have ever met. . . . Seth genuinely cares about YOU and what YOU have to say, all while hiding his pain and discomfort with his sweet smile. Seth shows the most incredible grace and patience every day of his challenging life."

Liz addressed hundreds of donors at a local country club as she championed her vision for helping adults with disabilities who had aged out of the public school system. The day program she envisioned would be individualized and support adults from ages eighteen to ninety-nine. The school motto was "Endless Opportunities for Extraordinary Adults." Seth couldn't wait to be a part of the first class of this unusual, custom-designed school.

Seth was proud to raise funds and awareness for this new educational opportunity. And people who knew him were just as thrilled to join his efforts. Seth has always had a soft spot for those who aren't as able as he is and felt called to help and bring joy to others. Seth's joy was–and still is–contagious and many wanted to be a part of it. Several people who cared deeply for Seth actually quit their full-time jobs and joined the staff.

Matthias considered Seth an "Eagle." He was humbled to find a silver plaque hung on the brick wall just inside the front entrance etched with the words, "I can do all things through Christ who strengthens me. Philippians 4:13 Seth Bayles." It gave him a tangible reminder of the source of his strength, joy, purpose, and contentment.

At Matthias, Seth didn't have to explain his medical conditions, cognitive impairment, or medications. He didn't fear what would happen if he had a seizure. A full-time nurse handled all of his medical supplies and would flush his feeding tube lines for him. His catheters

GRIEVING THE LOSSES, EMBRACING THE CALLING 347

were in the bathroom cabinet. No one ever stared or made him feel uncomfortable. He received physical and recreational therapy personalized for his specific needs from a professional who worked with his medical team. That professional, named Sharon, was also one of his regular myTEAM TRIUMPH Angels. Because she has known him so well for years, she knows how to motivate him to reach his goals by making therapy fun for him.

DRUMBEATS OF JOY

One day, Seth decided to bring his drum set to Matthias for music class. The drums and accessories filled our entire car. When I went to pick him up, I expected to reload the set to take back home, but when Seth got in the car, he promptly announced the drum set would be staying. I was shocked. Seth loved that drum set and always looked forward to playing it.

"Mom, you wouldn't believe the smiles on their faces, the laughter, the joy! I couldn't take it away from them."

After leaving the drum set there for several days, he said on the way home, "I'd like to fundraise to get Matthias their own drum set."

And so, he did. Within four days we had to close the campaign because we had more than enough money–over four thousand dollars in four days!

With the music teacher Joel's guidance, Seth had the thrill of looking through a catalog and choosing instruments that would serve the students. He was able to purchase needs and wants. Seth not only picked out a drum set, but he was able to choose one in his favorite color, royal blue. They purchased a sound system that the school needed for special events. In addition, kettle drums, bongos, handbells, and a high-quality wooden xylophone were also selected. Joel labeled the keys in braille. Seth rejoiced as a visually impaired fellow student played her favorite Christmas music.

Seth's heart overflowed when he saw how much the students used and enjoyed the items. Students with sensory issues loved being in control of making sounds. They not only heard the sound as they hit the drumhead but felt the release and vibration. Seth purchased all different types of drumsticks to accommodate the students' unique needs. Hot sticks, light-up sticks, and rubber sticks that could be bent around clenched hands helped the students beat out their woes and worries to create drumbeats of joy.

After several weeks of holding drum lessons, the students came alive with positive feedback–all except for Ceci, who never wanted to try. Seth encouraged her.

"Come on, Ceci, you can do this. You got this. I'll be right here."

One day, she allowed him to put drumsticks in her hands and hit the drums on her own. It made Seth's week.

"Mom, you should have seen the joy on her face!"

Seth said Joel later told him, "She tried because of you."

Another favorite student of Seth's was Daniel, who had little use of his hands. Seth configured rubber drumsticks in and around his hands, and voila! Daniel was able to thump the drum. Seth squealed with delight as he told me the story on the way home. Daniel spoke with such soft, labored breath that Seth couldn't understand what he was trying to say. Seth said he leaned in as Daniel spoke again.

"I-love-you-Seth!"

Seth was so moved. There was now no doubt in his mind that Matthias Academy was exactly where God had called him to be. This was his ministry. Seth had found his place, his people, and his calling. Matthias Academy felt like home. It was and is a place where everyone can be themselves. Seth loved being an encouragement to his fellow students, especially if they were having a difficult day. Together they celebrated victories and hardships like family. As a mom, I cherish the words I heard others say about our son.

"Encouragement flows out of Seth like breathing."

"Seth is such an amazing young man with a loving soul and natural leadership ability and tends to naturally slip into a mentor-type role for other students—"

"Others look forward to Seth's hugs and smiles."

One day, Seth's professor approached him and asked if he would be willing to lead a Bible study with a small group of students. When I picked him up from school that day, he shared this news with me with more excitement than I had ever seen before.

"Mom, you are not going to believe this."

"Tell me! What?"

"Kenny asked me to lead a Bible study! He said he thought I'd be great at it."

"Are you serious? Oh, my goodness, that's amazing!"

"This is what I've felt called to do, but I have such a hard time remembering things."

"Seth, God has called you to this. He's not going to leave you. He's going to equip you."

I let our church know the supplies Seth needed, and they immediately purchased them. Seth was realizing that God could do anything, at any time, anywhere he wanted, and through anyone he chose. We thought back to when Seth realized a hospital chaplaincy career was out of reach. But God–did not deny Seth the desire of his heart to encourage others. He often uses ordinary people to do extraordinary things. In a podcast interview a year earlier, the host asked Seth what he hoped to do in the future. When Seth said he would like to be a chaplain, the host replied, "Seth, I believe you already are." Seth's drumming and Bible classes affirmed his calling.

Liz is another hero that has helped shape our lives. She said yes to a vision for a special place for extraordinary adults. She stepped out in faith and cast a stone. Her ripple effect blessed families beyond measure and inspired a community. Seth also said yes to a new challenge. Both lives created ripples that continue to expand larger and farther than anyone could have ever imagined.

Seth's physical body continued to deteriorate. The long commutes to Mayo became more complicated. After a year of waiting and navigating the pandemic, Seth finally secured a consultation with an upper GI doctor. This was the appointment that the doctor had previously canceled.

Tests revealed a new motility disorder, now of the esophagus. This was likely the cause of the random choking, gagging, and throat issues. This meant Seth's body was losing yet another ability with no known treatment options. We depended on God one day at a time as we grieved the losses and helped our son bear these new realities.

Throughout this journey, we've been told a number of times that Seth has made a difference in the medical community. Modern medicine is advancing with the help of all that has been learned from Seth and other patients with rare conditions. I find comfort in knowing that my son's suffering is not in vain. I trust that others will not have to wait so long for answers. I pray someday they will get that lightbulb moment that we never did. But Seth was not the only family member through whom God showed His power. God was working in our family all along. Here is one example.

GOD HAS THE FINAL SAY

Matthew 19:26 revealed to me an astounding truth: "Jesus looked at them intently and said, 'Humanly speaking, it is impossible. But with God everything is possible'." Seth's brother Drew is sixteen months older than him. He is closest in age as well as relationally. Drew has always protected Seth, been his advocate, and has provided respite care, so Donnie and I can have an occasional date night out. Seth looks up to him, laughs at his jokes, and has a healthy respect for the man Drew has become.

By worldly standards, this relationship should not be possible. It's nothing short of miraculous. They have something in common beyond having the same parents. When things looked bleak for these boys, doctors told us to plan for the worst. But God had the final say.

The year was 1999. I was sent to the hospital for preeclampsia to have my labor induced. Thankfully, a diligent nurse discovered umbilical cord prolapse. This means the umbilical cord has dropped through the cervix into the birth canal ahead of the baby. This complication is a rare medical emergency. Staff called code over the intercom, and doctors and nurses came running. There was no time to spare as equipment was pulled from the wall and tossed onto the gurney, and the nurse riding on the side rail held the umbilical cord up inside me. All this happened as I was wheeled to the OR for an immediate cesarean. The last word I heard from a nurse before they put an oxygen mask over my nose and mouth was *stillbirth*. They were unable to obtain vitals on my baby or know how long the cord had been compressed. The next thing I remember was waking up after general anesthesia.

"Is my baby alive?"

"Yes."

"Praise God." I started to weep.

"We were able to revive him, but don't get your hopes up. He's got a long way to go, and even if he does survive, he could very well be in a vegetative state."

"Can I see him?"

"No. He's too fragile. Plus, he has machines, tubes, and wires everywhere. You don't want to see him like that."

"I just want to see him and have him hear my voice."

"He's too fragile. Even the sound of your voice could send him into cardiac arrest."

I refused to be discouraged. My faith and praise to God remained steady and unwavering. I was overwhelmed with gratitude that my son's life was spared. He was alive! Nothing would steal my joy. Our previous child, just two years earlier, died in my womb at fifteen weeks. I couldn't go through that grief again.

The medical team, thankfully, didn't give up and neither did those who joined us in prayer. Our church held round-the-clock prayer vigils for baby Drew. In addition, our pastors visited the hospital day and night to pray over Drew's incubator. Each day after the pastors left, the staff of the Neonatal Intensive Care Unit (NICU) said they saw signs of improvement. We were seeing God move mountains.

A stream of staff came into my room day and night to tell me they had heard about the events of how this baby shouldn't be alive.

Many said, "You are so lucky."

"Luck has nothing to do with it," I responded. "We are blessed."

I shared God's goodness to anyone who would listen. I trusted God's plan, whatever that was, however difficult the road ahead. Miraculously, Drew was discharged only eight days later. Everyone was shocked. He went home with no restrictions, no machines, nothing. His stats were textbook perfect!

Later, I became aware of the over three hundred pages of medical documentation from Drew's entry into the world. It made me sob. The assessment of baby Drew's condition as he was born by emergency cesarean: blue-gray, limp, lifeless, Apgar score of 0, meaning there were no signs of life, no heartbeat, no breathing, no response to stimulation. The documentation verified the miracle.

But God didn't just enable him to survive. He gave him life to thrive. After Drew's discharge from the NICU, he never had one health issue. He was remarkably healthy. To this day, he continues to defy the odds. He graduated at the top of his college class and lives with purpose serving his community.

I am grateful to God and the medical professionals who saved and sustained Drew's life. I brought Drew back to the hospital on his first and second birthdays to celebrate with the staff and encourage them never to give up hope. At the time, medical professionals gave their best-educated guesses based on evidence, experience, and statistics.

But God has the final say on how each of our stories plays out, and little did we know how God would use Drew over twenty years later in a life-saving episode for his brother Seth.

CHAPTER THIRTY-ONE
SORROWFUL YET ALWAYS REJOICING

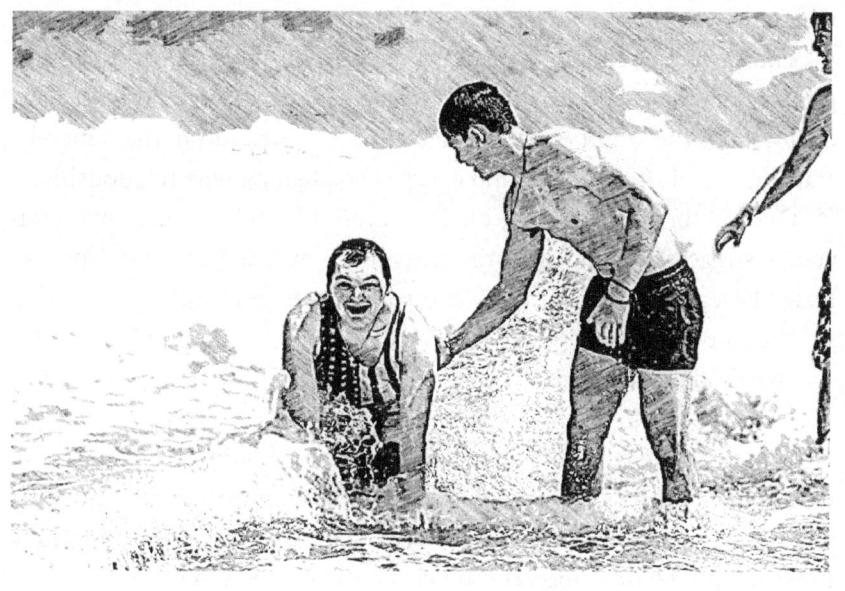

Suffering is unbearable if you aren't certain
that God is for you and with you.
–Tim Keller

Seth's rheumatologist decided to retire. He graciously gave us two years' notice and committed to vetting potential doctors to take over Seth's rare and complex case. It was hard to let go of this thirteen-year relationship. However, it made us feel better knowing he was working to find a good fit. He searched for an adult internist who worked with the compassion of a pediatric specialist. He was brilliant in his specialty and had a great bedside manner, always going above and beyond to explain things in layman's terms. Each visit, I had a million questions about the lab work and the roles that blood cells play in the immune system. I probably drove him crazy, but he never let on and we never felt rushed. He seemed to genuinely care. God, in the smallest of details, brought him on board. A fellow Mountaineer, he graduated from college in Donnie's home state of West Virginia, and he was a Steelers fan. Seth always looked forward to the visits where they detailed their projections for the Pittsburgh season.

Things were changing rapidly at the hospital. Two of Seth's primary doctors were leaving. We needed to start over and with new doctors on the adult side of the clinic. It was more than merely starting over, it meant time and energy establishing new relationships.

One doctor tactfully suggested, "Maybe this isn't the best place for you. I suggest looking into the possibility of the Rare and Undiagnosed Disease network at the National Institute of Health."

"I don't even know where that's located."

"Bethesda, Maryland."

"Oh, my."

"I'll be honest. There's no guarantee he would be accepted. It would be a process. It would involve compiling a medical summary and obtaining a referral from a medical facility. Seth's case would need to be accepted based upon certain criteria, interest, and funding."

He gave me something to think about, but like my unending pile of laundry at home, the pileup of changes and decisions was daunting. *Was it time to move on and leave Mayo Clinic? Should we look closer to home again? What should we do?*

A small glimmer of hope showed up in a letter we received. Seth was selected to be part of a clinical trial for patients with stomach paralysis (gastroparesis). Since there was currently no cure for this condition, I was excited. The thought that something could aid Seth's digestive system would be a game-changer. I immediately called and spoke extensively with the team conducting the trial. I didn't tell Seth because I knew how clinical trials work. Still, the mother in me waited with high hopes. After a board of physicians reviewed his case, the clinical research coordinator called me back. Due to several medical factors, she told me Seth would not benefit from the study - another heartbreaking disappointment.

To add insult to injury, Seth's pain management doctor and I had been talking about his recent debilitating headaches and dizzy spells. We both worked toward a gradual taper of a long-term medication Seth took for headaches. It did not go well, and the headaches increased at a debilitating level. His doctor voiced concern over ever weaning Seth off any medications in the future. He mentioned the possibility of trying cannabidiol, a component of medical marijuana. I was shocked. Mayo? Really?

He told me Mayo had a doctor who specialized in this. After I wrapped my brain around it, hope returned. At this point, we were open to a lot more than we had been in the past simply out of desperation. I had a ton of questions and had to be assured he could monitor Seth closely until he reached a therapeutic level. He contacted the specialist to see if he could set up a consultation to discuss this further.

He called back shortly thereafter to say they had to deny us the opportunity because we lived out of state. The laws were different across state lines, so he could not help us from Minnesota. When I broke the news to Seth, he took it in stride. He was used to the roller coaster of hope followed by disappointment.

Although we were getting great doctors to help, the options continued to be limited. It was hard for me not to get discouraged. I prayed, *God, are we supposed to stay here? God, show me what we're to do!*

Maybe we are supposed to go to the National Institute of Health. I was growing weary under the weight of it all. I had to prepare for three more appointments that day. I needed to go to a restroom, splash some water on my face, and gather my thoughts.

I was on a side of the clinic that patients rarely enter. Pretty sure I ended up in the employee restroom. As I headed to the sink, one of Seth's doctors, whom we hadn't seen in years, was washing her hands. We excitedly and warmly greeted each other. I thought that would be the end of it, but she lingered.

"You sent me a card a while back. I don't even know if you remember. It said, 'Be still–'"

"and know that I am God," I finished.

"Yes! I have that on my desk, and I refer to it often. I want you to know it meant so much."

She went on to explain some stresses she often dealt with, and those words brought her peace. We embraced, and she headed out. I smiled as I watched her leave. I knew that meeting wasn't an accident. I believe God steered me to cross paths with her. He used that doctor to encourage me and see things through a new lens. Maybe God wasn't moving us from here just yet . . .

February 2021

Mayo doctors suspected Seth had an autonomic dysfunction and scheduled a series of tests. As I understood it, our body's nervous system automatically regulates functions we don't think about as we move and live and breathe. God designed the human body to operate in such detailed harmony via unconscious, involuntary functions. We were here to test some of those functions for Seth.

As his name was called, we both headed toward the door where a gentleman held a clipboard. He stopped me as I walked beside Seth.

"He will be out after he's done. You can have a seat."

"I would like my mom to go back with me."

"She will be here when you are done."

Seth started to panic. He looked at me to plead his case.

I told the gentleman, "I don't need to go in for his testing. I just need to go over his medications. He cannot pronounce them. They are extensive. Plus, there was a medication I held for this particular test which I need to discuss with the technician."

He became more insistent. "We will call you if we need you. The new COVID restrictions and small rooms prohibit us from letting you back."

We were still in the waiting room filled with people. I didn't want to draw unnecessary attention to Seth, especially to explain his shortcomings and private medical information. Again, we were put in an uncomfortable situation. The gentleman stood at the doorway as people looked on. It was awkward, so I told Seth to go ahead.

I headed to the front desk and explained the situation. They told me they would have someone come out and talk to me. I waited, but no one came. When Seth returned, he was visibly shaken and more frustrated than I had ever seen him.

He said, "They asked me questions I didn't know the answer to. It was so embarrassing. I needed you there! They wouldn't let me get you. They kept asking about my medications. I told them, 'I don't know.' I didn't know! They said, 'We need to know what pills you took this morning.' I said, 'You would have to ask my mom, I don't know the names.' Then they said, 'I will say a medication name and you tell me if it sounds familiar.' I didn't know what to say!"

He was talking a mile a minute. He had a splitting headache from the test process, and now he was frustrated with me because I didn't fight to go back in the room with him. It was chaos.

"Can we just leave now!"

He was frustrated, in pain, embarrassed, exhausted, and angry at me. On our way home, I called the woman I had gotten to know quite well in the office of patient experiences. She expressed concern that *once again* Seth was denied access to his support person.

I asked, "How is this keeping anyone safe?"

She agreed with my frustration.

"The facility has my son's cognitive impairment on file. The doctors who performed the neuropsych evaluations are from this facility. The information is there. I don't understand why we have to be put in this position and cause Seth stress every single time. We had already proven he is justified in having access to his support person. It's unfair to have to openly share my adult son's cognitive shortcomings with every single person we come in contact with, in every department, at every appointment, in front of all who can hear."

She had empathy for our dilemma, and I'm sure this was a difficult situation on all sides compounded by coronavirus restrictions. "I'm not trying to take this out on you. But we need a better plan."

"I am so sorry you both have had to endure this. Unfortunately, I fear this may be our new normal. I think guardianship may be the best option. But even with that, I can't make any guarantees."

After we arrived back home, I checked Seth's patient portal to read the results of his test. The autonomic response test measured how his nervous system worked to control things like breathing, heart rate, and sweating. All three of those were abnormal.

Trying to put the puzzle pieces together with multisystem dysfunction is not an easy task. *Were all of Seth's issues, the headaches, dizziness, visual disturbances, hands going numb, dropping things, heat intolerance, blood pressure, heart rate, bladder, and digestive problems a result of this dysfunction?* We had gotten quite used to having more questions than answers.

Two more words on a radiology report sucker-punched me: "Brain Atrophy." I felt sick to my stomach. I was all too familiar with the term atrophy, the wasting away, that had occurred with the onset of this rare disease journey. *But now his brain? Oh, God, help me understand.*

The brain MRI from seven years ago when he was thirteen years old was normal. In simple terms, his latest brain scan at age twenty revealed both sides of his brain had diminished. Even if the atrophy was mild, these results were disconcerting. At this rate, I wondered what his brain would be like as he aged.

My mind reeled. It was a tough blow.

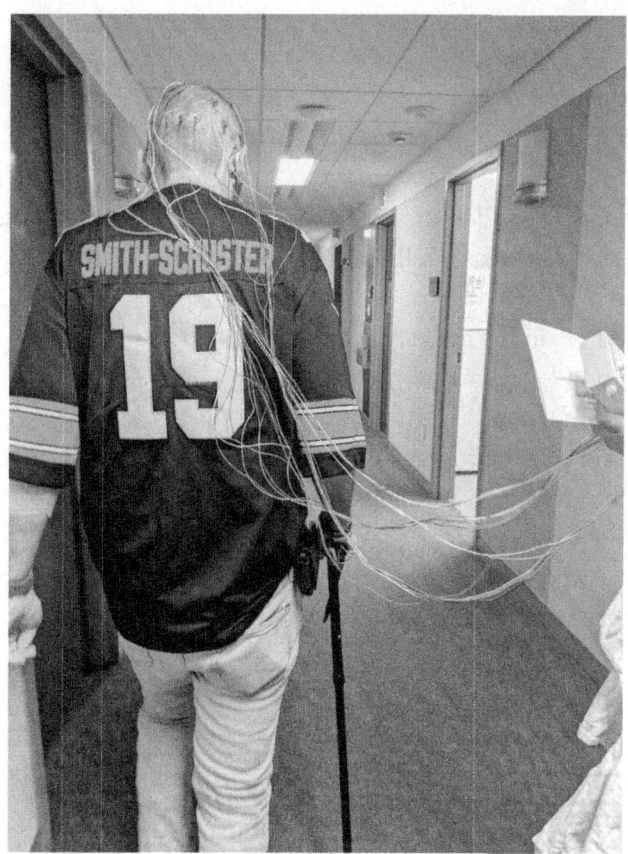

Setting aside all the medical jargon about brain atrophy, we needed to focus on the limitations affecting his daily life. Although most changes were subtle, we noticed Seth was losing cognitive abilities. He struggled with short-term memory, reasoning, problem-solving, etc. Some days were worse than others. This new reality was hard for all of us.

One night in the hospital, I couldn't sleep. I felt renewed sympathy as I looked at my son. His head was wrapped in gauze, covering the electrodes cemented all over his scalp. The monitors tracked brain activity while a CPAP machine kept his airway open. While he slept, I journaled these words to him.

THOUGHTS FROM 3:00 A.M.

Suffering is inevitable in this life . . . the struggle is real.

Pain, frustration, despair, challenges, disappointments, fatigue, sickness, and disease, tell us we cannot go on like this.

But God . . . in his grace and mercy gives hope, rest, and restoration.

Jesus said, "Come to me, all of you who are weary and carry heavy burdens, and I will give you rest." Matthew 11:28

What a sweet gift rest is . . .a sweetness not fully appreciated until received when you're exhausted and got nothing left.

For a time . . . all is right.

Nocturnal seizures, sleep apnea, nighttime tube feeding issues, and unrest threaten to overshadow the blessing

Rest gives us an opportunity to lay down our sword from the valiant fight of the day.

The Lord himself will continue to fight for you . . . rest well.

Cheer up faint-hearted warrior.

"Weeping may last through the night, but joy comes with the morning." Psalm 30:5

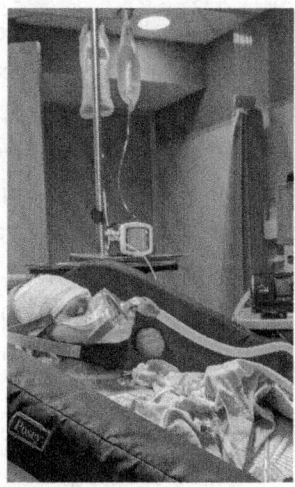

GUARDIANSHIP–FINALLY

The day had finally arrived to go before a judge to obtain guardianship. Seth was advised that he didn't need to be there, but I thought it was important for him to be a part of the entire process. The virtual court took place in the comfort of our home. Seth sat between Donnie and me on the sofa as others joined the live feed. Due to more than sufficient evidence presented, and agreed upon by multiple professionals, the proceedings didn't take long. Guardianship was granted, and Seth was relieved and happy to have this issue finally behind us.

Many professionals commented that Seth and I shouldn't have had to endure this grueling legal process on top of everything else. If I had it to do over again, I would have pursued guardianship sooner, but I didn't know what I didn't know.

LIFTING EACH OTHER UP

In 2021, Seth turned twenty-one on the twenty-first day in the twenty-first century. Seth may not reflect back on all of the medical fiascos he had that year as positive, but one thing's for sure–he was grateful for the gift of another year! We had so many reasons to celebrate.

Because Seth enjoyed water in all forms since he was a baby, one of the joys most difficult to abstain from (per doctor recommendations) was swimming in lakes, rivers, ponds, and hot tubs, all filled with germs and bacteria. In an effort to help Seth live life despite risks, we purchased a drysuit which allowed him to enjoy lake days with the family while reducing the risk of contaminants and infection. One day while we were talking, I mentioned the ocean. I told him salt water was healing, and he could go in it without the dry suit. Ever since then, the ocean called his name. Seth longed to feel the ocean against his skin.

We decided as a family that we would take a trip to the Atlantic Ocean. It would be several days of driving, but it would be worth it. It surpassed all of Seth's expectations. Just seeing the vast, foamy turquoise water put a *huge* smile on his face. Seth couldn't wait to seize the rare opportunity and get in the water. Even though the waves were pounding, in his mind, he was invincible. I snapped many photos that day, but one, in particular, spoke to me. It seemed a fitting representation of Seth's journey.

Because the people who cared about him were right by his side, Seth entered the unknown of the vast, intimidating ocean without fear. He wasn't worried *if* he fell. He knew that was inevitable, but *when* he fell, those who cared for him would be there to help him back up. As the immense waves beat against him and even after several painful falls, Seth's unmistakable joy was still evident. The obvious parallel to his life was unmistakable.

Even though Seth didn't want to leave, we knew we had to limit his time and exposure to the sun due to the medications he was on. We enjoyed the rest of the time in Florida inland with extended family. Several days later, we started the drive home. All seemed well, until a couple of states later. Seth's legs turned dark red and began to swell. He could no longer put on his leg braces. We thought the swelling may have resulted from being stationary in the truck for so long. We tried moving his legs more and elevating them. After we got home, his legs got far worse. They turned purple, blistered, and split wide open.

I couldn't understand what was happening. It was as if he was burning and continuing to burn.

I took him to the emergency room, but no one had seen a case like it. They prescribed antibiotics because his skin was open and oozing. I applied silver burn cream and wrapped him with gauze every few hours as he cried out in agony. The doctor had to do some research.

We found out it was a rare phenomenon that can happen with or without sun exposure for patients who have had chemo and/or radiation treatments. It's a delayed reaction and reactivation of sunburn by methotrexate and can occur long after the treatment is complete. Since Seth received the methotrexate weekly, I was told with each injection, the process essentially retriggered the burn and started the process over again. Even though it was documented in medical literature, the doctors we saw had never seen a case.

Seth couldn't sleep. His skin was on fire. He had severe burns, chills, and intense pain. He couldn't get in or out of bed, so he slept in a recliner. Anything brushing against his deep red, inflamed legs was excruciating, but he didn't complain. This process seemed to re-awaken the inflammatory peripheral sensory neuropathy in his legs from the rare disease process years prior. I walked into his room to check on him in the middle of the night. He was wide awake, wincing in intense pain. I felt so bad, I got down on my knees and started to gently unwrap the gauze on his legs.

"I'm sorry, Seth. I don't know that going to Florida was such a good idea."

"Mom, it was wonderful! I'm so glad we went. To experience the ocean like I dreamed was worth it all."

Even though things didn't go as planned, and he would pay for it later, he had no complaints and no regrets. As I lightly rubbed on the burn cream, he leaned back in the recliner and continued.

"I will remember it forever!"

In the midst of sorrow, he was rejoicing over the good. My eyes filled with tears realizing the indomitable joy that Seth possessed despite his current affliction. *Sorrowful, yet always rejoicing. Lord God, I want to live like that!* Reasons abounded to be sorrowful. But God . . .

THE REASON WHY

"Mom, I wish I had something I could give to people to offer them hope. It's too complicated for me to explain. Can you write down my story, so I can give it to them when they ask me why I'm at the clinic?" Seth saw a need with people he met but struggled to communicate his story in brief encounters.

For years, I shared Seth's journey on Facebook. Although not a writer by nature, positive feedback from followers urged me to compile those writings into a book. So I wrote a rough draft, but I knew little about the steps between a manuscript and the final publication. One day, our small group leader from church told me about a writer's conference. For lots of reasons, I brushed it off.

However, God cleared a path of opportunity and opened the door in a way that affirmed I was meant to go. Donnie requested vacation days to free me from my commitments while he and the kiddos cared for Seth and held down the fort. I received a scholarship of several hundred dollars to cover my registration, meals, and lodging. A whole tribe of loving, supportive people stepped up, so I could attend.

Feeling intimidated and inadequate without a clue of what to expect or bring, I set out alone to an area I had never before traveled. I arrived at the beautiful campus of Wheaton College just outside of Chicago, nervous, excited, and grateful for this opportunity. The architecture on the old campus intrigued me. I checked into the conference, eager to soak in everything I could about the publishing industry. I received information about the conference events and was assigned to a room in Fischer Hall.

Seth's favorite pediatrician, Dr. Fischer, came to mind. *Hmm. Fischer with a "c,"* I thought as I unpacked the hot pink tote bag that had seen countless trips to Mayo Clinic. I pondered the long journey that had gotten us to this point. Out of curiosity, I emailed Dr. Fischer and asked if he happened to be connected in some way to Fischer Hall. Even though his lifelong service to children had him working on the other side of the world, his prompt reply brought tears to my eyes.

There was a connection beyond what I could have ever anticipated. God used several members of his family as vessels to make Wheaton College what it is today. From "founding" the college in the 1800s, i.e., taking over a failing college, to the donation responsible for building Fischer Hall, his family was, indeed, connected. Some may brush it off as mere coincidence, but I chose to see the divine details that only God can orchestrate.

At the conference, I learned, among other things, the importance of the beginning and ending of a story. I would have loved nothing more than to write a triumphant ending that revealed a miraculous cure with all the warm fuzzy feels. But I realized, whether or not God chose to heal Seth this side of heaven was not our *only* hope for a happily ever after. Since God was still writing our story, I had no words to tie up Seth's journey in a neat little bow.

During a discussion group, someone asked me, "So, if there's a chance your son won't get better, *why* would you write a book?" I asked myself the same question. *Why would a mom of seven, who doesn't enjoy writing, spend so much time and effort writing a book?* If they only knew my struggles with ADHD and dyslexia. Long hours of writing and rewriting in front of a screen felt like shards of glass in my eyes. The process was brutal.

Later that evening, I retreated to my room in Fischer Hall. I sat in front of my laptop staring at the blinking cursor, grappling for words. *Even if–healing never comes, my son wants his story to be told*, I thought, as the "why" echoed through my mind.

I would spend the next year polishing the manuscript with no ending—until one day *the why* behind all of this became crystal clear. It was communicated by Seth himself, who had found his voice. His words were simple, yet profound.

One afternoon, my editor stopped by the house. After finishing our work, she wanted to say hi to Seth. As she stepped into his living quarters, she was taken aback by the amount of medical supplies. She stared at the wall of shelves filled with bins and drawers five feet high labeled like a medical supply room.

After taking it all in, she asked, "Seth, can I ask you something personal?" Seth nodded. "So, what do you make of all this, this long journey of yours? All the medical stuff, the hospital visits, the emergencies, the long pain. I mean, this is your life."

With barely a pause, Seth replied,

"I think God wants to use it for His glory."

EPILOGUE

We continue living life on the family farm, where there's plenty of activity year-round. No matter where our journey takes us, home is our favorite place. Uncle Bill, who lives on an adjoining property, remains my constant.

Donnie continues to hold down the fort whenever Seth and I need to travel for appointments, which will likely continue for the rest of his life. Donnie works hard and exudes sacrifice for his family, lives simply, and can fix just about anything. He serves our church full-time as the building manager.

Our two oldest sons have left the nest, gotten married, and have families of their own. Donnie and I have seven grandchildren and happily embrace our growing clan.

Our third oldest son, Drew, serves as a full-time first responder. His strength and bravery are evident while remaining humble and others focused. He gives back in various ways, including coaching youth sports.

Our daughter, Janae, is the toughest young woman I have ever known. She is training with our local fire department while continuing her education with Firefighter/EMT classes. Her calm spirit in emergencies and desire to help others affirm her calling.

Our two youngest sons, Gabriel and Luke, are in their last years of high school. They are busy training, playing tackle football, working multiple jobs, and moving forward in their own God-given paths. These two young men, who were babies when all of this began, are overcomers!

As for me? I'm "just the mom" grateful for our tribe, coffee, dry shampoo, and God's lavish love poured over our family. It's been quite a journey, and I can't imagine what the future holds, but trust the one who holds our future. His will be done, not mine.

Lastly, Seth, now in his early twenties, is living his life goals. He enjoys family time, reading and copying Scripture, and watching football. Seth attends Matthias Academy two days per week, where he teaches percussion to fellow students. He also leads a Bible study, not at a seminary level, but on a personal one. Seth encourages those facing hardships to trust God always.

On June 11, 2023, after leaving a baseball game, Seth had a grand mal seizure, turned blue, and went into sudden cardiac arrest. By the grace of God and the quick action of his brother Drew, this was not the end of Seth's story. Seth woke up in an ambulance without fear and filled with peace. He was ready for eternity with God.

Are you?

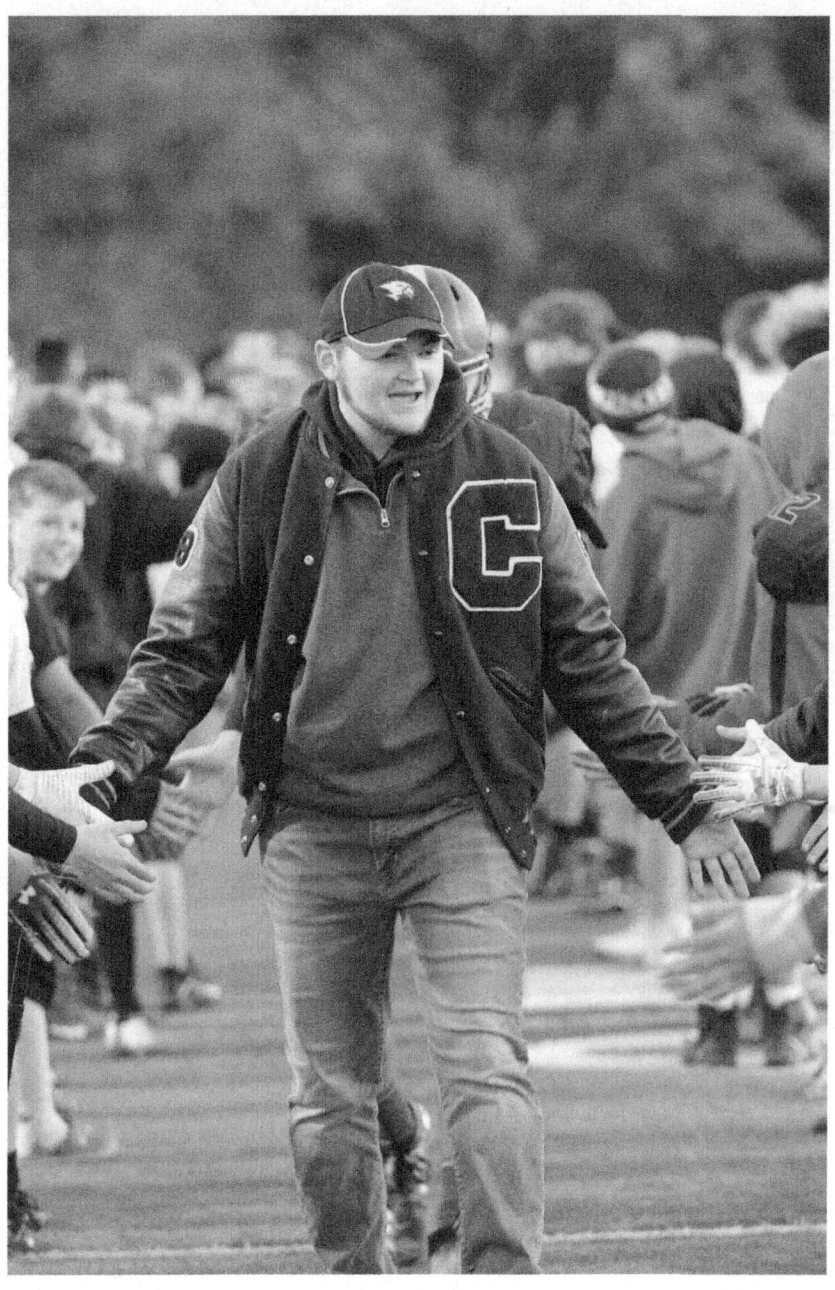

AFTERWORD

SHE COULD RUN, BUT SHE COULD NOT HIDE

Ecclesiastes 4:9-10, "Two are better than one, because they have a good reward for their toil. For if they fall, one will lift up his fellow. But woe to him who is alone" (ESV).

FROM JULIE

It's impossible to count all the people God brought into our lives who helped carry our burdens on this journey, but this book wouldn't be complete without mentioning one more person God used to help support us. She recalls the first time we met; I recall the second.

She invited me to her home. I walked in the door to see a large, framed canvas hanging over the fireplace mantle directly in front of me. The oxygen left my lungs. When I recovered, I managed to say, "That–that is my favorite painting!" I had the exact same masterpiece placed on the bookshelf next to my desk where I could see it daily as I wrote. Around the time that Seth was born, someone gave me a greeting card with a print of this painting on the front. From the moment I laid eyes on it, I loved it so much that I framed it. It spoke to my heart and soul. It was one of the few treasures I brought to Wisconsin when we moved from South Florida nearly twenty years ago.

The painting depicted a woman kneeling on a brightly striped blanket with her feet tucked up under her sundress. The sun shone on top of her silhouette as her head bowed over an open Bible. Until this moment, I had never seen another copy. I didn't even know the name of the artist, but this new friend, Cathy, did. More importantly, we both knew the greatest artist of all–our Heavenly Father, the One who flung the planets into place and painted the skies with his magnificent palette. His presence was here, in the smallest details, connecting two girls from the Midwest for mutual encouragement.

After reading my manuscript Cathy said, "You have a diamond here. It just needs to be polished." She offered to help me navigate the grueling work that lay ahead. I had no idea what that would entail. She put her book project on hold to help me with mine. Who would do that? I quickly realized it was far more than editing help–it was the beginning of a beautiful friendship.

We hobbled along, calling ourselves Frick and Frack, laughing, praying and praising, sometimes crying, as we learned together the art and craft of writing and the workings of the publishing industry. She was my mentor, cheerleader, confidant, and burden-lifter. God used her investment of time, talent, and encouragement, to make this finished product possible. She taught me more than I can measure, and I am better for having met her.

We really are stronger together!

I'll let Cathy write her part of the book journey for herself.

FROM CATHY

I saw her from the back at a writers conference. She was tall with spiky jet-black hair and big, dangly earrings. My roommate met her earlier and insisted, "You *have* to meet this lady and hear her story! Her name is Julie."

I tried to back out from meeting "this lady" because I had other things in mind for my time at the conference. The next afternoon, I happened to be standing behind Julie as she spoke to one of the acquisition editors. She was boisterous and cheerful. The aura of positive energy emanating from her was almost visible, like heat waves on a hot day. It was more than I could absorb, and I literally backed up two steps to shield myself from it. I could tell by things Julie said to the editor that she was new to the world of writing and didn't understand the publishing industry. *Too much work*, I thought as she chatted with the professionals remembering my timid first time seventeen years earlier. I still got nervous showing my work to agents, so I could sympathize with her first steps.

Still, I tried to politely decline my roommate's insistence that I meet this Julie. I already had a writers critique group and didn't have time to join another. My roommate was standing nearby pointing Julie toward me for an introduction. It was too crowded to run and hide as I tried to figure out how to disengage from this whirlwind of energy. Julie turned toward me, and her bright spirit was magnetic. After my roommate introduced us, Julie insisted we exchange phone numbers. How does one politely decline someone so chipper and well-meaning? We exchanged phone numbers, and I thought, *I'm not doin' a thing with that number. It's gonna sit unused in my contacts*. We parted and that was that–so I thought.

Two weeks after the conference, my cell phone rang. When I answered, that same energy of hers bounded right through the phone! She was so positive about her writers group, I agreed to visit. The group was lively and intentional, but I knew immediately it was not realistic for me to join a second group. As she and I spoke one-on-one, she revealed more of her book journey and that she was looking for editorial help.

The Holy Spirit whispered to my heart, "Help her write her proposal–and don't charge her." It's hard to explain the still, small voice of the Holy Spirit in my life. I only know that I have been walking not perfectly, but faithfully, for over fifty years, and I know the voice of my Shepherd. As it turned out, not only did Julie and I have some unusual things in common (like the painting), but she lived an easy fifteen-minute drive straight up the road from me. I had passed her house every day for nine years on my way to work wondering who lived on that large corner farm property.

So, like Pooh and Piglet on an explore, we started down the path together. She, a beginner writer, and I, a step ahead guiding her through the tough work of rewrites and "ferocious self-editing," as one of my mentors had taught me. She had three hundred pages of a first draft. As I read it one night during a storm, the power went out, so I continued by candlelight, unable to put it down.

God helped us learn from so many people and resources. We refused to be blocked by things that were hard to do. We determined *difficult* did not mean *impossible*. It only meant it took a little more time and a few more steps than easy. We plodded on day after day in between wife and mother duties, and what jubilant satisfaction we felt when Julie sent off her proposal and started receiving replies.

During my quiet time the morning after, the Holy Spirit whispered, "You can't leave Julie now, high and dry to tackle the entire book by herself! Keep helping her." I had about a two-second hesitation, but I knew that voice all too well. There was no point in hesitating or doing the usual, "Really, Lord? You really want me to do that?" I kept trying to run away from Julie, but God kept spinning me around like a boomerang to run right back into her.

And that is how God works. He networks. He nudges. He moves, breathes, and controls what happens. What a rich experience I would have missed had I run away and not obeyed his Spirit. I would have missed the up-close and personal view of her story and the influence of her faith. She showered me with gifts of thanks though I wanted none. She was the gift. Her example of joy, her generosity, and her lavish love toward everyone, not to mention getting to know her family, strengthened my own faith.

I do not have many heroes because I don't want to idolize anyone, but I do have a few women of the faith whose lives inspire me. They are people who shared the gospel despite terrible hardships. People like Corrie ten Boom (*The Hiding Place*), Elisabeth Elliot (*Through Gates of Splendor, The Savage My Kinsman*) . . . and now, Julie Bayles. What an honor to see her in action managing their busy household, to walk beside her and help edit and polish her story. I am better for having met *her*. Frick and Frack, stronger–and better–together, for sure.

To God be the glory, great things He has done!

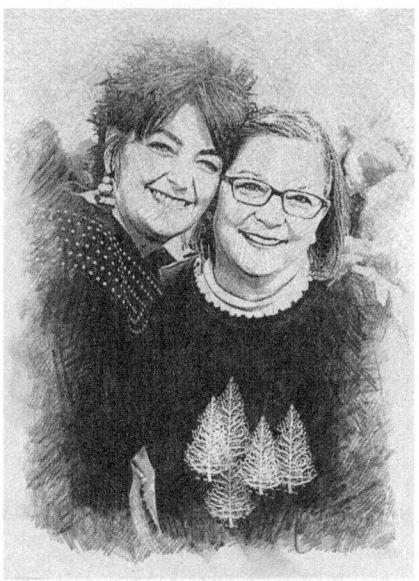

Julie and Cathy

LIST OF REFERENCES

Abrahams, Jim, The Charlie Foundation to Cure Pediatric Epilepsy. George, Paulette. Good Morning, Beautiful: Winning The Battle Over Seizures (Ambassador, International, Greenville, SC, 2010), page 124.

AccuWeather By Mark Puleo, 'It was literally pouring snow': On this one fateful Groundhog Day,
https://www.accuweather.com/en/winter-weather/2011-groundhog-day-blizzard-in-chicago-10-years-later/891018#:~:text=The%20Groundhog%20Day%20Blizzard%20of,on%20any%20given%20Tuesday%20afternoon.

Big Ben 7, The Official Web site of Super Bowl Champion Ben Roethlisberger, "Two Special Gifts for Two Special People." September 3, 2018
http://bigben7.com/two-special-gifts-for-two-special-people/

Carol Bradley Bursack, "Long-term Caregiving May Shorten Life Up To Eight Years." May 14, 2014.
https://www.healthcentral.com/article/longterm-caregiving-may-shorten-life-up-to-eight-years

Clary, Mike. "Cancer Cluster Frightens Palm Beach County Community," South Florida Sun Sentinel, February 16, 2010. https://palmbeach.floridahealth.gov/programs-and-services/infectious-disease-services/acreage/_documents/acreage-cancer-investigation-informational-timeline.pdf.

CSBroadcast, CSB President & CEO Scott Huedepohl "Feel Good Friday." December 10, 2020

"Disease Clusters In Florida," NRDC, March 2011. www.nrdc.org/health/diseaseclusters

ESPN, Jeremy Fowler, "Ben Roethlisberger comes through with signed footballs." September 3, 2018
https://www.espn.com/nfl/story/_/id/24566151/ben-roethlisberger-comes-autograph-patient

Ephesians 3:20 Holy Bible scripture paraphrased - chapter 13.
https://www.biblegateway.com/passage/?search=Ephesians%203%3A20&version=NLT

Epilepsy Foundation SUDEP Program, "What is SUDEP?" August 05, 2013 https://www.epilepsy.com/complications-risks/early-deathsudep

Groeschel, Craig (@craiggroeschel). "If it's not God's time, you can't force it. If it is God's time, you can't stop it." Instagram, July 12, 2023. https://www.instagram.com/p/CundxX7so9r/

Kenosha News, Jill Tatge-Rozell, "Campaign funds musical instruments for Matthias Academy in Bristol." April 5, 2021
https://www.kenoshanews.com/news/local/watch-now-campaign-funds-musical-instruments-for-matthias-academy-in-bristol/article_36382f66-ecaa-50c6-b5a7-549208c670fe.html

KROC 106.9, "The 3 Most Tissue Worthy, Heartwarming Rochester Stories of 2017." December 28, 2017
https://kroc.com/the-3-most-tissue-worthy-heartwarming-minnesota-stories-of-2017/

Mayo Clinic, In the Loop "Blanket Drive Is About More Than Keeping Patients Warm" December 20, 2018
https://intheloop.mayoclinic.org/2018/12/20/blanket-drive-is-about-more-than-keeping-patients-warm/

Mayo Clinic, In The Loop "Handoff Redux – Memorable Moment Magnified for Young Patient." September 13, 2018
https://intheloop.mayoclinic.org/2018/09/13/handoff-redux-memorable-moment-magnified-for-young-patient/?utm_source=twitter&utm_medium=sm&utm_content=post&utm_campaign=mayoclinic&geo=national&placementsite=enterprise&mc_id=us&cauid=100503&linkId=56980825

Mayo Clinic, In the Loop "Memorable moment magnified for young patient" September 25, 2018
https://newsnetwork.mayoclinic.org/discussion/in-the-loop-memorable-moment-magnified-for-young-patient/

Mayo Clinic, In the Loop "16-Year-Old Collects More Than 1 Million Pop Tabs for The Ronald McDonald House" July 7, 2017
https://intheloop.mayoclinic.org/2017/07/11/16-year-old-collects-more-than-1-million-pop-tabs-for-ronald-mcdonald-house/

LIST OF REFERENCES

Mayo Clinic, "Favorite Mayo Clinic Stories of 2018: "It Belongs with Him" –Mayo Surgeon Gives Patient Signed Football-February 14, 2019 https://news.mayocliniclabs.com/2019/02/14/favorite-mayo-clinic-stories-of-2018-it-belongs-with-him-mayo-surgeon-gives-patient-signed-football-throwbackthursday/

Minyard, Mary Garrison. "Alzheimer's, Dementia Takes Toll on Caregivers Too," Marshall County Daily, January 11, 2018. https://www.marshallcountydaily.com/2018/01/11/alzheimers-dementia-takes-toll-on-caregivers-too/

National Geographic, Yurt/Mongolian Ger https://education.nationalgeographic.org/resource/yurt/
Piper, John. *Don't Waste Your Life*. Wheaton, IL: Crossway, 2003.
Piper, John. "Embrace the Life God Has Given You." Two-Minute clip on Grief. MARCH 10, 2017. https://www.desiringgod.org/embracethe-life-god-has-given-you
Piper, John. "God is always doing 10,000 things in your life, and you may be aware of three of them." Desiring God, Twitter (X), 11:41 AM · Dec 19, 2014. Available: https://twitter.com/desiringGod/status/545982148235116544?lang=en.

Piper, John. "You Have One Life, Don't Waste It" https://www.youtube.com/watch?v=mfpmbmsvu3A

"Ripple effect." oxfordlearnersdictionaries.com, 2023. https://www.oxfordlearnersdictionaries.com/us/definition/english/ripple-effect?q=ripple+effect

Schulz, R. & S. R. Beach. "Caregiving as a risk factor for mortality: the Caregiver Health Effects Study," NIH National Library of Medicine, December 15, 1989. https://pubmed.ncbi.nlm.nih.gov/10605972

"The Acreage Cancer Investigation Informational Timeline," Palm Beach County Health Department, November 9, 2010. https://palmbeach.floridahealth.gov/programs-and-services/infectious-diseaseservices/acreage/_documents/acreage-cancer-investigation-informational-timeline.pdf

Thompson, Katie. "More Americans Than Ever Serving as Caregivers for Ailing, Aging Loved Ones," WCVB ABC February 17, 2023. https://www.wcvb.com/article/more-americans-caregivers-ailingaging-loved-ones/4295420

TMJ-TV-4 Milwaukee, "Local football manager battling autoimmune disease designs play from hospital." October 11, 2019
https://www.tmj4.com/news/local-news/local-football-manager-battling-auto-immune-disease-designs-play-from-hospital

U-Haul Stories, "Seth Bayles is Simply Amazing." January 02, 2015
https://myuhaulstory.com/2015/01/02/seth-bayles-simply-amazing/

West of the I, Darren Hillock, "Central HS homecoming football game dedicated to Seth Bayles." October 4, 2018
https://www.westofthei.com/2019/10/04/central-hs-homecoming-football-game-dedicated-to-seth-bayles/72392

WQAD Channel 8-ABC-Mark Puleo (AccuWeather) February 2, 2021- Looking back on a blizzard that stranded thousands of commuters in Chicago,
https://www.wqad.com/article/weather/accuweather/2011-groundhog-day-blizzard-chicago-commuters-photos/507-fa23b28a-c6d5-40fd-96a6-12842c7761f9

QR Code links:

A Journey to Healing, Samaritan's Purse, February 12, 2016
https://www.samaritanspurse.org/article/a-journey-to-healing/

Pop Tab Program – Ronald McDonald House, Rochester, MN October, 2017
https://d1q3agiwlaj31r.cloudfront.net/rmdh-pop-tab-program.mp4

Seth's Story - Ronald McDonald House - Rochester, MN, October 12, 2017
https://d1q3agiwlaj31r.cloudfront.net/rmdh-seth-bayles-story.mp4

Website: www.sethsjourney.com
Seth's Journey, LLC
P.O Box 593
Bristol, Wisconsin, 53104
Email: Julie@sethsjourney.com

Please follow us on Facebook and Instagram @sethsjourney9 and try and keep up. There's never a dull moment in this unexpected, blessed, messy, and beautiful life.

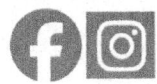

POP TABS FOR SETH

If you would like to be part of Seth's continuing effort to collect tabs for the work of the Ronald McDonald House, we would be ecstatic to have you join hands with us. You may drop off or mail tabs to:

Bristol Fire and Rescue
(Pop Tabs in honor of Seth Bayles)
8312 198th Avenue
Bristol, WI 53104

OR

Ronald McDonald House Charities
(Pop Tabs in honor of Seth Bayles)
850 2nd St NW
Rochester, MN 55902

ACKNOWLEDGEMENTS

An astounding number of people have helped us along the way. This book is a tribute of heartfelt gratitude to those who invest in the lives of others. Over twenty-five pages of stories were painstakingly moved to "the cutting room floor" to finalize an optimal length. If I didn't list you by name, you know who you are. Seth and I know who you are, and more importantly, God knows . . .

The following are some of those who had a direct part in making the book possible. We ARE Stronger Together!

Cathy Harvey, my editor, grammarian, and writing coach extraordinaire–and now, a special friend forever. Besides teaching me the difference between "forward" and "foreword," we plowed through a thousand pages of grammar rules. I can't even begin to calculate how many hours you invested in this project, and I will never be able to sufficiently thank you.

Donnie and the rest of the Bayles Bunch, there are no adequate words to express how much love and gratitude I have for you all! Your regular sacrifices do not go unnoticed. While Seth required my time and attention, you continued to fight the good fight. To Seth's siblings, although this book is primarily about your brother's health journey, I am beyond proud of the six of you–and I am honored to be your mom!

I'm grateful for my three sisters. Donna, my penny-shopping bestie, thank you for taking my hours at the family business, so I could finish this. Kris, thanks for your encouragement and for recommending the best illustrator ever! Trisha, whose sudden death during the editing of this book, prompted within me a renewed sense of the frailty of life.

I am indebted to our church family, especially our small group, who prayed for this project for years. For as long as I can remember, you have held us up in our weakest and affirmed we were in this together. To all prayer warriors, you are a treasured gift.

To my writer's group: You took me in, shared the craft of writing, and encouraged this calling. Your prayers and suggestions spurred me on toward the finish line!

Dear beta readers: Kathy Vojnar, Christy Hoff, Carol and Terry Flaningam, Caryssa Christian, Jeff and Allison Cabalka, and Kim Allen. Thank you for the huge sacrifice of your time to give your input. Your feedback, support, and encouragement had me in tears of joy and relief that this was a story that needed to be told.

I want to give special thanks to Phil Fischer, Cindy Bonsall, and John Stulak. I join countless others who have so much respect and admiration for your life's work of serving others. To have your endorsement of this book was especially meaningful. Seth and I are honored to call you friends.

Scott Anderson, Nick Mueller, Joseph Bergs, and Molly Fay, I will always remember what you contributed to this project. You all spoke encouragement and affirmation, wrote letters and emails, gave the go-ahead with approvals, and/or allowed me to use your commendations. I am truly grateful.

Mindy Cooling, you have stood behind every single one of Seth's endeavors. The day Donnie and I sat in your office at Mindy Cooling State Farm, and you said, "Seth's story needs to be told, and I want to help make that possible right now," was a day we will never forget. Thank you for making this possible and for loving our family and community.

To my amazing formatter/layout designer, Catherine Posey, who did the impossible in record time. Thank you for taking on such a unique and complex project with grace and understanding. Through repeated revisions, you responded with patience.

To Lauren Hengeveld, thank you for your patience in converting a hundred photo files so I could visually tell our story.

A huge thank you to the illustrator, photographers, videographers, producers, and organizations who allowed us to share their incredible works of art, photos, and short film projects. Seth and I are indebted to you for helping our journey come alive for those with special needs who may not be able to read this book.

Nick Collins, you generously shared your knowledge of technology, coding, web design, marketing, security, and business. You are not only brilliant in the above fields but humble and kind. Thank you for solving the technical issues and being a huge blessing to our family over the years.

To Lisa Metcalfe, Terri Penz, and Sue Weber, as well as all those committed to supporting this book and its distribution, thank you. Together, we can do so much!

To Lauren Woolard, from the first *very* rough draft, your regular encouragement about my writing gave me the push I needed to move forward and stick with it.

Cathy Hamilton, for your overview assessment, input, citations/reference section, and encouragement. Thank you for your patience with my newbie learning curve.

Thank you Julie-Allyson Ieron, for your excellent suggestions during the proposal stage and to Zena Dell Lowe, as well, for nailing the purpose and idea for the cover photo, character development, and story arc.

Sherry Costello, thank you for using your God-given creativity to design and construct our beautiful web page, logo, and so much more. You exceeded my expectations with your vision and skills, attention to detail, and great love.

To experts who made learning the publishing industry possible, offered advice, answered my questions, and poured encouragement into me: Cecil Murphey, Lin Johnson, Terry Whalin, Cynthia Ruchti, Jill Holler, Delores Liesner, Chelsea Stanley, James C. Magruder, Elizabeth Daghfal, Paulette George, Diane Nienas, Sherri Gallagher, Joey Christensen, Renee Bollas, Karen Sytsma, Letticia Callies, Mary Kerkman, and Emily Conrad. You all were a godsend!

Dr. Edmonson and Dr. Arroyo, who agreed to help so long ago. You gave my little boy a fighting chance. We will never be able to adequately thank you for the countless hours you both invested trying to unravel this medical mystery.

We commend Seth's long-standing physicians, some for over a decade, whose names were not mentioned in the book. Dr. Mason II, Dr. Moir, Dr. Wilder, Dr. Hand, Dr. Grothe, Dr. Bergs, Dr. Renaud, Dr. Cofer, Dr. Durbin, Dr. Codipilly, and Dr. Boesch, to name a few.

I am at a loss as to how to highlight every individual who has been and is a part of this complex care journey–thanks to all of you, and by God's grace, Seth's life and care is still ongoing.

To the thousands, near and far, who encouraged us and took the time to pray for us, you are invaluable! God has worked through you as His vessel. I could easily fill another book with the names of those who, in one form or another, have become a part of our journey. Still, I would only have scratched the surface because there are so many friends and fellow warriors whose faith and tenacity helped inspire the book's theme. We love you all!

Finally, I thank our great God, who gave me the strength and endurance to finish this project. To Him be the glory!

> "But my life is worth nothing to me unless I use it for finishing the work assigned me by the Lord Jesus–the work of telling others the Good News about the wonderful grace of God."
> Acts 20:24

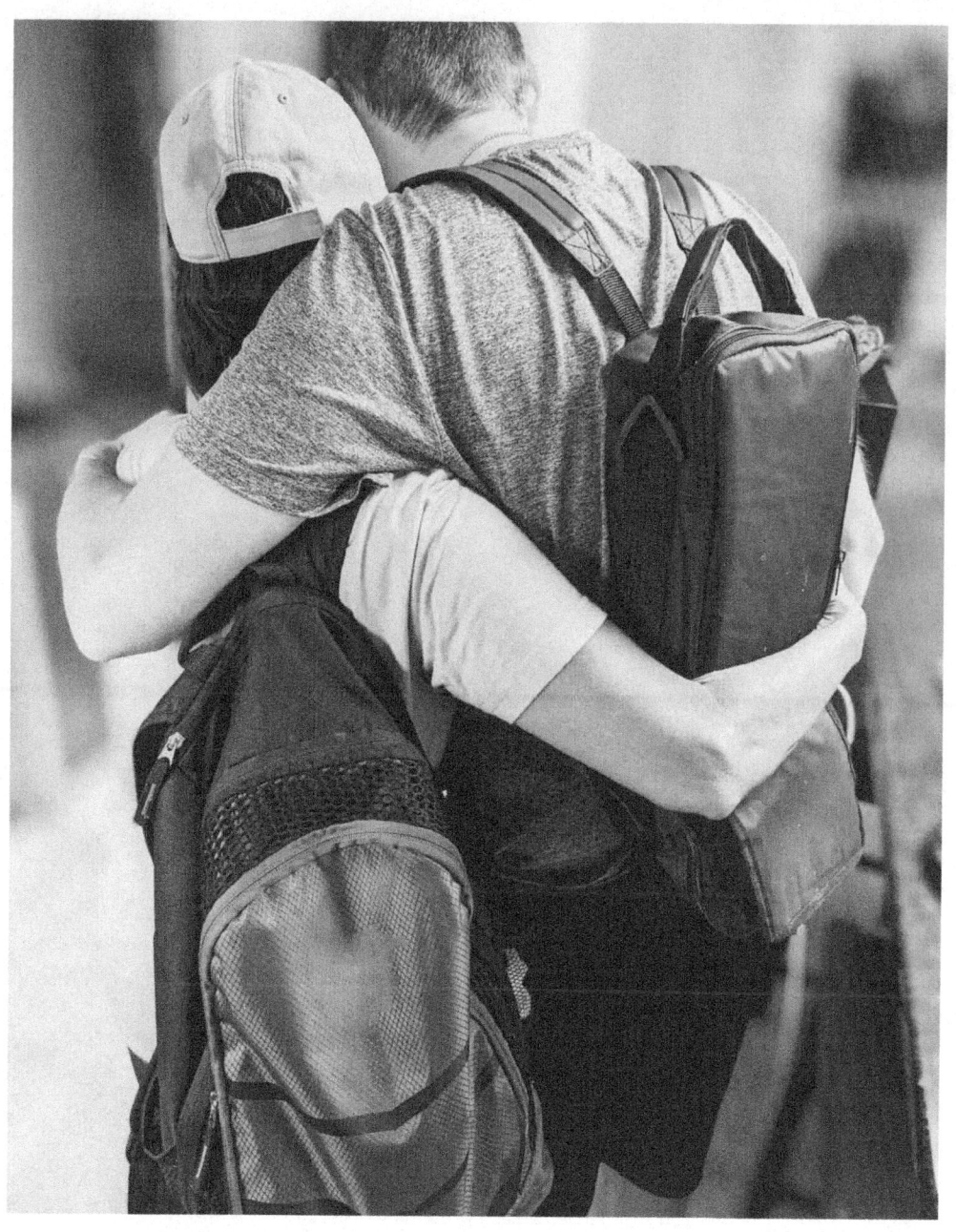

Made in the USA
Coppell, TX
29 December 2025

67539690R00223